Use R!

Series Editors
Robert Gentleman
Kurt Hornik
Giovanni Parmigiani

More information about this series at
http://www.springer.com/series/6991

Frans Willekens

Multistate Analysis of Life Histories with R

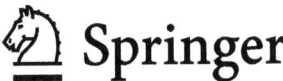

Frans Willekens
Max Planck Institute for Demographic Research
Rostock
Germany

ISSN 2197-5736　　　　　　　ISSN 2197-5744 (electronic)
ISBN 978-3-319-08382-7　　　ISBN 978-3-319-08383-4 (eBook)
DOI 10.1007/978-3-319-08383-4
Springer Cham Heidelberg New York Dordrecht London

Library of Congress Control Number: 2014950218

© Springer International Publishing Switzerland 2014
This work is subject to copyright. All rights are reserved by the Publisher, whether the whole or part of the material is concerned, specifically the rights of translation, reprinting, reuse of illustrations, recitation, broadcasting, reproduction on microfilms or in any other physical way, and transmission or information storage and retrieval, electronic adaptation, computer software, or by similar or dissimilar methodology now known or hereafter developed. Exempted from this legal reservation are brief excerpts in connection with reviews or scholarly analysis or material supplied specifically for the purpose of being entered and executed on a computer system, for exclusive use by the purchaser of the work. Duplication of this publication or parts thereof is permitted only under the provisions of the Copyright Law of the Publisher's location, in its current version, and permission for use must always be obtained from Springer. Permissions for use may be obtained through RightsLink at the Copyright Clearance Center. Violations are liable to prosecution under the respective Copyright Law.
The use of general descriptive names, registered names, trademarks, service marks, etc. in this publication does not imply, even in the absence of a specific statement, that such names are exempt from the relevant protective laws and regulations and therefore free for general use.
While the advice and information in this book are believed to be true and accurate at the date of publication, neither the authors nor the editors nor the publisher can accept any legal responsibility for any errors or omissions that may be made. The publisher makes no warranty, express or implied, with respect to the material contained herein.

Printed on acid-free paper

Springer is part of Springer Science+Business Media (www.springer.com)

Preface

Suppose you are asked to describe an individual. You probably list age, sex, marital status, presence of children and number of children, main occupation, education level, ethnicity, place of residence, place of work, main source of income, religious denomination and some lifestyle features. You probably add years of major transitions: when the person graduated from school, got married, entered the current job and moved to the current address. If the person has children, you may add the name, age and sex of each child. When you are asked to describe a population, you may mention size, age structure, distribution by level of education, employment status, marital status and health status. It describes the population at a point in time. If asked to describe population change, you may mention changes in size and distribution. Population change is an outcome of changes in people's lifestyle and life course. An ageing population is a result of people having fewer children and living longer. A declining married proportion is an outcome of fewer people marrying, postponement of marriage and marriages being less stable. Fewer marriages may be linked to changes in the meaning of the institution of marriage. An increase in the proportion of unemployment is an outcome of more people losing their job and/or decreased likelihood of finding a job when unemployed, resulting in longer unemployment spells. The description of population change in terms of changing lives is referred to as the biographical method. The method emphasizes personal attributes, life events and life histories.

An individual may be characterized by a set of attributes such as marital status, employment status, health status, place of residence and income level. If attributes are represented by discrete variables with finite numbers of categories, a combination of categories defines a state of existence and an individual with given values of attributes is said to occupy a state. Individuals with the same values of attributes occupy the same state. The state space is the set of possible states. In practice, one or a few attributes are selected to define the state space. Which attributes are selected depends on the research question. Other attributes that are relevant but not of primary importance are treated as covariates.

As life unfolds, an individual moves between states. The sequences of states and transitions between states describe life histories or careers. Employment histories, marital histories and residential histories are examples of careers. In studies of life histories, two approaches are distinguished (Abbott 2001). The first views a life path as a whole and tries to find typical patterns. The approach is generally known as sequence analysis. The second views a life history as a realization of a stochastic process and aims at the description, explanation and prediction of life histories. Probability models are used to represent stochastic processes and to model the life histories that they generate. This book is about the second approach. Life histories are viewed as realizations of continuous-time Markov processes that depend on rates of transition between states. The rates are estimated from longitudinal data.

The multistate methods that are presented in this book are included in the software package *Biograph*, a package in R that implements the biographical method. The packages can be downloaded from the Comprehensive R Archive Network (CRAN) (http://cran.r-project.org/). *Biograph* retrieves useful information from life history data. It estimates transition rates and computes useful life history indicators. A particularly useful feature of *Biograph* is the set of utilities that connect the package to R packages for multistate modeling including *mstate*, *msm*, *mvna*, *etm*, *Epi*, and the package *TraMineR* for sequence analysis. *Biograph* produces input data in the right format and basic R objects for the packages.

The motivation to write the book was to stimulate the use of multistate modeling among social science students and researchers with basic knowledge of survival analysis and event history analysis. The methods presented in the book are illustrated using two data sets. The first is a subsample of the German Life History Survey. Blossfeld and Rohwer (2002) and Blossfeld et al. (2007) used the data to illustrate the statistical modeling of time-to-event data. By using the same data set, the multistate analysis of life histories is presented as a logical extension of the analysis of time-to-event data. At the end of the book, another data set is considered: the Netherlands Fertility and Family Survey of 1998. The data sets are included in the *Biograph* package.

The book should appeal to anyone interested in how populations change and how the change is related to the lifestyle and life course of individuals. The changes include today's major societal challenges: ageing, population decline, migration and integration, population diversity, population health, labour market dynamics and the role of education and skills in the modern knowledge society. The book should be of particular interest to demographers, epidemiologists and students of population health, sociologists, criminologists, economists and historians. The book is suitable as a textbook for graduate courses on event history analysis. It may also be used as a self-study book provided the reader has a basic knowledge of survival analysis and multistate modeling. The R code used on the book is available online.

The preparation of the book has been a long but exciting journey. Most of the work was done while I was with the Netherlands Interdisciplinary Demographic Institute (NIDI) in The Hague. The book was completed at the Max Planck Institute for Demographic Research in Rostock, Germany. I would like to thank Hans-Peter Blossfeld for allowing me to use the subsample of the German Life History Survey that he used in his book with Götz Rohwer, *Techniques of Event History Modeling* (Blossfeld and Rohwer 2002). James Raymer, Jutta Gampe, Sabine Zinn and Arthur Allignol provided useful comments on the manuscript. I am grateful for their help.

Rostock, Germany Frans Willekens
May 2014

Contents

1	**Introduction**	1
2	**Life Histories: Real and Synthetic**	7
	2.1 Introduction	7
	2.2 Transition Rates	10
	2.3 Transition Probabilities and State Occupation Probabilities	28
	2.4 Expected Waiting Times and State Occupation Times	40
	2.5 Synthetic Life Histories	46
	2.6 Conclusion	51
3	**The Biograph Object**	53
	3.1 Introduction	53
	3.2 Description of a *Biograph* Object	54
	3.3 How to Create a *Biograph* Object?	57
	3.4 Data Restructuring	59
	3.5 Other Data Formats	62
	3.6 A Note on Dates	74
	3.7 Conclusion	78
4	**Exploratory Data Analysis**	81
	4.1 Introduction	81
	4.2 The Multistate System and Its Measurement	82
	4.3 Episodes and Transitions	89
	4.4 State and Event Sequences: Individual and Aggregate	91
	4.5 State Occupancies, Transitions and State Occupation Times	95
	4.6 Covariates	103
	4.7 Conclusion	106
5	**Visualisation of Life Histories**	109
	5.1 Introduction	109
	5.2 Points of Departure	110
	5.3 Basic Graphics with *ggplot2*	112

	5.4	The Lexis Diagram	120
	5.5	State Distribution and State Sequences	130
	5.6	Conclusion	133

6 Statistical Packages for Multistate Life History Analysis ... 135
6.1 Introduction ... 135
6.2 The *Survival* Package ... 135
6.2.1 The Survival Object ... 136
6.2.2 Kaplan-Meier Estimator ... 137
6.2.3 Exponential Transition Rate Model ... 138
6.2.4 The Cox Model ... 141
6.2.5 Nelson-Aalen Estimator ... 153
6.3 The *eha* Package ... 153
6.3.1 Transition Rate Models ... 154
6.3.2 The Cox Model with Parametric Baseline Hazard ... 157
6.3.3 Change Observation Window ... 162
6.4 The *mvna* and *etm* Packages ... 165
6.4.1 mvna: Nelson-Aalen Estimator in Multistate Models ... 165
6.4.2 etm: Aalen-Johansen Estimator in Multistate Models ... 172
6.5 The *mstate* Package ... 173
6.5.1 Illness-Death Model ... 175
6.5.2 Reversible Markov Chain ... 189
6.6 The *msm* Package ... 195
6.6.1 Multistate Transition Rate Models ... 196
6.6.2 Synthetic Individual Life Histories ... 202

7 The Multistate Life Table ... 205
7.1 Introduction ... 205
7.2 Transition Rates ... 206
7.3 The Multistate Survival Function ... 208
7.4 Expected State Occupation Times ... 210
7.5 Synthetic Individual Life Histories ... 212
7.6 Summary ... 215

8 Application to the Netherlands Family and Fertility Survey ... 217
8.1 Introduction ... 217
8.2 Data and Preparation of *Biograph* Object ... 217
8.3 Exploratory Analysis ... 223
8.3.1 Summary Indicators ... 223
8.3.2 State Sequences ... 227
8.3.3 Age Profiles ... 237
8.3.4 Occurrence-Exposure Rates ... 239
8.4 Transition Rate Models ... 244
8.4.1 Data Preparation ... 244
8.4.2 Cumulative Transition Rates ... 246
8.4.3 Regression Models ... 251
8.5 The Multistate Life Table ... 256
8.6 Conclusion ... 264

9 Summary... 267

Annexes... 271
    Annex A: How to Create a *Biograph* Object.................. 271
    Annex B: List of Biograph Functions and Data................ 292
    Annex C: Biograph Functions and the Functions They Depend On.... 294

References.. 299

Index.. 305

List of Figures

Fig. 2.1	Employment career of respondent with ID 76	14
Fig. 3.1	Labour market data: state space and transitions. GLHS	55
Fig. 4.1	State occupancies by age. GLHS	100
Fig. 4.2	Trellis plot of age distribution at labour market entry, by birth cohort and sex. GLHS	106
Fig. 5.1	Scatter plot of ages at labour market entry, by birth cohort and sex. GLHS	113
Fig. 5.2	Scatter plot of ages at labour market entry by cohort, sex and level of education. GLHS	115
Fig. 5.3	Bar charts of age distribution at labour market entry, by sex, level of education and birth cohort. Facet grid of GLHS data	117
Fig. 5.4	Aesthetic mapping of lengths of episodes in months, by type of episode and state occupied. GLHS	120
Fig. 5.5	Lexis diagram: scatter plot of calendar years and ages at labour market entry by sex. GLHS	123
Fig. 5.6	Lexis diagram: scatter plot of calendar years and ages at labour market entry by birth cohort and sex. GLHS	124
Fig. 5.7	Lexis diagram: employment careers of selected GLHS respondents. Display A, using *Epi* package	125
Fig. 5.8	Lexis diagram: employment careers of selected GLHS respondents. Display B, using *ggplot2* package	126
Fig. 5.9	Lexis diagram: job exits and exposure times by calendar period and age: exposure times, transition counts and occurrence-exposure rates. GLHS	128
Fig. 5.10	State occupancies by age and sex, using *TraMineR*. GLHS	131
Fig. 5.11	Frequency plot of state sequences, by sex, using *TraMineR*. GLHS	132
Fig. 6.1	Kaplan-Meier estimator of job duration, by sex. GLHS	138
Fig. 6.2	Probabilities that job spells exceed given durations based on the stratified Cox model with single covariate (sex). GLHS	144

Fig. 6.3	Cumulative hazard based on the stratified Cox model with a single covariate (sex). GLHS	145
Fig. 6.4	Scaled Schoenfeld residuals for effect of education on job exit rate by job duration. GLHS	147
Fig. 6.5	Predicted job survival for individuals with given characteristics based on the Cox model. GLHS (confidence intervals omitted)	151
Fig. 6.6	Predicted job survival for individuals with given characteristics based on the Cox model. GLHS (with confidence intervals)	152
Fig. 6.7	Trellis plot of cumulative hazard rates, produced by *mvna*. GLHS	169
Fig. 6.8	Cumulative hazard rates. GLHS	170
Fig. 6.9	Age-specific transition rates from NoJob to Job (NJ) and from Job to NoJob (JN): Nelson-Aalen estimates and occurrence-exposure rates. GLHS	172
Fig. 6.10	Illness-death model of job change. GLHS	176
Fig. 6.11	Survival functions for J1J, J1N and J2N transitions, by sex. GLHS	182
Fig. 6.12	Cumulative hazards of J1J, J1N and J2N transitions. GLHS	184
Fig. 6.13	Multistate survival curve for male, born in 1939–1941 and with lower secondary school with vocational training. GLHS	188
Fig. 6.14	The reversible Markov chain model.	190
Fig. 6.15	Cumulative job entry and job exit rates of females, predicted by Cox model with predictors gender and marital status, using the msfit function of the *mstate* package. GLHS	193
Fig. 6.16	Observed and predicted state occupation probabilities by age. GLHS	200
Fig. 7.1	Cumulative NJ and JN transition rates by age: Nelson-Aalen estimator and cumulative occurrence-exposure rates. GLHS	208
Fig. 7.2	The multistate survival function: state occupation probabilities in N and J, predicted by the multistate life table from empirical transition rates. GLHS	212
Fig. 8.1	Schematic representation of pathways to the first child	220
Fig. 8.2	Lifelines for selected subjects. OG	230
Fig. 8.3	Lexis diagram: leaving parental home for marriage, by age and calendar year. OG	231
Fig. 8.4	State occupancies by age. OG	232
Fig. 8.5	State sequences of selected respondents, produced by *TraMineR*. OG	234
Fig. 8.6	Observed state occupancies by age, produced by *TraMineR*. OG sample population	235
Fig. 8.7	Observed state occupancies by age and cohort, produced by *TraMineR*. OG sample population	235
Fig. 8.8	Trellis plot of age at first marriage, by birth cohort and level of education. OG	240
Fig. 8.9	Trellis plot of cumulative transition rates (Nelson-Aalen estimator), 13 transitions. OG	249

Fig. 8.10	Multistate survival function: state occupation probabilities by age. OG	257
Fig. 8.11	Multistate survival function: state occupation probabilities for women born before 1960 and with a religion other than Roman Catholic or Protestant. Produced by *mstate* package. OG	263
Fig. A.1	State space and transitions. Hypothetical case B	276

List of Tables

Table 2.1	Subsample of German Life History Survey (GLHS)	13
Table 2.2	Nelson-Aalen estimator and Aalen variance of cumulative transition rates. GLHS, subsample of ten respondents	20
Table 2.3	Piecewise-constant exponential model: occurrences, exposures and transition rates. GLHS, 201 respondents	27
Table 2.4	State occupancies and state occupation times. Individual with ID 76.	28
Table 2.5	Aalen-Johansen estimator of transition probabilities. GLHS subsample of ten individuals.	36
Table 2.6	Probabilities of being with/without a job at selected ages: non-parametric method. GLHS, 201 respondents	38
Table 2.7	Employment histories in virtual population, based on GLHS aggregate transition rates.	48
Table 2.8	Employment histories in observed population and virtual population, based on age-specific GLHS transition rates	50
Table 3.1	*Biograph* object: GLHS data	54
Table 3.2	GLHS input data for Blossfeld and Rohwer's TDA programme (rrdat)	58
Table 3.3	*Biograph* object: GLHS data with intrastate transitions removed	60
Table 3.4	*Biograph* object: GLHS data with observation window starting at labour market entry	61
Table 3.5	*Biograph* object: GLHS data with observation window starting at birth and ending at labour market entry	62
Table 3.6	*Biograph* object: GLHS observations from CMC 600 to CMC 800	62
Table 3.7	GLHS data in *TraMineR* extended format: states occupied at birthdays	65
Table 3.8	GLHS data in *TraMineR* compressed format	65
Table 3.9	GLHS data in episode format	66

Table 3.10	Lexis object: GLHS data	67
Table 3.11	GLHS data in *mvna* format	70
Table 3.12	GLHS data in `msdata` format for *mstate* package	71
Table 3.13	GLHS data in long format, produced by `reshape` function of *stats* package	73
Table 3.14	GLHS data in *msm* format	73
Table 3.15	Calendar dates of transitions in GLHS	78
Table 4.1	Types of episodes. GLHS	90
Table 4.2	State occupation times by type of episode. GLHS	90
Table 4.3	Transitions and censoring, by state of origin and destination. GLHS	91
Table 4.4	Mean ages at transition and censoring. GLHS	91
Table 4.5	Selected individual state sequences. GLHS	94
Table 4.6	Most frequent state and event sequences. GLHS	94
Table 4.7	Individual state occupation times by age. Respondent with ID 188. GLHS	98
Table 4.8	Observed aggregate state occupation times at selected ages. GLHS	99
Table 4.9	Number of transitions by origin and destination and mean ages. GLHS.	101
Table 4.10	Number of transitions at selected ages. GLHS.	101
Table 4.11	Data for calculation of transition rate, selected ages. GLHS	102
Table 4.12	State and event sequences, by birth cohort. GLHS.	104
Table 5.1	Lexis object: data on episodes between birth and labour market entry. GLHS	122
Table 6.1	Sample population at risk, by age, and transitions, by age, produced by *mvna*. GLHS	167
Table 6.2	Sample population at risk, by age, and transitions, by age, produced by *Biograph*. GLHS	168
Table 6.3	GLHS data in wide format to be used as input in *mstate*	176
Table 6.4	GLHS data in long format to be used as input in *mstate*	177
Table 6.5	GLHS data in expanded format of *mstate*	178
Table 6.6	Expanded data set for reversible Markov chain model, with selection of covariates. GLHS	191
Table 6.7	Number of transitions between states, reported by *msm* package. GLHS	196
Table 6.8	NJ and JN transition rates, estimated by *msm*. No covariates and time unit is month. GLHS	197
Table 6.9	NJ and JN transition probabilities for periods of 12 months, estimated by *msm*. GLHS	198
Table 6.10	NJ and JN transition rates. No covariates and time unit is year. GLHS	199
Table 6.11	NJ and JN transition rates of birth cohort 1949–1951, by sex, predicted by exponential transition rate model (*msm*). GLHS	201

List of Tables   xix

Table 6.12	Expected state occupation times, by sex, predicted by exponential transition rate model (*msm*). GLHS	202
Table 6.13	Simulated individual employment career, generated by *msm* based on aggregate GLHS transition rates	203
Table 7.1	Data for generation of employment careers of synthetic individuals	213
Table 7.2	State sequences: observed and simulated. GLHS	215
Table 8.1	*Biograph* object: selection of NLOG98 data	222
Table 8.2	Overview of episodes observed in OG data	225
Table 8.3	Number of transitions and mean ages, by origin and destination. OG	226
Table 8.4	Aggregate yearly transition rates. OG	227
Table 8.5	Event and state sequences in OG	228
Table 8.6	Pathways in OG, by birth cohort	229
Table 8.7	State occupancies by age. Selected ages. OG	232
Table 8.8	Rates (probabilities) of transition between marital status/living arrangement, produced by *TraMineR*. OG	236
Table 8.9	Probabilities of transition between marital status/living arrangement, derived from occurrence-exposure rates. OG	237
Table 8.10	Data for estimation of occurrence-exposure rates, by age. OG	241
Table 8.11	Occurrence-exposure rates (M-matrix: age-cohort rates). OG	243
Table 8.12	Risk set and transition count for estimating (cumulative) rate of leaving parental home to live independently at age 28. Data produced by *mvna*. OG	248
Table 8.13	One-year probabilities of transition between marital status/living arrangement for females aged 20. Comparison of Nelson-Aalen estimator and occurrence-exposure rates. OG	260
Table 8.14	Ten-year probabilities of transition between marital status/living arrangement for females aged 20, based on Nelson-Aalen estimator combined with assumption of time-invariant rates. OG	260
Table A.1	Transition dates for three hypothetical individuals	273
Table A.2	Data on three hypothetical individuals	273
Table A.3	Object produced by the *Biograph* function Sequences.ind.0	274
Table A.4	*Biograph* object: hypothetical data A	274
Table A.5	*Biograph* object: data types	275
Table A.6	*Biograph* object with dates in CMC	276
Table A.7	Hypothetical survey data: multiple transitions	277
Table A.8	*Biograph* object: hypothetical data B	278
Table A.9	*Biograph* object: data types	279
Table A.10	Changes in living arrangements. SHARELIFE. A selection of respondents	282
Table A.11	Sorted transition dates. Selection of respondents	283
Table A.12	Biograph object (transposed) with SHARELIFE data. Selected respondents	283

Table A.13	*Biograph* object: NFHS-AP	286
Table A.14	Data frame with event dates in days since transplantation. EBMT	289
Table A.15	*Biograph* object: EBMT data	290
Table A.16	*Biograph* object: simulated life histories	291

List of Boxes

Box 4.1	Sample Paths for Selected Subjects. GLHS	93
Box 6.1	Basic Exponential Transition Rate Model with Covariate Sex. GLHS	139
Box 6.2	Basic Exponential Model with Covariates Sex and Birth Cohort. GLHS	140
Box 6.3	Basic Exponential Model with Several Covariates (Full Model). GLHS	141
Box 6.4	Cox Proportional Hazard Model. GLHS	142
Box 6.5	Cox Proportional Hazard Model with Several Covariates. GLHS	146
Box 6.6	Terms of Cox Model Used to Predict Length of the First Job Episode for Respondent with ID 2. GLHS	150
Box 6.7	Predicted Cumulative Job Exit Rate with Confidence Intervals. Selection of Hypothetical Individuals. GLHS	153
Box 6.8	Weibull Regression Model (*eha*), Without Covariates. GLHS	155
Box 6.9	Weibull Regression Model (*eha*), with Covariates. GLHS	156
Box 6.10	Impact of Gender on Job Exit Rate: Cox Regression Model. GLHS	158
Box 6.11	Impact of Several Covariates on Job Exit Rate: Cox Model (*eha*). GLHS	158
Box 6.12	Impact of Several Covariates on Job Exit Rate: Cox Proportional Hazard Model with Weibull Baseline Hazard (*eha*). GLHS	159
Box 6.13	Weibull Model of Job Exit Rates; Null Model Without Covariates. GLHS	160
Box 6.14	Numbers of Job Exits, Exposure Times and Job Exit Rates, by Duration Intervals of 1 Year. GLHS	161
Box 6.15	Transitions, Exposure Times and Occurrence-Exposure Rates of Respondents Who Are Aged 20–30 Years During the Period 1970–1980. GLHS	164
Box 6.16	The Effect of Gender on Transition Rates. Cox Model. GLHS	179

Box 6.17	Effect of Gender on J1J, J1N and J2N Transition Rates. Cox Model with Stratification by Destination State. GLHS	184
Box 6.18	Effect of Gender, Birth Cohort and Level of Education on Timing of Job Change. Cox Model. GLHS	186
Box 6.19	Transitions in the Reversible Markov Chain Model. GLHS	190
Box 6.20	Cox Proportional Hazard Model for the NJ and JN Transitions. GLHS	191
Box 6.21	Effect of Gender and Marital Status on NJ and JN Transition Rates. GLHS	193
Box 8.1	Life Path of Respondent with ID 8. OG	229
Box 8.2	Effect Reason for Leaving Home on Rate of Leaving Parental Home. Cox Competing Risks Model. OG	252
Box 8.3	Effect of Birth Cohort and Religion on First Birth Rate for Cohabiting and Married Women. Cox Model, Using *mstate* Package. OG	255

Chapter 1
Introduction

In this book, a particular class of models is considered: multistate models. Multistate models are ideally suited to model life histories. At a given instant, an individual has a set of attributes, such as marital status, employment status, living arrangement, health status and place of residence. In multistate analysis, a person with a given set of attributes is said to occupy a given state, and persons with the same attributes occupy the same state. When an attribute changes, the person moves to a different state. Most personal attributes change in the life course, implying transitions between states. Marriage, marriage dissolution, birth of a child, job change, migration, onset of disability and death are events that imply a transition between states. The set of possible states is the state space. The state variable is the state an individual occupies at a given time or age. If individuals are combined in cohorts or populations, the state variable is the number of individuals in a state at a given time or age. *The life course is operationalised as a sequence of states and transitions between states.* Two types of states are distinguished: states that can be entered and left (transient states) and states that can be entered but not left (absorbing states). Age is not a personal attribute; it is a time scale. Different time scales may be used to measure time to transition, calendar time and age being the most common time measurements.

The multistate model is approached from a *survival analysis* perspective. Survival analysis is a subfield of statistics that studies the occurrence and timing of events. An event is an outcome of a stochastic process. The occurrence of the event and the waiting time to the event are random variables with characteristic distributions. A stochastic process model implies a parametric model of the waiting time to the event. For instance, a model that assumes that the event occurs at a constant rate implies an exponential waiting time distribution. A model that assumes that the rate declines exponentially with duration leads to a Gompertz distribution of time-to-event. Instead of using a model, the empirical distribution of waiting times may be used directly to estimate event rates. In that case, no stochastic process model and associated waiting time distribution are assumed. The method is known as the non-parametric approach.

It is often useful to distinguish event types. For instance, upon completion of college education and receipt of a bachelor degree, a person may move on to graduate school, get a job, take time off for travel or get involved in another activity. These activities are competing for the individual's time. They are competing destinations and competing risks. Another example: Marital dissolution is an event caused by death of the spouse or a divorce. Death of the spouse and divorce are competing causes of marriage dissolution. They compete to be the reason for marriage dissolution. In multistate analysis, competing risks are everywhere, and the modelling of competing risks is an important part of multistate modelling.

In multistate modelling, the life course is modelled as a continuous-time Markov process, which may be written as a system of differential equations. The parameters of the model are instantaneous transition rates, also referred to as hazard rates. They are estimated from data by tracking event occurrences and persons at risk of the event. To experience an event, a person has to be at risk. For example, only married persons are at risk of divorce. Partners who are not married may separate, and a separation may be perceived as a divorce, but it is not a divorce. The risk concept is central to the study of life histories. To determine the probability of an event at a given age, event occurrences at that age and persons at risk need to be recorded. Tracking events and persons is complicated when (a) people can enter, leave and re-enter the population at risk any time during a period of observation, (b) people may leave for reasons unrelated to the study or (c) observations do not cover the entire sequence of entries and exits but only a segment of that sequence: the segment in the observation period or observation window. The third complication implies that the observation starts after some people have already experienced the event or ends before all people included in the observation have experienced the event. The statistical theory for estimating hazard rates and probabilities by counting events and tracking exposure times is the counting process theory (Andersen et al. 1993; Aalen et al. 2008). It is the main theory applied in this book. A *counting process* tracks event occurrences and an *at risk process* keeps track of who is exposed. Occurrences are related to exposures (population at risk and exposure times). Transition counts, risk sets and exposure times provide the necessary information to derive transition rates. One approach is to update and cumulate the transition rate each time a transition is recorded. Life history measures are computed from cumulated hazards. In the book, the method is contrasted with an alternative method, which also counts events and tracks exposure times. Instead of estimating hazard rates each time an event occurs, the rates are estimated for time periods. During a period of 1 year, say, the event count and exposure time are determined and the hazard rate is computed as the ratio of occurrences and exposures. This approach to estimating occurrence-exposure rates is common in demography, epidemiology and other disciplines. Both methods are covered in this book. The first method is implemented in statistical packages for multistate modelling discussed in this book. The second method is implemented in *Biograph*.

Biograph tracks transitions and the population at risk of a transition. The package relies on life history data, collected retrospectively in cross-sectional surveys or prospectively in follow-up studies. Life history data come in a variety of formats. Most empirical studies organise data by life domain, e.g. employment, partnership and marriage, family and fertility, health and migration. For the study of life histories, events need to be ordered chronologically by time of occurrence, and populations at risk at these times must be determined. *Biograph* uses a particular chronological format, known as the wide format (see later). Other authors use a different format. For that reason, a number of functions are included in *Biograph* that convert one data format into another. The *Biograph* format is the data structure of a *Biograph* object.

The graphics capabilities of R motivated the visualisation of life histories. The methods presented in the book should be considered as a first step towards visualisation of life history data. In the demographic tradition, individual lifelines are presented in an age-time diagram with age on the y-axis and calendar time on the x-axis. In several textbooks, the diagram is used to show how measurement and estimates vary by age, period and cohort. The diagram is known as the Lexis diagram. *Biograph* uses two packages to display life histories in the Lexis diagram: the *Epi* package that includes functions to produce Lexis diagrams and the *ggplot2* package. Some functions in *Biograph* include functions of another package in CRAN with considerable graphics capabilities: *TraMineR*.

Biograph was designed to make life history data analysis accessible to a large group of students and researchers. The package includes a step-by-step method for tracking event occurrences and populations at risk and for calculating rates of transition between states. The rates are then used to predict the probability of a particular transition (transition probability), the probability of being in a given state at a given age (state probability) and the expected time spent in each of the states (state occupation times).

Biograph produces several life history indicators. They include state and transition probabilities and expected state occupation times. Indicators are generated for individuals, groups of individuals with similar characteristics or experiences (e.g. birth cohorts) and the entire population. They are derived from transition rates that are estimated from data. The aim of the exploratory analysis is to help comprehend the data before engaging in advanced statistical analysis. *Biograph* visualises data in a way that should simplify the exploratory analysis of life histories and facilitate the detection of cases that need special attention. *Biograph* predicts life paths for groups and individuals. Predicted life paths are synthetic biographies because they are obtained using a model and estimating the model parameters by pooling biographic information from different individuals.

In the literature on multistate modelling, the estimation of transition rates receives considerable attention. The Comprehensive R Archive Network (CRAN) includes several contributed packages that estimate transition rates from data, e.g. *survival*, *eha*, *mvna*, *mstate* and *msm*. *Biograph* contains functions that convert a *Biograph* object into input data for these packages.

Observations on the life course may be recorded retrospectively or prospectively during a period of time. The observation period is referred to as the *observation window*. In a cross-sectional retrospective survey, subjects are asked to recall events between birth and survey date or, more often, during a brief period (e.g. 5 years) prior to the survey. In a longitudinal survey or follow-up study, subjects are followed for a number of years, and events are recorded upon occurrence (in continuous time) or indirectly by recording for the same individual the states occupied at consecutive points in time (panel). Changes in the observation window may influence the estimates of transition rates because they influence event counts, persons at risk and durations at risk. *Biograph* allows the imposition of different observation windows on the same data set to assess how sensitive results are to variations in observation period. The observation window may be defined by age and/or by calendar time. For instance, you may want to consider not the entire period for which you have data but only the most recent 3 years. Or you may want to restrict the analysis to individuals between ages 20 and 30. By tracking transitions and persons at risk between ages 20 and 30, transition rates may be obtained that apply to that age group. To obtain the transition rate for one age, 21 say, transitions and persons at risk should be considered between the 21st and the 22nd birthday. *Biograph* monitors transitions and exposure times for observation windows you specify. For each individual in the (sample) population and for any observation window you specify, it determines the precise dates of entry in each of the states and the dates of exit. It determines whether the exit is due to the transition of interest, another transition (competing event) or because observation ends (censoring). That flexibility is an important feature of the package.

In life history data analysis, data storage and data structure have occupied researchers for many years (see, e.g. Alter and Gutmann 1999). In *Biograph*, all data pertaining to an individual are stored in one record. The data format is known as the wide format and the file structure as person file. To use *Biograph*, the data must be in the proper format. A first step in any data analysis involving *Biograph* is to create a *Biograph* object, which has data in the format required by *Biograph*. The package includes utilities for preparing *Biograph* objects from raw data. It also has functions that convert data in wide format to a long format and vice versa. In the long format, a record contains information on a transition or an episode. In that file structure, the life history of an individual with several transitions is distributed over multiple records.

Two data sets are used to illustrate *Biograph*. The first data set is a subsample of the German Life History Survey (GLHS). The GLHS was organised in 1981–1983 and provides information on the life histories of more than 5,000 men and women from three birth cohorts: 1929–1931, 1939–1941 and 1949–1951. Blossfeld and Rohwer (2002) and Blossfeld et al. (2007) used a subsample of 201 respondents for training purposes. The 201 respondents experienced 600 job episodes. The data are used to illustrate hazard rate modelling of the job episodes with TDA (Transition Data Analysis) (2002 publication) and Stata (2007 publication). The same subsample of 201 respondents is used in this book. This book considers 201 *employment careers*, consisting of a total of 600 job spells and 382 episodes without a job. Dates of job entry and job exit are given in Century Month Code (CMC). Personal attributes are the date of birth and five covariates: sex, level of education, date of marriage, date of labour market entry and birth cohort. The GLHS subsample is used throughout the book, except in Chap. 7. In that chapter, another date set is considered to illustrate *Biograph*: the Netherlands Family and Fertility Survey of 1998.

The book consists of nine chapters. In Chap. 2, I present an overview of the methods used in the book. The *Biograph* object and the *Biograph* data format are described in Chap. 3. In the chapter, I also present several functions to change the observation window and to convert a *Biograph* object to objects that are recognised by other packages in the Comprehensive R Archive Network (CRAN). Chapters 4 and 5 cover descriptive and exploratory analysis. The computation of life history indicators from the sample data is presented in Chap. 4. Visualisation of event histories and state sequences is the subject of Chap. 5. The Lexis diagram and the visualisation of state and event sequences represent the main methods. Chapters 6 and 7 go beyond descriptive analysis. Chapter 6 covers the estimation of multistate models from data using specialised statistical packages. The following packages in CRAN are covered:

- *survival* (Therneau 2014; Therneau and Grambsch 2000)
- *eha* (Broström 2012, 2014)
- *mstate* (Putter et al. 2007, 2011; De Wreede et al. 2011; Putter 2014)
- *mvna* (Allignol 2013) (see also Allignol et al. 2011)
- *etm* (Allignol 2014) (see also Allignol et al. 2011)
- *msm* (Jackson 2011, 2014a)

Several of these packages for multistate analysis are described in a special issue of the Journal of Statistical Software (Putter 2011a).

Methods for constructing synthetic biographies are presented in Chap. 7. The chapter builds on two complementary developments. The first is the multistate life table (MSLT) developed in demography. The second is microsimulation. In Chap. 8, an illustrative analysis of data from the Netherlands Family and Fertility Survey 1998 (NLOG98) demonstrates the added value of *Biograph*. The chapter addresses a particular research question: what is the effect of the age of leaving the parental home and the sequences of partnerships and living arrangements on the age at first birth? Chapter 9 provides a summary and a conclusion.

In Annex A, additional data sets are presented to illustrate how to create a *Biograph* object. The first and the second are hypothetical data. The third is the Survey of Health, Ageing and Retirement in Europe (SHARE). SHARE is a panel survey of more than 45,000 individuals aged 50 and over in more than 10 European countries. The survey started in 2004. The third wave of data collection, SHARELIFE, collected detailed retrospective life histories in 13 countries in 2008–2009. SHARELIFE data are used in this book. The fourth is the National Family Health Survey (NFHS) of India. The survey is a repeated cross-section, organised in 1992–1993, 1998–1999 and 2005–2006. The NFHS is comparable to the Demographic and Health Surveys (DHS) organised in a large number of countries to collect information on family formation and family dynamics. The fifth has data from the European Registry for Blood and Marrow Transplantation, maintained by the European Group for Blood and Marrow Transplantation (EBMT). The population covered are patients who have undergone a haematopoietic stem cell transplantation (HSCT) procedure, patients with bone marrow failures receiving immunosuppressive therapies and patients receiving non-haematopoietic cell therapies. The sixth data set is the output of a microsimulation that generates individual life histories from transition rates. For this application, I use the msm.sim function of the *msm* package. By storing the life histories in a *Biograph* object, the virtual population resulting from the microsimulation can be investigated using *Biograph* and other packages for life history data analysis.

Annex B is a list of *Biograph* functions and data included in the package. For each function, the dependencies on other functions are listed in Annex C.

Chapter 2
Life Histories: Real and Synthetic

2.1 Introduction

Life history data are generally incomplete. Usually, they do not cover for each individual in the study the entire life span or the life segment of interest. If data are collected retrospectively, observation ends at interview date, and no information is available on events and experiences after the date. Data collected prospectively are incomplete because events and other experiences are recorded during a limited period of time only. To deal with data limitations, models are introduced. The model that is considered in this chapter describes life histories. The model is based on the premise that life histories are realisations of a continuous-time Markov process. A Markov process is a stochastic process that describes a system with multiple states and transitions between the states. The time at which a transition occurs is random but the distribution of the time to transition is known. In the continuous-time Markov process, the transition time has an exponential distribution. The rate of transition out of the current state (exit rate) is the parameter of the exponential distribution. It depends on the current state only and is independent of the history of the stochastic process. In a system with multiple states, an individual who leaves the current state may enter one of several states. In competing risks models, states in the state space are viewed as competing destinations and transition rates are destination-specific. The Markov process is a first-order process: the destination state depends on the current state only and is independent of states occupied previously.

The Markov model predicts[1] the probability that an individual of a given age occupies a given state. The Markov model may also be used to predict the number of transitions during a given interval and the number of times an individual

---

[1] Prediction is used in the statistical meaning. Prediction is a statement about an outcome. A model is often used to predict an outcome, e.g. an event that occurs in a population or that is experienced by an individual in a population. The parameter(s) of the model are estimated from observations on

occupies a given state. The stochastic process that describes the transition counts or the state occupancy counts is a Markov counting process (see below). It belongs to the class of counting processes. The most elementary counting process is the Poisson process. It is a stochastic process that counts the number of transitions without considering origin and destination states. In a Poisson process, the time between two consecutive transitions has an exponential distribution.

The parameters of the Markov model are estimated from data. By pooling data on different but similar individuals, models can be estimated that describe the entire life histories. The life history that is based on pooled data is a *synthetic* life history. It is a virtual life history; it is not observed. It does not say anything about a specific individual in a sample but tells something about the sample the individual is part of. A synthetic biography summarises information on several individuals. It is the life course that would result if an individual lives a life prescribed by the collective experience of similar individuals under observation. The collective experience is summarised in *transition rates*. These rates play a key role in generating synthetic biographies. Transition rates are estimated from life history data and used to generate synthetic biographies. Maximum likelihood estimates of transition rates are used to generate expected life histories and expected values of life history indicators. Individual life histories are distributed randomly around an expected life path. Microsimulation is used to generate individual life histories from empirical transition rates.

In life history analysis and life history modelling, age is the main time scale. Age is a proxy for stage of life. Other useful time scales are calendar time and time since a reference event. Birth, marriage, labour market entry and entry into observation are examples of reference events. The standard approach in survival analysis is to use time since the baseline survey or (first) entry into the study (time-on-study). Time-on-study has no explanatory power, which is acceptable if time dependence of a transition rate is not of interest, such as in the Cox model with free baseline hazard. Korn et al. (1997) argue that time-on-study is not appropriate for predicting transition rates. They recommend age as the time scale (see also Pencina et al. 2007 and Meira-Machado et al. 2009). Rates of transition between states generally vary with age. The Markov process that accommodates changing rates is the time-inhomogeneous Markov process. The model of that process is discussed in this chapter.

To characterise life histories, a set of indicators is usually used, including state occupancies at consecutive ages, durations of stages of life and ages at significant transitions. The indicators are sometimes combined in a table, known as the *multistate life table*. The multistate life table originated in demography (Rogers 1975), but it is currently used across disciplines. The model that produces the values of the indicators summarised in the multistate life table is the Markov process model.

---

a selection of individuals. Prediction is part of statistical inference. It should not be confused with forecasting.

2.1 Introduction

Two examples may clarify the concept of synthetic biography. The first relates to the length of life and the second to marriage and fertility:

(a) Suppose we are interested in the life expectancy of a 60-year-old. The empirical evidence consists of a 10-year follow-up of 1,000 individuals aged 60 and over. At the beginning of the observation period, some individuals are relatively young (60 years, say), while others are already old (over 90, say). During the observation period of 10 years, some individuals die. The oldest old are more likely to die than other individuals under observation. To determine the expected remaining lifetime for a 60-year-old, one could calculate the mean age at death of those who die during the observation interval. The observed mean age at death provides a wrong answer, however. It depends on the age composition of the population under observation. If the group under observation consists of many old persons, the mean age at death will be higher than for a group that consists mainly of persons in their sixties and seventies. To remove the effect of the age composition, death rates are calculated by age. The distribution of ages at death is obtained by applying a piecewise exponential survival model, with parameters the age-specific mortality rates. The expected age at death is 60 plus the expected remaining lifetime or life expectancy. The life expectancy of a 60-year-old is the number of years that the individual may expect to live if at each age over 60 he experiences the age-specific mortality rate estimated during the 10-year follow-up of 1,000 individuals. At young ages, he experiences the mortality rates of individuals who were 60 recently. At older ages, the mortality rates are from old persons who turned 60 many years ago. The life expectancy is adequate if the age-specific mortality rates do not vary in time.

(b) The second illustration considers marriage and fertility. Suppose we want to know at what age women start marriage and at what duration of marriage they have their first child. It is not possible to follow all women until they have their first child since some will remain childless. Suppose the data are from a 5-year follow-up survey of girls and women aged 15–35 at the onset of observation. At the end, they are 20–40. During the follow-up, the age at marriage and the age at birth of the first child are recorded. At the start of observation, some individuals are already married. Other individuals remain unmarried during the entire period of observation. They may marry after observation is ended or they may not marry at all. To determine the age at marriage and the duration of marriage at time of birth of the first child, marriage and childbirth are described by a continuous-time Markov process with transition rates the empirical marriage rates and marital first birth rates. The model describes the marriage and first birth behaviour of hypothetical and identical individuals of age 15 assuming that at consecutive ages, they experience the empirical rates of marriage and first birth. Transition rates may depend on covariates and other factors.

This chapter consists of two parts. The first part (Sect. 2.2) is devoted to the estimation of transition rates from data. The second part (Sects. 2.3, 2.4 and 2.5) focuses on life histories derived from transition rates. Section 2.3 shows how transition probabilities and state occupation probabilities are computed from transition rates. The computation of expected occupation times is covered in Sect. 2.4. The generation of synthetic life histories is discussed in Sect. 2.5. Section 2.6 is the conclusion.

The methods presented in this chapter are illustrated using employment data from a subsample of 201 respondents of the German Life History Survey (GLHS) (see Chap. 1). Two states are distinguished: employed (**Job**) and not employed (**Nojob**). Transitions are from employed to not employed (JN) and from not employed to employed (NJ). Dates of transition are given in months; it is assumed that transitions occur at the beginning of a month. In the chapter, references are made to R packages for multistate modelling and analysis, in particular *mvna* (Allignol 2013; Allignol et al. 2008), *etm* (Allignol 2014; Allignol et al. 2011), *msm* (Jackson 2011, 2014a), *mstate* (Putter et al. 2011; de Wreede et al. 2010, 2011), *dynpred* (Putter 2011b), ELECT (van den Hout 2013) and *Biograph* (Willekens 2013a).

2.2 Transition Rates

Transition rates are the parameters of the Markov process that underlies the multistate life history model. In this section, two broad approaches for estimating transition rates are covered. Age, which is the time scale, is treated as a continuous variable. Transitions may occur at any age. Transition rates are estimated by relating transitions to exposures. In the first approach, transition rates may vary freely with age. The age profile is not constrained in any way. In the second approach, transition rates are restricted to follow an age profile described by a parametric model. The first approach is non-parametric; the second is parametric. The two approaches are covered by, e.g. Aalen et al. (2008).

In the non-parametric analysis of life history data, cumulative transition rates are estimated for ages at which transitions occur. Without any parametric assumptions, the transition rate can be any nonnegative function, and this makes it difficult to estimate. The cumulative transition rate is easy to estimate. This is akin to estimating the cumulative distribution function, which is easier than estimating the density function (Aalen et al. 2008, p. 71). At ages at which transitions occur, the cumulative transition rate jumps to a higher value. Therefore, the function that describes cumulative transition rates is a step function. It implies that between observations, the cumulative transition rate is the one estimated at the last observation. The shape of the function is entirely free, not influenced by an imposed age dependence. The cumulative transition rate is said to be empirical. In the second approach, the age dependence is restricted to follow an imposed pattern. A convenient and simple restriction is a constant transition rate. If the transition rate is constant, the cumulative transition rate increases linearly with age and the survival function is exponential. The restriction of constant rate may be relaxed by keeping the rate constant within relatively narrow age intervals and let the rate vary freely between age

2.2 Transition Rates

intervals. Because of the imposed age dependence, there is no need to estimate the cumulative transition rate each age a transition occurs. It suffices to estimate the cumulative transition rate at the end of each age interval. The cumulative hazard function is not a step function. It is a piecewise linear function: linear within age intervals with slopes varying between intervals. The two approaches differ, but at the limit when the age interval becomes infinitesimally small, they coincide. The first approach is common in biostatistics, while the second is common in the life table method of demography, epidemiology and actuarial science. Covariates may be introduced in each approach. The cumulative transition rates may be estimated at each level of covariate or a regression model may be used. A (piecewise) constant transition rate is only one of the many possible restrictions imposed on the age dependence of transition rates. In demography, biostatistics, epidemiology and other fields, a large number of models are used to describe age dependencies of rates. These models are beyond the scope of this chapter.

A few software packages in R implement the non-parametric method. They include *mvna* and *mstate*. The packages *eha*, *msm* and *Biograph* implement the parametric method, more particularly the piecewise constant transition rate model: the transition rate varies freely between age intervals and is constant within age intervals.

Transition rates are estimated by relating transitions to exposures. At a given age, the rate of transition is estimated by dividing the number of transitions and the risk set, which is the population under observation and at risk just before a transition occurs. In multistate modelling, a risk set is the number of individuals under observation and occupying a given state. That basic principle allows complex observation schemes. Individuals may be at risk but not under observation. It is not practical to track every individual from birth to death to record occurrences and monitor risk sets and periods at risk. When the period of observation does not cover the entire life span, observations are incomplete. Individuals may enter and leave the population at risk during the observation period. They may leave the population at risk because the transition of interest occurs or another, unrelated, transition removes them from the population at risk. Individuals who leave the population at risk may return later and be at risk again. Counting transitions and tracking exposures necessarily take place during periods of observation. Transitions and exposures outside the observation period are not recorded. The nonoccurrence of a transition during a period of observation to persons at risk of that transition is however useful information that should not be omitted. The proportion of individuals under observation and at risk that experiences a transition is an estimator of the likelihood of a transition. The proportion that does not experience a transition is an estimator of the survival probability.

Dates of transition are usually measured in the Gregorian calendar. For reasons of computation, calendar dates are often converted into Julian dates, which are days since a reference date. Sometimes, calendar months are coded as number of months since a reference month. The Century Month Code (CMC) is a coding scheme with reference month January 1900. The reference month is month 1. In life history analysis, dates are often replaced by ages. In this chapter, dates (in CMC) and ages are used, but age is the main time scale. Hence, most of the time reference is made to age. Transitions may occur at any time and age. Hence, time at transition and age at transition are random variables. T will be used to denote time and age, and X will be used to denote age only. A realisation of T is t and a realisation of X is x. Continuous time is approximated by dividing a period in very small time intervals. A small interval following t is denoted by $[t+\mathrm{d}t)$, where $\mathrm{d}t$ is the length of the interval. The brackets indicate the type of interval: [means that t is not included in the interval and) means that $t+\mathrm{d}t$ is included in the interval. A small interval following age x is $[x, x+\mathrm{d}x)$. When is an interval small? An interval is considered small when at most one transition occurs in the interval.

In the employment data used for illustrative purposes (GLHS), two states are distinguished (J and N) and two transitions: NJ and JN. In this chapter, transitions between jobs are not considered. Individuals in state N are at risk of the NJ transition and individuals in J are at risk of the JN transition. Labour market entry (first jobs) is selected as onset of the observation. The original GLHS data include transitions between jobs, and dates at transition are expressed in CMC. Two *Biograph* functions are used to prepare the desired data file from the original data. The function Remove.intrastate is used to remove transitions between jobs. The function ChangeObservationWindow.e is used to select observation periods between labour market entry and survey date. Table 2.1 shows the data for a selection of ten respondents. Two variants are presented. The first shows calendar dates at transition. The second shows ages, except for the birth date, which is given in CMC. Calendar dates and ages are derived from CMC using *Biograph*'s date_b function.

```
d <- Remove.intrastate(GLHS)
dd <- ChangeObservationWindow.e (Bdata=d,
            entrystate="J",
            exitstate=NA)
d3.a <- date_b (Bdata=dd,
            selectday=1,
            format.out="age")
```

The ten individuals experience 33 episodes (20 job episodes and 13 episodes without a job). They experience 23 transitions during the observation period (13 JN transitions and 10 NJ transitions). Individual 2 is born in September 1929 and enters the labour market (first job) in May 1949 at age 19. She leaves the first job in May 1974 at age 44 and remains without a paid job until the end of the observation period in November 1981, when she is at age 52. Individuals 1, 5 and 7 are employed throughout the observation period. They move between jobs, but they do not experience a period without a job. Individuals 3, 4, 6, 8, 9 and 10 have several jobs, separated by periods without a job. Observation periods differ between individuals. In this chapter, we estimate transition rates for the JN and NJ transitions, transition probabilities, state occupation probabilities and expected state occupation times for the subsample of 201 respondents. For illustrative purpose, a selection of the ten respondents shown in Table 2.1 is also used. The focus is on the method and not on the application.

2.2 Transition Rates

Table 2.1 Subsample of German Life History Survey (GLHS)

```
a. Calendar dates
    ID born  start end   sex    path  Tr1   Tr2   Tr3   Tr4
1    1 Mar29 Mar46 Nov81 Male    J    <NA>  <NA>  <NA>  <NA>
2    2 Sep29 May49 Nov81 Female JN    May74 <NA>  <NA>  <NA>
3   67 Dec39 Feb55 Nov81 Female JNJN  Sep58 Aug70 Mar80 <NA>
4   76 Jun51 Oct69 Nov81 Male   JNJNJ Apr70 May72 Jan76 Apr76
5   82 Jun51 Aug74 Nov81 Female  J    <NA>  <NA>  <NA>  <NA>
6   96 Feb39 Apr57 Nov81 Female JNJNJ Apr62 Apr64 Feb65 Nov68
7   99 May40 Sep58 Nov81 Male    J    <NA>  <NA>  <NA>  <NA>
8  180 Aug40 Aug54 Nov81 Male   JNJNJ Apr56 Apr59 Jul61 Jan63
9  200 Nov50 Sep68 Dec81 Male   JNJNJ Apr70 Jan72 Jan74 Jan79
10 208 May40 Jul59 Nov81 Female  JNJN May61 Nov61 Dec62 <NA>

b. Ages
    ID born  start  end    sex    path  Tr1    Tr2    Tr3    Tr4
1    1 351  17.000 52.667 Male    J     NA     NA     NA     NA
2    2 357  19.667 52.167 Female JN    44.667  NA     NA     NA
3   67 480  15.167 41.917 Female JNJN  18.750 30.667 40.250  NA
4   76 618  18.333 30.417 Male   JNJNJ 18.833 20.917 24.583 24.833
5   82 618  23.167 30.417 Female  J     NA     NA     NA     NA
6   96 470  18.167 42.750 Female JNJNJ 23.167 25.167 26.000 29.750
7   99 485  18.333 41.500 Male    J     NA     NA     NA     NA
8  180 488  14.000 41.250 Male   JNJNJ 15.667 18.667 20.917 22.417
9  200 611  17.833 31.083 Male   JNJNJ 19.417 21.167 23.167 28.167
10 208 485  19.167 41.500 Female  JNJN 21.000 21.500 22.583     NA
```

Individual 4 (with ID 76) will be singled out for a detailed description. He gets his first job in October 1969 at age 18 and remains employed until April 1970. He is not employed for about 2 years, until he gets another job in May 1972. From January to April 1976, he experiences another period without employment. At the end of the observation, i.e. at survey date, the person is 30 years of age and employed. The employment career is JNJNJ. The lifeline is shown in Fig. 2.1. The figure is a Lexis diagram, which is a diagram with calendar time on the x-axis and age on the y-axis. The transitions are displayed, as well as the job and no job episodes. The Lexis diagram is discussed in detail in Chap. 5. During the observation period, the individual experiences the JN transition two times, in April 1970 at age 18 and in January 1976 at age 24. Transitions are assumed to occur at the beginning of a month. From 1 October 1969 to 31 March 1970, he is at risk of the first occurrence of the JN transition, and from 1 May 1972 to 31 December 1975, he is at risk of the second occurrence. From 1 April 1976, he is at risk of a third occurrence but does not experience the JN transition before the end of the observation on 1 November 1981. The individual experiences three job episodes, two end in a JN transition and one ends because observation is terminated (censored). In addition, the respondent experiences two episodes without a job. They end with a new job.

The estimation of transition rates involves counting transitions and persons at risk. Let k denote an individual. Transitions are denoted by origin state and destination state. The number of states is I and any two states are denoted by i and j. Let $_kN_{ij}(t_1,t_2)$ denote the number of (i,j)-transitions individual k experiences during a period of observation from t_1 to t_2. Without loss of generality, in this

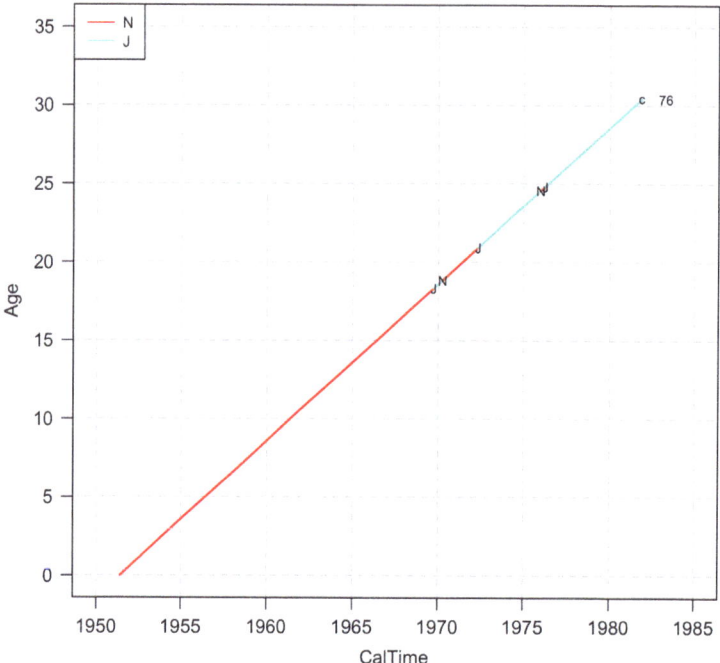

Fig. 2.1 Employment career of respondent with ID 76

section, I assume that $t_1 = 0$ and represent t_2 by t. The observation interval is therefore from 0 to t. The variable $_kN_{ij}(0, t)$ is denoted by $_kN_{ij}(t)$. Data on numbers of transitions are *count data*. Transition counts cannot be predicted with certainty; hence, $_kN_{ij}(t)$ is a random variable. The distribution of transition counts is described by a stochastic process model. A widely used model is the Poisson process model, where changes ('jumps') occur randomly and are independent of each other (Çinlar 1975). The sequence of random variables $\{_kN_{ij}(t); t \geq 0\}$ is a random process, known as a *counting process* (Aalen et al. 2008, p. 25). The counting process is a continuous process. The increment in $_kN_{ij}(t)$ during the small interval between t and $t + dt$ is denoted by $d_kN_{ij}(t)$. It is a binary variable with possible values 0 (no transition) and 1 (transition). Individual counting processes are aggregated to obtain the aggregated process: $N_{ij}(t) = \sum_{k=1}^{K} {_kN_{ij}(t)}$, where K is the number of individuals in a (sample) population. If dt is sufficiently small to make the counting process absolutely continuous, at most, one transition occurs in the interval dt.

A main issue in survival analysis, and in multistate modelling in particular, is to determine who is at risk or exposed at time (age) t and who is not. Individuals may experience a transition between t and $t + dt$ if and only if they are at risk at t, i.e. just before the interval $[t, t + dt)$. If individual i is at risk at t, he/she is at risk during the infinitesimally small interval from t to $t + dt$. To be at risk of the (i,j)-transition, an individual should be in state i. Let $_kY_i(t)$ be a binary variable, which takes the value of 1 if individual k is in state i at t and 0 if the individual is not. The binary random

2.2 Transition Rates

variable $_kY_i(t)$ indicates the exposure status. The number of individuals in state i just before t, and at risk of the (i,j)-transition, is $Y_i(t) = \sum_{k=1}^{K} {_kY_i(t)}$. It is the *risk set*. The sequence of risk sets $\{Y_i(t), t \geq 0\}$ is the *at risk process* or *exposure process*. The risk set in state i at time (age) t, $Y_i(t)$, changes when an individual enters state i or leaves the state and when the observation starts or ends. In many studies, $Y_i(t)$ is large relative to the numbers of (i,j)-transitions. That empirical observation will be used for estimating the variance of the transition rate.

During the observation period from 0 to t, individual k is at risk of experiencing the (i,j)-transition during the time (age) segments he occupies state i. The state occupation time measures the duration at risk. It is $_kL_i = \int_0^t {_kY_i(\tau)}\, d\tau$. The total duration at risk may be spread over multiple 'at risk' episodes. This approach, in which a counting process and an at risk process are distinguished, is known as the counting process approach to the study of life histories and event histories. The approach is very flexible. It allows late entry, exit and re-entry in state i during the observation period.

The counting process is a random process. It can be modelled by a Poisson process. The parameter of the model is the transition rate. The transition rate in the small time (age) interval $[t, t+dt)$ is referred to as the instantaneous transition rate and is denoted by $_k\mu_{ij}(t)$. The counting process approach to the Poisson process describes the intensity of the process in terms of the instantaneous transition rate and exposure status. It adds exposure status to the conventional description of the Poisson process in probability theory. Aalen et al. (2008) write the intensity at t as the product of the instantaneous transition rate and the indicator function $_kY_i(t)$, which is equal to 1 if individual k is at risk just before t and 0 otherwise: $_k\lambda_{ij}(t) = {_k\mu_{ij}(t)}{_kY_i(t)}$. The intensity function is the transition rate function weighted by the exposure status. If individual k is not at risk at t, the intensity is zero although the transition rate may be positive. The product $_k\lambda_{ij}(t)dt$ is the probability that individual k experiences the (i,j)-transition during the small time (age) interval from t to $t+dt$, provided that just prior to the interval k is at risk of the (i,j)-transition, i.e. is in state i. It is the product of the intensity and the length of the interval. The probability is conditioned on being at risk. In survival analysis, that condition is usually imposed by the statement 'provided that the event has not occurred yet'. That condition applies in case of a single event because an individual is at risk as long as (1) the event has not occurred yet and (2) the individual is under observation. In the case of repeatable transitions or different types of transitions, an individual may be under observation but not at risk. In the example of employment, an individual in state N is under observation but not at risk of the JN transition.

If at most one transition occurs during the interval dt, the probability of occurrence may be expressed in different but equivalent ways. It is the probability that $_kN_{ij}(t)$ changes to $_kN_{ij}(t)+1$; the probability that the transition occurs at t, $\Pr(d_kN_{ij}(t)=1)$ and the probability that the transition time (age) $_kT_{ij}$ is in the $[t, t+dt)$ interval: $\Pr(t \leq {_kT_{ij}} < t+dt)$. The probability that $d_kN_{ij}(t)$ is one, $\Pr(d_kN_{ij}(t)=1)$, is equal to the expected value of $d_kN_{ij}(t)$, hence $_k\lambda_{ij}(t)\,dt = E[d_kN_{ij}(t)]$. Note that $_kN_{ij}(t)$ and its increment $d_kN_{ij}(t)$ are observations, whereas

$_k\lambda_{ij}(t)$ is a model of the increment $d_k N_{ij}(t)$ (Poisson process model that satisfies the two conditions listed above). $_k\lambda_{ij}(t)$ is the *intensity process* of the counting process $_k N_{ij}(t)$.

If individuals are independent of each other, the intensity process of the aggregated counting process $N_{ij}(t)$ is $\lambda_{ij}(t) = \sum_{k=1}^{K} {_k\lambda_{ij}(t)}$. If in addition all individuals are assumed to have the same hazard rate, i.e. $_k\mu_{ij}(t) = \mu_{ij}(t)$ for all k, then the survival times are independent and identically distributed. The aggregate intensity process may be written as $\lambda_{ij}(t) = \sum_{k=1}^{K} {_k\lambda_{ij}(t)} = \mu_{ij}(t) \sum_{k=1}^{K} {_k Y_i(t)} = \mu_{ij}(t) Y_i(t)$, where $Y_i(t)$ is the number of individuals in state i just before t. It is the population at risk. The model $\lambda_{ij}(t) = \mu_{ij}(t) Y_i(t)$ is the multiplicative intensity model for a counting process (Aalen et al. 2008, p. 34). In the multiplicative intensity model, the at risk process $Y_i(t)$ does not depend on unknown parameters (Aalen et al. 2008, p. 77). That condition is satisfied if the population at risk is large relative to the number of transitions. The same condition was introduced by Holford (1980) and Laird and Olivier (1981) in the context of estimating (piecewise constant) transition rates with log-linear models. The transition rates $\mu_{ij}(t)$ are key model parameters, and a main aim of statistical analysis is to determine how they vary over time (age) and depend on covariates.

The observed increment $dN_{ij}(t)$ of the counting process $N_{ij}(t)$ generally differs from the model estimate $\lambda_{ij}(t)dt$ because observations do not meet the conditions imposed by the Poisson process. Aalen et al. (2008, p. 27) refer to the difference as noise and to the probability of a transition during the interval dt as signal. The noise cumulated up to time (age) t is the martingale $M_{ij}(t)$, and $dM_{ij}(t)$ is the increment in noise during the small interval following t: $dM_{ij}(t) = dN_{ij}(t) - \lambda_{ij}(t)\,dt$. The intensity process and the noise process are stochastic processes, whereas $N_{ij}(t)$ represents observations. Note that $N_{ij}(t) = \int_0^t dN_{ij}(\tau)$, $\Lambda_{ij}(t) = \int_0^t \lambda_{ij}(\tau)\,d\tau$ and $M_{ij}(t) = \int_0^t dM_{ij}(\tau)$, where $\Lambda_{ij}(t)$ is the cumulative intensity process, that is, the expected number of transitions up to t, predicted by the Poisson model. The martingale is the difference between the counting process and the cumulative intensity process. It can be interpreted as cumulative noise. The intensity process is central to the statistical modelling of event occurrences and transitions between states. Note that the intensity process depends on the transition rate and the at risk process.

A frequently used measure in multistate modelling is the cumulative hazard $A_{ij}(t) = \int_0^t dA_{ij}(\tau)$, where $dA_{ij}(\tau)$ is equal to the increment in the cumulative hazard during an infinitesimally small interval. In case of a continuous process, $dA_{ij}(\tau) = \mu_{ij}(\tau)\,d\tau$. The reason for using the cumulative hazard is given above. The transition rates $\mu_{ij}(t)$ and the cumulative transition rates $A_{ij}(t)$ are estimated from the data. The estimation method is determined by the assumed underlying stochastic process. In this chapter, two methods are described. In the first method, no assumption is made about the process. The method is known as the

2.2 Transition Rates

non-parametric method because of the absence of a parametric model that describes the time (age) dependence of transition rates. The second method assumes that transition rates are (piecewise) constant. As a consequence, the duration to the next transition and the time between two consecutive transitions follow a (piecewise) exponential distribution. In the remainder of this chapter, I use age as time scale.

(a) Non-parametric Method

Recall that $N_{ij}(t)$ is the number of (i,j)-transitions experienced by individuals in the (sample) population during the observation interval from 0 to t, and T_{ij} is the age at an (i,j)-transition. For the estimation of empirical transition rates (non-parametric), transitions are ordered by age of occurrence. Let T_{ij}^n denote the age of the n-th occurrence of the (i,j)-transition experienced in the (sample) population. The number of individuals at risk just before T_{ij}^n is $Y_i(T_{ij}^n)$. Consider the age interval $[t, t+dt)$. If in a population no event occurs in the interval, the natural estimate of $\mu_{ij}(t)\,dt$ is zero. If a transition is recorded during the interval, the natural estimate is 1 divided by the number of individuals at risk, that is, $1/Y_i(t)$ or the proportion of individuals at risk that experiences a transition. Aggregating these contributions over all age intervals at which transitions occur, up to age t, gives the estimator $\hat{A}_{ij}(t)$ of $A_{ij}(t)$. A natural estimator of the cumulative transition rate at age t is $\hat{A}_{ij}(t) = \int_0^t \frac{dN_{ij}(\tau)}{Y_i(\tau)}$, where numerator and denominator are aggregations over all individuals. If transition ages are T_{ij}^n, then the estimator is

$$\hat{A}_{ij}(t) = \sum_{T_{ij}^n \leq t} \frac{1}{Y_i(T_{ij}^n)},$$

where T_{ij}^n is the age at the n-th occurrence of the (i,j)-transition. The estimator is known as the Nelson-Aalen estimator. The estimator was initially developed by Nelson and extended to event history models and Markov processes by Aalen, who adopted a counting process formulation (see Aalen et al. 2008, pp. 70ff). The Nelson-Aalen estimator corresponds to the cumulative hazard of a discrete distribution, with all its probability mass concentrated at the observed ages at transition. The matrix $\hat{\mathbf{A}}(t)$ is a matrix of step functions with jumps at ages at transition.

The variance of the Nelson-Aalen estimator is $\hat{\sigma}_{ij}^2(t) = \sum_{T_{ij}^n \leq t} \frac{1}{[Y_i(T_{ij}^n)]^2}$ (Aalen variance). The variance increases with t. The increment is $\Delta \hat{\sigma}_{ij}^2(T_{ij}^n) = \frac{1}{[Y_i(T_{ij}^n)]^2}$. In large samples, the Nelson-Aalen estimator at age t is approximately normally distributed. Therefore, the 95 % confidence interval is $\hat{A}_{ij}(t) \pm 1.96 \, \hat{\sigma}_{ij}(t)$. If the sample size is small, the approximation to the normal distribution is improved by using a log-transformation giving the confidence interval $\exp\left[\ln \hat{A}_{ij}(t) \pm 1.96 \hat{\sigma}_{ij}(t)/\hat{A}_{ij}(t)\right]$ (Aalen et al. 2008, p. 72).

Consider the employment careers of the ten individuals, shown in Table 2.1. To track individuals at risk, ages at entry into observation and exit from observation and ages at transition should be ordered. Individual 8 enters observation at age 14.00, followed by individual 3 at age 15.16. The first transition occurs at age 15.67 when individual 8 enters a period without a job. At that age, 2 individuals are at risk of the JN transition (3 and 8). The Nelson-Aalen estimator of the cumulative transition rate at that age is ½. The next event is at age 17.00 when individual 1 enters observation. Just before that age, individual 3 is at risk in J and individual 8 in N. At age 17.00, individual 1 joins 3 in J. The next event is at age 17.83 when individual 9 enters observation. When individual 6 enters observation at age 18.17, three individuals are in J and one in N. Individuals 4 and 7 enter observation at age 18.33. At age 18.67, individual 8 enters J again. Just before that age, he is the only person in N and at risk of the NJ transition, while 6 individuals are in J. Hence, the estimator of the hazard is 1. The next event is at age 18.75, when individual 3 leaves J and enters a period without a job. At that age 7 individuals are in J and at risk of the JN transition (1, 3, 4, 6, 7, 8, 9). The cumulative JN transition rate $1/2 + 1/7 = 0.64$. The Aalen variance is $(1/2)^2 + (1/7)^2 = 0.270$. At that age, three individuals have not yet entered observation and do not contribute to the cumulative hazard estimation (2, 5 and 10). The cumulative transition rate increases to age 44.67 when individual 3 enters a period without a job. At that age, the cumulative transition rate is 2.696 and the Aalen variance is 0.764. Table 2.2 shows the Nelson-Aalen estimator based on data of the ten respondents. The columns are: (1) age at entry into observation, exit from observation or transition, (2) the population at risk just prior to the transition (`nrisk`), (3) occurrence of a transition (`nevent`), (4) censoring (`ncens`), (5) the Nelson-Aalen estimator of the cumulative transition rate (`cumhaz`) at the indicated age, (6) the Aalen estimator of the variance (`var`) and (7) increment in the cumulative hazard (`delta`). The information is shown each time a transition occurs or a respondent enters or leaves observation. The number of events is less than the number of entries (10) + the number of exits (10) + the number of JN transitions (13) + the number of NJ transitions (10), because individuals 3 and 7 enter observation at the same time, individual 5 enters observation when individuals 6 and 9 experience a JN transition, and individuals 4 and 5 leave observation at the same age, as do individuals 7 and 10. The table is produced by the `mvna` function of the *mvna* package. The last column is produced by the `etm` function of the *etm* package (see below). The object `d.10` is the *Biograph* object for a selection of ten respondents, and `D$D` is an object with data of ten respondents in *mvna* format. The following code is used:

2.2 Transition Rates

```
# Select 10 respondents and create Biograph object
idd <- c(1,2,67,76,82,96,99,180,200,208)
d.10 <- d3.a[d3.a$ID%in%idd,]
D<- Biograph.mvna (d.10)
library (mvna)
library (etm)
tra <- matrix(ncol=2,nrow=2,FALSE)
tra[1, 2] <- TRUE
tra[2,1] <- TRUE
na <- mvna(data=D$D,c("J","N"),tra,"cens")
etm.0 <- etm(data=D$D,c("J","N"),tra,"cens",s=0)

gg.1 <- data.frame (
    round(na$"J N"$time,4),
    na$n.risk[,1],
    unname(aperm(na$n.event,c(3,2,1))[,2,1]),
    na$n.cens[,1],
    round(na$"J N"$na,4),
    round(na$"J N"$var.aalen,3),
    round(aperm (etm.0$delta.na,c(3,2,1))[,2,1],4))
dimnames (gg.1) <- list
 (1:37,c("age","nrisk","nevent","ncens","cumhaz","var","delta
 "))
gg.2 <- data.frame (
    round(na$"N J"$time,4),
    na$n.risk[,2][na$time %in% na$"N J"$time],
    unname(aperm(na$n.event,c(3,2,1))[,1,2])[na$time %in%
     na$"N J"$time],
    na$n.cens[,2][na$time %in% na$"N J"$time],
    round(na$"N J"$na,4),
    round(na$"N J"$var.aalen,3),
    round(aperm (etm.0$delta.na,c(3,2,1))[,1,2][na$time %in%
     na$"N J"$time],4))
dimnames (gg.2) <- list
 (1:nrow(gg.2),c("age","nrisk","nevent","ncens","cumhaz","var
 ","delta"))
```

The ten respondents enter observation at ages 14.00 (ID 180), 15.67 (ID 67), 17.00 (ID 1), 17.83 (ID 200), 18.17 (ID 96), 18.83 (ID 99), 19.17 (ID 208), 19.67 (ID 2) and 23.17 (ID 82) (see Table 2.1). They experience 13 JN transitions and 10 NJ transitions. At time of survey, 7 respondents had a job and 3 were without a job. The youngest age at job exit is 15.67 years (ID 180). The youngest age at survey is 30.42 (ID 76 and 82) and the highest is 52.67 (ID 1). Two respondents are 41.50 years at survey date, one (ID 99) has a job and one (ID 208) is without a job.

The time-continuous model of the counting process $\{N_{ij}(t), t \geq 0\}$ assumes that not more than one transition occurs in an interval. In practice and in particular in large samples, more than one individual may experience a transition in the same time interval (e.g. same day). If multiple transitions occur in the same interval, their times of occurrence are referred to as *tied transition times*. Tied transition times may be a consequence of (a) grouping and rounding or (b) time (age) intervals that are genuinely discrete. For instance, if instead of days or months, seconds are used as time units, it is unlikely that more than one transition occurs at the same time (age). If tied transition times are due to grouping and rounding, the interval may be

Table 2.2 Nelson-Aalen estimator and Aalen variance of cumulative transition rates. GLHS, subsample of ten respondents

```
Transition JN
      age nrisk nevent ncens cumhaz   var delta
 1  14.0000    1      0     0 0.0000 0.000 0.0000
 2  15.1667    1      0     0 0.0000 0.000 0.0000
 3  15.6667    2      1     0 0.5000 0.250 0.5000
 4  17.0000    1      0     0 0.5000 0.250 0.0000
 5  17.8333    2      0     0 0.5000 0.250 0.0000
 6  18.1667    3      0     0 0.5000 0.250 0.0000
 7  18.3333    4      0     0 0.5000 0.250 0.0000
 8  18.6667    6      0     0 0.5000 0.250 0.0000
 9  18.7500    7      1     0 0.6429 0.270 0.1429
10  18.8333    6      1     0 0.8095 0.298 0.1667
11  19.1667    5      0     0 0.8095 0.298 0.0000
12  19.4167    6      1     0 0.9762 0.326 0.1667
13  19.6667    5      0     0 0.9762 0.326 0.0000
14  20.9167    6      1     0 1.1429 0.354 0.1667
15  21.0000    6      1     0 1.3095 0.382 0.1667
16  21.1667    5      0     0 1.3095 0.382 0.0000
17  21.5000    6      0     0 1.3095 0.382 0.0000
18  22.4167    7      0     0 1.3095 0.382 0.0000
19  22.5833    8      1     0 1.4345 0.397 0.1250
20  23.1667    7      2     0 1.7202 0.438 0.2857
21  24.5833    6      1     0 1.8869 0.466 0.1667
22  24.8333    5      0     0 1.8869 0.466 0.0000
23  25.1667    6      0     0 1.8869 0.466 0.0000
24  26.0000    7      1     0 2.0298 0.486 0.1429
25  28.1667    6      0     0 2.0298 0.486 0.0000
26  29.7500    7      0     0 2.0298 0.486 0.0000
27  30.4167    8      0     2 2.0298 0.486 0.0000
28  30.6667    6      0     0 2.0298 0.486 0.0000
29  31.0833    7      0     1 2.0298 0.486 0.0000
30  40.2500    6      1     0 2.1964 0.514 0.1667
31  41.2500    5      0     1 2.1964 0.514 0.0000
32  41.5000    4      0     1 2.1964 0.514 0.0000
33  41.9167    3      0     0 2.1964 0.514 0.0000
34  42.7500    3      0     1 2.1964 0.514 0.0000
35  44.6667    2      1     0 2.6964 0.764 0.5000
36  52.1667    1      0     0 2.6964 0.764 0.0000
37  52.6667    1      0     1 2.6964 0.764 0.0000

Transition NJ
      age nrisk nevent ncens cumhaz   var delta
 1  17.0000    1      0     0 0.0000 0.000 0.0000
 2  17.8333    1      0     0 0.0000 0.000 0.0000
 3  18.1667    1      0     0 0.0000 0.000 0.0000
 4  18.3333    1      0     0 0.0000 0.000 0.0000
 5  18.6667    1      1     0 1.0000 1.000 1.0000
 6  18.8333    1      0     0 1.0000 1.000 0.0000
 7  19.1667    2      0     0 1.0000 1.000 0.0000
 8  19.4167    2      0     0 1.0000 1.000 0.0000
 9  19.6667    3      0     0 1.0000 1.000 0.0000
10  20.9167    3      1     0 1.3333 1.111 0.3333
11  21.0000    3      0     0 1.3333 1.111 0.0000
12  21.1667    4      1     0 1.5833 1.174 0.2500
13  21.5000    3      1     0 1.9167 1.285 0.3333
14  22.4167    2      1     0 2.4167 1.535 0.5000
15  22.5833    1      0     0 2.4167 1.535 0.0000
16  23.1667    2      0     0 2.4167 1.535 0.0000
17  24.5833    4      0     0 2.4167 1.535 0.0000
18  24.8333    5      1     0 2.6167 1.575 0.2000
19  25.1667    4      1     0 2.8667 1.637 0.2500
20  26.0000    3      0     0 2.8667 1.637 0.0000
21  28.1667    4      1     0 3.1167 1.700 0.2500
22  29.7500    3      1     0 3.4500 1.811 0.3333
23  30.4167    2      0     0 3.4500 1.811 0.0000
24  30.6667    2      1     0 3.9500 2.061 0.5000
25  31.0833    1      0     0 3.9500 2.061 0.0000
26  40.2500    1      0     0 3.9500 2.061 0.0000
27  41.2500    2      0     0 3.9500 2.061 0.0000
28  41.5000    2      0     1 3.9500 2.061 0.0000
29  41.9167    1      0     1 3.9500 2.061 0.0000
30  52.1667    1      0     1 3.9500 2.061 0.0000
```

2.2 Transition Rates

divided in even smaller intervals and the transition times (ages) ordered. The increment in the Nelson-Aalen estimator of the cumulative hazard at age T_{ij}^n may be written as $\Delta \hat{A}_{ij}\left(T_{ij}^n\right) = \sum_{k=0}^{d_n-1} \dfrac{1}{Y_i\left(T_{ij}^n\right) - k}$ (Aalen et al. 2008, p. 84). If the age intervals are genuinely discrete, the increment in the Nelson-Aalen estimator at age T_{ij}^n is $\Delta \hat{A}_{ij}\left(T_{ij}^n\right) = \dfrac{d_n}{Y_i(T_{ij}^n)}$, where $Y_i(T_{ij}^n)$ is the population at risk just prior to the interval and d_n is the number of transitions recorded at age T_{ij}^n. In the presence of tied transition times, the variance of the Nelson-Aalen estimator needs to be adjusted. When tied event times are a consequence of grouping or rounding, the increment in the variance is $\Delta \hat{\sigma}_{ij}^2\left(T_{ij}^n\right) = \sum_{k=0}^{d_n-1} \dfrac{1}{\left[Y_i\left(T_{ij}^n\right) - k\right]^2}$. In case of discrete age intervals, the increment in the variance is estimated by $\Delta \hat{\sigma}_{ij}^2\left(T_{ij}^n\right) = \dfrac{\left[Y_i(T_{ij}^n) - d_n\right] d_n}{\left[Y_i(T_{ij}^n)\right]^3}$. Aalen et al. (2008, p. 85) report that the numerical difference between the two approaches to tie correction is usually quite small, and it is not very important which of the two one adopts.

(b) Parametric Method: Exponential and Piecewise Exponential Models

The Nelson-Aalen estimator is non-parametric. The shape of the hazard function is not constrained in any way. In a parametric counting process model, the age dependence of the transition rate is constrained, and consequently the waiting times to a transition are constrained. It is assumed that there is a continuous-time process underlying the data. In addition, the transition rate may depend on covariates. Covariates are not considered in this chapter. Two models are considered in this chapter. The first is the exponential model, which imposes a constant transition rate and an exponential waiting time distribution. The second model is a piecewise exponential model, which imposes piecewise constant transition rates. Transitions rates are assumed to be constant in age intervals of usually 1 year. The transition rates of consecutive age groups are unrelated, i.e. no restrictions are imposed on how the piecewise constant rates vary with age. The estimation method therefore combines a parametric approach (within intervals) and a non-parametric approach (between intervals). Individuals are assumed to be independent and to have the same instantaneous transition rate. In other words, transition times of the individuals in the (sample) population are assumed to be independent and identically distributed. The estimation of piecewise exponential models and occurrence-exposure rates received considerable attention in the literature (see, e.g. Hoem and Funck Jensen 1982; Tuma and Hannan 1984; Hougaard 2000; Blossfeld and Rohwer 2002; Aalen et al. 2008; Van den Hout and Matthews 2008; Li et al. 2012). Mamun (2003) and Reuser (2010), who study the effect of covariates on disability and mortality, impose the restriction that the piecewise constant transition rates (occurrence-exposure rates) increase exponentially with age. The result is a Gompertz model with piecewise constant transition rates. The choice of model is determined by the age profile of transition rates (exponential increase) and data limitations. Parametric models of transition rates covering the entire age range in multistate models have been estimated too. Van den Hout and Matthews (2008) estimate a multistate model in which the age dependence of transition rates is described by a Weibull model, and Van den Hout et al. (2014) use a Gompertz model. In demography, a variety of models are specified to describe age profiles of transition rates in multistate models. For an overview of models, see Rogers (1986).

In the counting process approach, the likelihood function is written in terms of the counting process $_kN_{ij}(t)$ and the intensity process $_k\lambda_{ij}(t)$, where t represents age. The intensity process at age t is $_k\lambda_{ij}(t) = {}_k\mu_{ij}(t)\,_kY_i(t)$. The indicator function $_kY_i(t)$ is 1 if individual k is under observation and in state i at t and 0 otherwise. The total occupation time in state i is $_kY_i = \int_0^\omega {}_kY_i(\tau)\,d\tau$, with ω the highest age. If individuals are independent, the intensity process at age t is $\lambda_{ij}(t) = \sum_{k=1}^K {}_k\lambda_{ij}(t)$, and $\lambda_{ij}(t)dt$ is the number of (i,j)-transitions between t and $t+dt$, given the instantaneous transition rate and the exposure function. If in addition all individuals have the same hazard rate, i.e. $_k\mu_{ij}(t) = \mu_{ij}(t)$ for all k, then the survival times are independent and identically distributed. The aggregate intensity process may be written as $\lambda_{ij}(t) = \sum_{k=1}^K {}_k\lambda_{ij}(t) = \mu_{ij}(t) \sum_{k=1}^K {}_kY_i(t) = \mu_{ij}(t)\,Y_i(t)$, where $Y_i(t)$ is the number of individuals under observation and in state i just before t. If the transition rate is constant, then $_k\mu_{ij}(t) = {}_k\mu_{ij}$ for all t and the intensity process at t is $_k\lambda_{ij}(t) = {}_k\mu_{ij}\,_kY_i(t)$. If the transition rate is piecewise constant during the age interval from x to $x+1$, $_k\mu_{ij}(t) = {}_k\mu_{ij}(x)$ for $x \leq t < x+1$ and the intensity process at t is $_k\lambda_{ij}(t) = {}_k\mu_{ij}(x)\,_kY_i(t)$ for $x \leq t < x+1$. The intensity of leaving state i at age t, irrespective of destination, is $_k\lambda_i(t) = \sum_{j \neq i} {}_k\lambda_{ij}(t)$, which may be written as $_k\lambda_i(t) = {}_k\mu_i(t)\,_kY_i(t)$, with $_k\mu_i(t) = \sum_{j \neq i} {}_k\mu_{ij}(t)$.

Let ω denote the highest age in the study. A transition is observed if it occurs before ω. Individual k experiences $_kN_{ij}(\omega)$ occurrences of the (i,j)-transition from 0 to ω. In addition, the observation is censored in state i or in another state. Hence, the number of episodes of exposure is the number of transitions plus one. The contribution of individual k to the likelihood function is:

$$\left[\prod_{n=1}^{{}_kN_{ij}(\omega)} {}_k\lambda_{ij}^n\left({}_kT_{ij}^n\right)\exp\left[-\int_0^\omega {}_k\lambda_i^n(\tau)d\tau\right]\right]\exp\left[-\int_0^\omega {}_k\lambda_i^c(\tau)d\tau\right]$$

where $_kT_{ij}^n$ is the age at the n-th occurrence of the (i,j)-transition. Since the intensity depends on the instantaneous transition rate and exposure, the likelihood function is written in terms of the counting process $_kN_{ij}(t)$ and its intensity process $_k\lambda_{ij}(t)$ (Aalen et al. 2008, p. 210). Notice that $_k\lambda_{ij}^n({}_kT_{ij}^n) = \mu_{ij}\,_kY_i^n({}_kT_{ij}^n)$, with the at risk function equal to one if individual k is in state i just before the transition and 0 otherwise, and $_k\lambda_i^n(\tau) = \mu_i\,_kY_i^n(\tau)$, with the at risk function equal to one if k is in i at τ. The last term is the probability of surviving in state i between the age at last entry and age at censoring. The intensity $_k\lambda_i^c(\tau)$ depends on the instantaneous rate of leaving i and the at risk function, which is zero except for τ larger than or equal to the age of the last transition and less than the age at censoring. In the traditional approach,

2.2 Transition Rates

integration is from the beginning of the period during which individual k is at risk of the (i,j)-transition to the end of that period. In the first term, the end is the age at the next occurrence; in the last term, it is the age at censoring. Hougaard (2000, p. 181) derives the likelihood function following the traditional approach:

$$\left[\prod_{n=1}^{_kN_{ij}(\omega)+1} {}_k\lambda_{ij}^n\left({}_kT_{ij}^n\right)^{_k\delta_{ij}^n}\right] \exp\left[-\int_0^\omega {}_k\lambda_i(\tau)d\tau\right]$$

where ${}_k\delta_{ij}^n$ is one if the at risk period ends in an (i,j)-transition and zero if it ends because the observation is discontinued (censored). The counting process approach to the likelihood function is (Aalen et al. 2008, p. 210):

$$\left[\prod_{0\le t<\omega} {}_k\lambda_{ij}(t)^{\Delta_k N_{ij}(t)}\right] \exp\left[-\int_0^\omega {}_k\lambda_i(\tau)d\tau\right]$$

with ${}_k\Delta N_{ij}(t)$ the increment of ${}_kN_{ij}$ at age t.

The full likelihood is

$$\left\{\prod_{k=1}^{K}\left[\prod_{0\le t<\omega} {}_k\lambda_{ij}(t)^{\Delta_k N_{ij}(t)}\right]\right\} \exp\left[-\int_0^\omega \lambda_i(\tau)d\tau\right]$$

with $\lambda_i(\tau)$ the intensity process of the aggregated process $N_i(t)$.

The log-likelihood is $\ell(\mu_{ij}) = \sum_{k=1}^{K}\sum_{t=0}^{\omega}\Delta_k N_{ij}(t) \ln[{}_k\lambda_{ij}(t)] - \int_0^\omega \lambda_i(\tau)\,d\tau$. The maximum likelihood estimator of μ_{ij} is the value of μ_{ij} for which the score function is zero: $U(\mu_{ij}) = \frac{\partial \ell}{\partial \mu_{ij}} = 0$. The score function is the first-order condition for maximising the likelihood that the model predicts the data. In the exponential model, ${}_k\lambda_{ij}(t) = \mu_{ij}\,{}_kY_i(t)$ and the first term of the log-likelihood is $\ln(\mu_{ij})\sum_{k=1}^{K}\sum_{t=0}^{\omega}\Delta_k N_{ij}(t) = \ln(\mu_{ij})\;N_{ij}(\omega)$. The second term is $\mu_{ij}\int_0^\omega Y_i(\tau)\,d\tau = \mu_{ij}\,R_i(\omega)$, with $R_i(\omega)$ the total exposure time in state i for all individuals in the (sample) population. The score function is $U(\mu_{ij}) = \frac{\partial \ell(\mu_{ij})}{\partial \mu_{ij}} = \frac{N_{ij}(\omega)}{\mu_{ij}} - R_i(\omega)$. The solution of the equation $U(\mu_{ij}) = 0$ gives the maximum likelihood estimator of the transition rate: $\hat{\mu}_{ij} = N_{ij}(\omega)/R_i(\omega)$. The estimator is the observed number of transitions (occurrences) divided by the total duration at risk (exposure). The estimator is an occurrence-exposure rate.

In large samples, the estimator $\hat{\mu}_{ij}$ is approximately normally distributed around the true value of μ_{ij}, with the variance estimator $\hat{\mu}_{ij}^2/N_{ij}(\omega) = \hat{\mu}_{ij}/R_i(\omega)$. To improve the distribution for $\hat{\mu}_{ij}$, the logarithmic transformation is used. Only ten transitions are needed for $\ln(\hat{\mu}_{ij})$ to be approximately normally distributed around $\ln(\mu_{ij})$ with variance estimator $1/N_{ij}(\omega)$ (Aalen et al. 2008, p. 215).

The cumulative transition rate under the exponential model (occurrence-exposure rate) increases linearly with duration. The empirical cumulative transition rate (Nelson-Aalen estimator) is a step function (Andersen and Keiding 2002,

p. 100). The two estimators are usually close. To improve the approximation, the age interval from 0 to ω may be partitioned in subintervals and the occurrence-exposure rate estimated for each subinterval. The exponential model turns into a piecewise exponential model with piecewise constant transition rates. That is the common approach in demography, where an age interval is usually 1 year. The estimator of the transition rate and the variance, given above, is applied to each subinterval. Consider the aggregate counting processes $N_{ij}(t)$ and $Y_i(t)$ and sub-intervals from exact age x to exact age y (y not included). Age intervals are usually 1 year, but a more general interval is chosen here. The transition rate, which is constant in the interval, is denoted by $\mu_{ij}(x, y)$. The observed number of (i,j)-transitions during the interval is $N_{ij}(x, y)$, and the observed exposure time in state i is $R_i(x, y)$. Following Aalen et al. (2008, pp. 220ff), the score function is solved. The score function is $U[\mu_{ij}(x,y)] = \frac{\partial \ell[\mu_{ij}(x,y)]}{\partial \mu_{ij}(x,y)} = \frac{N_{ij}(x,y)}{\mu_{ij}(x,y)} - R_i(x,y)$, where $N_{ij}(x,y) = \int_0^\omega I_{ij}(\tau) dN_{ij}(\tau) d\tau$ and $R_i(x,y) = \int_0^\omega I_{ij}(\tau) Y_i(\tau) d\tau$ with $I_{ij}(\tau)$ an indicator function taking the value of one in the interval from x to y and a value of zero otherwise.

The maximum likelihood estimator of the transition rate from i to j during the interval from x to y is the occurrence-exposure rate $\hat{\mu}_{ij}(x,y) = N_{ij}(x,y)/R_i(x,y)$. Occurrence-exposure rates are approximately independent and normally distributed around their true values, and the variance of $\hat{\mu}_{ij}(x,y)$ can be estimated by $\hat{\mu}_{ij}(x,y)/R_i(x,y)$ or the logarithmic transformation $\text{var}\{\ln[\hat{\mu}_{ij}(x,y)]\} = 1/N_{ij}(x,y)$. In demography, epidemiology and actuarial science, transition rates are usually occurrence-exposure rates and are determined by dividing occurrences by exposures. In the absence of exposure data, exposure is approximated by the product of the mid-period population and the length of the period, a method also used by Aalen et al. (2008, p. 222).

By way of illustration of the method, aggregate transition rates and age-specific transition rates are estimated from the subsample of 201 individuals, entering observation at labour market entry. The analysis focuses on transitions between job episodes and episodes without a job. Transitions between jobs are omitted. *Biograph* and some additional calculations produced the main results reported in this section. The results are compared to those generated by the *msm* package for multistate modelling. The 201 individuals experience 504 episodes (323 job episodes and 181 episodes without a job). The total observation time between first job entry and survey is 4,668 person-years (3,397 person-years in J and 1,271 person-years in N). The sample population experienced 303 transitions during the observation period (181 JN transitions and 122 NJ transitions). The JN transition rate is $181/3{,}397 = 0.0533$ per year and the NJ transition rate is $122/1{,}271 = 0.0960$ per year. To determine the 95 % confidence interval of the occurrence-exposure rate, the log-transformation of the estimator is used: $\exp\left[\ln(\hat{\mu}_{ij}) \pm 1.96 \sqrt{1/N_{ij}}\right]$. The confidence interval around the JN transition rate is $\exp\left[\ln(0.0533) \pm 1.96 * \sqrt{1/181}\right]$, which is (0.0461, 0.0617). The confidence

2.2 Transition Rates

interval around the NJ transition rate is $\exp\left[\ln(0.096) \pm 1.96 * \sqrt{1/122}\right]$, which is (0.0804, 0.1146). Bootstrapping, i.e. sampling the original 201 observations with replacement, with 100 bootstrap samples, produces a JN transition rate of 0.0535 with confidence interval (0.0452, 0.0636) and a NJ transition rate of 0.0977 with confidence interval (0.0701, 0.1264). Five hundred bootstrap samples yield a JN transition rate of 0.0534 with confidence interval (0.0.0451, 0.0629) and a NJ transition rate of 0.0973 with confidence interval (0.0729, 0.1254). Bootstrapping produces confidence intervals that are somewhat larger than the analytical method.

The package *msm* produces the same estimates and confidence intervals. The code is:

```
library (msm)
d <- Remove.intrastate(GLHS)
dd <- ChangeObservationWindow.e
        (Bdata=d,entrystate="J",exitstate=NA)
data <- date_b (Bdata=dd,selectday=1,format.out="age",
        covs=c("marriage","LMentry"))
Dmsm <-  Biograph.msm(data)
twoway2.q <- rbind(c(-0.025, 0.025),c(0.2,-0.2))
crudeinits.msm(state ~ date, ID, data=Dmsm,
        qmatrix=twoway2.q)
GLHS.msm.y <- msm( state ~ date,
        subject=ID,
        data = Dmsm,
        use.deriv=TRUE,
        exacttimes=TRUE,
        qmatrix = twoway2.q,
        obstype=2,
        control=list(trace=2,REPORT=1,
                abstol=0.0000005),
        method="BFGS")
```

The first line removes transitions between jobs. The second line changes the observation window: observation starts at labour market entry (first job) and ends at interview. The third line converts dates in CMC into ages. The fourth line converts the *Biograph* object data to the long format required by the *msm* package. The fifth and sixth lines generate initial values for transition rates. The next line calls the msm function for estimating the transition rates. Object GLHS.msm.y contains the estimates and the 95 % confidence intervals, with the row variable denoting origin and the column variable destination. State 1 is J and state 2 is N.

```
                   State 1                       State 2
State 1 -0.05328 (-0.06164,-0.04606)  0.05328 (0.04606,0.06164)
State 2 0.09602 (0.08041,0.1147)     -0.09602 (-0.1147,-0.08041)
```

As expected, the 95 % confidence intervals produced by the *msm* package are the same as computed above. The *msm* package includes a function (boot) that uses bootstrapping to produce estimates, standard errors and confidence intervals. Bootstrapping, with 100 bootstrap samples, produces the following estimates and confidence intervals: 0.0532 for the JN transition rate, with 95 % confidence interval (0.0453, 0.0621), and 0.0988 for the NJ transition rate, with 95 % confidence interval (0.0755, 0.1294).

Consider the piecewise constant exponential model with age intervals of 1 year. The input data are transition counts (occurrences) and exposures by single year of age for the 201 respondents. Transition counts and exposure times are shown in Table 2.3. Column JN shows the number of transitions from J to N and PY is the exposure time. The table also shows the state occupancies at birthdays (Occup) and the number of observations censured by age (cens). The estimate of the transition rate is r.est and the 95 % confidence interval is (r.L95, r.U95). The estimate and the confidence interval are obtained using the analytical method. Bootstrapping produces the estimate b.est and the confidence interval (b.L95, b.U95). The cumulative transition rate is cumrate. Consider age 30. Of the 201 individuals, 198 are under observation at that age; 138 have a job on their 30th birthday and 60 are without a job. For 3 individuals, the information is missing. Two did not reach age 30 yet when observation ended at age at interview (ID 45 and 115) and one entered labour force and observation after age 30 (ID 49). Together, the individuals spent 127.75 years in state J and 56.58 years in state N between the 30th and 31st birthdays. Notice that an individual in state J on his 30th birthday may spend some time in state N before reaching age 31. At age 30, 2 individuals experienced a JN transition and 3 an NJ transition. At that age, the JN transition rate is $2/127.75 = 0.0157$ and the NJ transition rate is $3/60.25 = 0.0530$. In Table 2.3, r.est denotes the estimator of the transition rate. The 95 % confidence interval around the JN transition rate at age 30 is $\exp\left[\ln(0.0157) \pm 1.96 * \sqrt{1/2}\right]$, which is (0.0039, 0.0626). The confidence around the NJ transition rate at age 30 is $\exp\left[\ln(0.0530) \pm 1.96 * \sqrt{1/3}\right]$, which is (0.0171, 0.1644). In the table, r.L95 denotes the lower bound and r.U95 the upper bound. The table also shows estimated transition rates (b.est) and confidence intervals (b.L95 and b.U95) obtained by bootstrapping with 100 bootstrap samples. The bootstrap standard errors are generally larger than the asymptotic standard errors, but it is not always the case in the table because of the relatively small number of bootstrap samples.

The cumulative JN transition rate at age 30 is 1.3455, and the cumulative NJ transition rate is 3.2957.

Biograph produced several of the figures in Table 2.3. The state occupancies at birthday are produced by the Occup function, the transitions by the Trans function and the transition rates and cumulative rates by the Rates.ac function.

Biograph tracks individual transitions and state occupancies (exposure times). The purpose of tracking individuals is to show an individual's contribution to transition counts and exposure times. Consider individual with ID 76. The data are shown in Table 2.1 and the employment career in Fig. 2.1. Table 2.4 shows the states occupied at all birthdays between first job and survey date and the exposure times by age. At exact age 18, the individual is not under observation yet (state -). He enters observation at age 18.333, when he gets his first job. Between the 18th

2.2 Transition Rates

Table 2.3 Piecewise constant exponential model: occurrences, exposures and transition rates. GLHS, 201 respondents

```
State J
Occup     PY  JN cens   r.L95   r.est   r.U95   b.L95   b.est   b.U95 cumrate
13     0   1.83   0    0 0.0000 0.0000 0.0000 0.0000 0.0000 0.0000 0.0000
14     6  20.42   2    0 0.0245 0.0979 0.3916 0.0000 0.0941 0.2255 0.0000
15    28  33.83   3    0 0.0286 0.0887 0.2750 0.0254 0.0893 0.2043 0.0979
16    37  43.17   6    0 0.0624 0.1390 0.3094 0.0480 0.1494 0.2830 0.1866
17    52  78.25   1    0 0.0018 0.0128 0.0907 0.0000 0.0125 0.0438 0.3256
18    95 111.67   9    0 0.0419 0.0806 0.1549 0.0344 0.0828 0.1332 0.3384
19   123 137.83  11    0 0.0442 0.0798 0.1441 0.0299 0.0763 0.1273 0.4190
20   146 138.17  24    0 0.1164 0.1737 0.2592 0.1022 0.1739 0.2409 0.4988
21   138 143.42  17    0 0.0737 0.1185 0.1907 0.0629 0.1157 0.1696 0.6725
22   141 150.17   9    0 0.0312 0.0599 0.1152 0.0294 0.0618 0.0933 0.7910
23   151 151.33  10    0 0.0356 0.0661 0.1228 0.0279 0.0669 0.1049 0.8510
24   151 145.00  15    0 0.0624 0.1034 0.1716 0.0536 0.1095 0.1668 0.9170
25   143 139.00  11    0 0.0438 0.0791 0.1429 0.0374 0.0811 0.1292 1.0205
26   135 134.25  14    0 0.0618 0.1043 0.1761 0.0588 0.1050 0.1660 1.0996
27   129 131.58   6    0 0.0205 0.0456 0.1015 0.0142 0.0453 0.0831 1.2039
28   135 133.75   8    0 0.0299 0.0598 0.1196 0.0264 0.0594 0.1062 1.2495
29   134 138.08   5    2 0.0151 0.0362 0.0870 0.0069 0.0343 0.0682 1.3093
30   138 127.75   2   19 0.0039 0.0157 0.0626 0.0000 0.0143 0.0335 1.3455
31   120 108.83   5   18 0.0191 0.0459 0.1104 0.0088 0.0483 0.0926 1.3612
32   102  90.33   4   14 0.0166 0.0443 0.1180 0.0104 0.0461 0.0977 1.4071
33    84  85.08   3    0 0.0114 0.0353 0.1093 0.0052 0.0335 0.0688 1.4514
34    86  84.83   3    0 0.0114 0.0354 0.1097 0.0000 0.0379 0.0915 1.4867
35    84  86.08   1    0 0.0016 0.0116 0.0825 0.0000 0.0138 0.0424 1.5220
36    87  86.83   1    0 0.0016 0.0115 0.0818 0.0000 0.0103 0.0368 1.5337
37    86  87.58   0    0 0.0000 0.0000 0.0000 0.0000 0.0000 0.0000 1.5452
38    88  88.08   2    0 0.0057 0.0227 0.0908 0.0000 0.0241 0.0573 1.5452
39    90  89.75   1    1 0.0016 0.0111 0.0791 0.0000 0.0101 0.0361 1.5679
40    88  83.17   1   17 0.0017 0.0120 0.0854 0.0000 0.0120 0.0448 1.5790
41    74  68.08   0   12 0.0000 0.0000 0.0000 0.0000 0.0000 0.0000 1.5910
42    62  57.17   2    8 0.0087 0.0350 0.1399 0.0000 0.0406 0.1301 1.5910
43    53  53.00   0    0 0.0000 0.0000 0.0000 0.0000 0.0000 0.0000 1.6260
44    53  52.00   2    0 0.0096 0.0385 0.1538 0.0000 0.0415 0.1085 1.6260
45    51  52.33   1    0 0.0027 0.0191 0.1357 0.0000 0.0180 0.0595 1.6645
46    52  52.00   0    0 0.0000 0.0000 0.0000 0.0000 0.0000 0.0000 1.6836
47    52  52.00   0    0 0.0000 0.0000 0.0000 0.0000 0.0000 0.0000 1.6836
48    52  52.00   0    0 0.0000 0.0000 0.0000 0.0000 0.0000 0.0000 1.6836
49    52  51.92   0    1 0.0000 0.0000 0.0000 0.0000 0.0000 0.0000 1.6836
50    51  37.25   2   26 0.0134 0.0537 0.2147 0.0000 0.0544 0.1249 1.6836
51    24  15.67   0   17 0.0000 0.0000 0.0000 0.0000 0.0000 0.0000 1.7373
52     7   3.33   0    7 0.0000 0.0000 0.0000 0.0000 0.0000 0.0000 1.7373
53     0   0.00   0    0 0.0000 0.0000 0.0000 0.0000 0.0000 0.0000 1.7373

State N
Occup     PY  NJ cens   r.L95   r.est   r.U95   b.L95   b.est   b.U95 cumrate
13     0   0.00   0    0 0.0000 0.0000 0.0000 0.0000 0.0000 0.0000 0.0000
14     0   0.33   0    0 0.0000 0.0000 0.0000 0.0000 0.0000 0.0000 0.0000
15     2   3.67   0    0 0.0000 0.0000 0.0000 0.0000 0.0000 0.0000 0.0000
16     5   8.25   2    0 0.0606 0.2424 0.9693 0.0000 0.2412 0.6905 0.0000
17     9   8.08   3    0 0.1197 0.3713 1.1512 0.0000 0.4121 1.0889 0.2424
18     7   9.92   3    0 0.0975 0.3024 0.9377 0.0000 0.2947 0.6461 0.6137
19    13  13.67  10    0 0.3936 0.7315 1.3596 0.3920 0.7578 1.1739 0.9161
20    14  26.83   6    0 0.1005 0.2236 0.4978 0.0928 0.2296 0.4226 1.6477
21    32  33.50  11    0 0.1818 0.3284 0.5929 0.1760 0.3322 0.5461 1.8713
22    38  33.75   9    0 0.1387 0.2667 0.5125 0.1203 0.2764 0.4944 2.1996
23    38  41.17   6    0 0.0655 0.1457 0.3244 0.0455 0.1488 0.2946 2.4663
24    42  48.92   6    0 0.0551 0.1226 0.2730 0.0421 0.1317 0.2440 2.6121
25    51  55.00   3    0 0.0176 0.0545 0.1691 0.0000 0.0564 0.1292 2.7347
26    59  60.42   6    0 0.0446 0.0993 0.2210 0.0449 0.1014 0.1646 2.7892
27    67  65.17   9    0 0.0719 0.1381 0.2654 0.0648 0.1457 0.2569 2.8886
28    64  66.00   6    0 0.0408 0.0909 0.2024 0.0297 0.0911 0.1569 3.0267
29    66  61.75  11    0 0.0987 0.1781 0.3217 0.0882 0.1783 0.2794 3.1176
30    60  56.58   3    0 0.0171 0.0530 0.1644 0.0000 0.0523 0.1221 3.2957
31    53  50.83   4    9 0.0295 0.0787 0.2097 0.0198 0.0824 0.1614 3.3487
32    45  45.75   0    3 0.0000 0.0000 0.0000 0.0000 0.0000 0.0000 3.4274
33    46  44.92   5    0 0.0463 0.1113 0.2674 0.0281 0.1060 0.1873 3.4274
34    44  45.17   1    0 0.0031 0.0221 0.1572 0.0000 0.0219 0.0730 3.5387
35    46  43.92   4    0 0.0342 0.0911 0.2427 0.0203 0.0917 0.2204 3.5609
36    43  43.17   0    0 0.0000 0.0000 0.0000 0.0000 0.0000 0.0000 3.6519
37    44  42.42   2    0 0.0118 0.0471 0.1885 0.0000 0.0458 0.1160 3.6519
38    42  41.92   4    0 0.0358 0.0954 0.2542 0.0085 0.0938 0.2038 3.6991
39    40  40.17   0    0 0.0000 0.0000 0.0000 0.0000 0.0000 0.0000 3.7945
40    41  36.25   4    5 0.0414 0.1103 0.2940 0.0263 0.1130 0.2514 3.7945
41    33  30.50   0    5 0.0000 0.0000 0.0000 0.0000 0.0000 0.0000 3.9048
42    28  24.50   1    7 0.0057 0.0408 0.2898 0.0000 0.0463 0.1723 3.9048
43    22  22.00   0    0 0.0000 0.0000 0.0000 0.0000 0.0000 0.0000 3.9457
44    22  23.00   0    0 0.0000 0.0000 0.0000 0.0000 0.0000 0.0000 3.9457
45    24  22.67   2    0 0.0221 0.0882 0.3528 0.0000 0.1051 0.3614 3.9457
46    23  23.00   0    0 0.0000 0.0000 0.0000 0.0000 0.0000 0.0000 4.0339
47    23  23.00   0    0 0.0000 0.0000 0.0000 0.0000 0.0000 0.0000 4.0339
48    23  23.00   0    0 0.0000 0.0000 0.0000 0.0000 0.0000 0.0000 4.0339
49    23  22.92   0    1 0.0000 0.0000 0.0000 0.0000 0.0000 0.0000 4.0339
50    22  17.92   1   10 0.0079 0.0558 0.3962 0.0000 0.0570 0.1755 4.0339
51    13   8.83   0    8 0.0000 0.0000 0.0000 0.0000 0.0000 0.0000 4.0897
52     5   2.00   0    5 0.0000 0.0000 0.0000 0.0000 0.0000 0.0000 4.0897
53     0   0.00   0    0 0.0000 0.0000 0.0000 0.0000 0.0000 0.0000 4.0897
```

Table 2.4 State occupancies and state occupation times. Individual with ID 76

	-	J	N	+	-	J	N	+
18	1	0	0	0	0.333	0.500	0.167	0.000
19	0	0	1	0	0.000	0.000	1.000	0.000
20	0	0	1	0	0.000	0.083	0.917	0.000
21	0	1	0	0	0.000	1.000	0.000	0.000
22	0	1	0	0	0.000	1.000	0.000	0.000
23	0	1	0	0	0.000	1.000	0.000	0.000
24	0	1	0	0	0.000	0.750	0.250	0.000
25	0	1	0	0	0.000	1.000	0.000	0.000
26	0	1	0	0	0.000	1.000	0.000	0.000
27	0	1	0	0	0.000	1.000	0.000	0.000
28	0	1	0	0	0.000	1.000	0.000	0.000
29	0	1	0	0	0.000	1.000	0.000	0.000
30	0	1	0	0	0.000	0.417	0.000	0.583
31	0	0	0	1	0.000	0.000	0.000	1.000

and 19th birthday, respondent with ID 76 spends 0.333 years before observation (in state -), 0.5 years in J and 0.167 years in N. At age 30, he spends 0.417 years in J and 0.583 years in the state 'censored'. The tracking of individual transitions and exposures is necessary for a correct estimation of transition rates and is a central aspect of the counting process approach. If $\hat{m}_{ij}(x)$ is an estimate of the rate of transition from i to j between exact ages x and $x+1$, then the contribution of the individual to the likelihood function is $\hat{m}_{ij}(x) \exp\left[-\hat{m}_{ij}(x)\right]$ if the individual experiences a transition between x and $x+1$ and $\exp\left[-\hat{m}_{ij}(x)\right]$ if he experiences no transition. The best estimate of $m_{ij}(x)$ is the one that maximises the likelihood function for all individuals combined.

2.3 Transition Probabilities and State Occupation Probabilities

In multistate modelling, distinct types of probabilities have been identified (see, e.g. Schoen 1988, pp. 81ff). Survival probabilities, transition probabilities and state occupation probabilities are well known. They relate to the state occupied at a given age or at given ages. An event probability is the probability that a given transition occurs at least once during a given period. The cumulative incidence, which is frequently used in epidemiology and health sciences, is an event probability. If the destination state is an absorbing state, e.g. dead, the transition probability and the event probability are the same. Otherwise they differ. The probability types are discussed in some detail. In this section and the following sections, age is denoted by x and y. State and transition probabilities are denoted by p and event probabilities by π. The matrix of transition probabilities between ages x and y is $\mathbf{P}(x,y)$, and the vector of state probabilities at x is $\mathbf{p}(x)$. The probability of a continuous stay in a

2.3 Transition Probabilities and State Occupation Probabilities

state between ages x and y will be denoted by $S(x,y)$. It is the survival probability in the state; it is the probability of nonoccurrence of an event (exit from the state).

The survival probability at age x is the probability of being alive at that age. In some fields, such as demography, dead is usually not a separate state in the state space. It is an absorbing state that is integrated in the diagonal of the transition matrix. The probability of being alive is the probability of being in any of the states of the state space. In medical statistics, the absorbing state of dead is usually a separate state of the state space. In that case, the survival probability is the probability of being in a transient state. Unless specified otherwise, the state occupation probability at age x is the probability of occupying a given state at age x, *conditional* on being in any of the states of the state space at x, i.e. conditional on still being part of the population. The transition probability is the probability of occupying a given state at age y, conditional on occupying a given state at age x with $y \geq x$. All probabilities are derived from transition rates. Before deriving probabilities from rates, probability types are discussed. Probabilities are defined for periods. A period may be delineated by two ages, two transitions or by an age and a transition. The delineation results in periods of fixed or variable length. Probabilities may be conditional on being in a given state or having experienced a transition.

Probabilities are computed at a *reference age*. The reference age indicates the position of the observer in the life course. The reference age is particularly relevant in the presence of mortality or when the probability is conditional on the state occupied at the reference age. For instance, the probability of experiencing a period without a job between ages 30 and 40 is likely to differ between persons employed at age 30 and persons employed at age 25, but not necessarily at age 30. At age 30, the latter category may have a job or may be without a job. The difference is due to competing events between ages 25 and 30. In medical statistics, the reference age x from which a transition probability is estimated is known as the landmark time point or age and the method to select a range of reference ages as the landmark method. Individuals who experience the transition of interest before the landmark time point or who leave the population at risk for another reason (e.g. censoring) are removed from the data (Van Houwelingen and Putter 2008; Beyersmann et al. 2012, p. 187). The landmark method is used for dynamic prediction (van Houwelingen and Putter 2011). The central idea of dynamic prediction is that, by increasing the reference age, time-varying covariates may be updated with more recent values and predictions adjusted.

If a period is delineated by two ages, the first age is denoted by x and the second by y ($y > x$). The probability of a transition, an event or a continuous stay in a given state between ages x and y depends on competing events before and during the period. To exclude the effect of competing events before x, the probability is computed at age x. If the impact of competing events before x needs to be accounted for, the probability is computed at an age lower than x. For instance, the probability of impairment after age 65 depends on the likelihood of surviving to 65. It is higher if computed at 65 than at age zero. Probabilities are computed for individual k, but the reference to k is omitted for convenience.

The probability that an individual who is in state i on his x-th birthday will be in state j at age y is the transition probability $p_{ij}(x,y)$. It may be written as $p_{ij}(x,y) = \Pr(X(y)=j|X(x)=i)$, where $X(x)$ is a random variable denoting the state occupied at age x. The transition probability depends on the life history. If the life history is represented by Θ, that dependence is denoted by $p_{ij}(x,y) = \Pr(X(y)=j|X(x)=i,\Theta)$. That dependence is omitted in this section on the derivation of probabilities. The time scale is continuous (t is a continuous variable). The process is time-homogeneous if the transition probability $p_{ij}(x,y)$ only depends on the age difference $y-x$ and not on age x. In life history data analysis with age as the time scale, the process is time-inhomogeneous. Age matters. Transition probabilities defined for the age interval from x to y are combined in a matrix of transition probabilities:

$$\mathbf{P}(x,y) = \begin{bmatrix} p_{11}(x,y) & p_{21}(x,y) & \cdots & p_{I1}(x,y) \\ p_{12}(x,y) & p_{22}(x,y) & \cdots & p_{I2}(x,y) \\ \cdot & \cdot & & \cdot \\ \cdot & \cdot & & \cdot \\ p_{1I}(x,y) & p_{2I}(x,y) & \cdots & p_{II}(x,y) \end{bmatrix}$$

where $p_{ii}(x,y)$ is the probability that an individual who is in state i at age x will also be in state i at age y. Between x and y, the individual may move out of i and return later but before y. The reason for using matrices is that, except for a few simple cases, transition probabilities depend on all transition intensities and that requires systems of equations, which are conveniently written as matrix equations.

The interval from x to y may be partitioned into smaller intervals: $x = x_0 < x_1 < x_2 \ldots < x_P = y$. The transition probability matrix $\mathbf{P}(x,y)$ may be written as a matrix product:

$$\mathbf{P}(x,y) = \mathbf{P}(x_0,x_1)\,\mathbf{P}(x_1,x_2)\,\mathbf{P}(x_2,x_3)\ldots\mathbf{P}(x_{P-1},x_P)$$

The equation is the Chapman-Kolmogorov equation for the Markov process. If the number of time points increases and the distance between them goes to zero in a uniform way, the matrix product approaches a limit termed a (matrix-valued) product integral. The product integral is a counterpart of the usual integral in classical calculus.

State occupation probabilities at age y are derived from transition probabilities $\mathbf{P}(x,y)$ and state probabilities at age x. Let $\mathbf{p}(x)$ denote the vector of state probabilities at exact age x. The state probabilities at age y are $\mathbf{P}(x,y)\,\mathbf{p}(x)$.

To show the link between transition probability and (cumulative) transition rate, consider the infinitesimally small interval from τ to $\tau+d\tau$ with $x \leq \tau < y$. The transition probability may be expressed in terms of increments of cumulative transition rates. The cumulative transition rates at age τ may be arranged in a matrix:

2.3 Transition Probabilities and State Occupation Probabilities

$$\mathbf{A}(\tau) = \begin{bmatrix} A_{11}(\tau) & -A_{21}(\tau) & . & . & -A_{I1}(\tau) \\ -A_{12}(\tau) & A_{22}(\tau) & . & . & -A_{I2}(\tau) \\ . & . & . & & . \\ . & . & & . & . \\ -A_{iI}(\tau) & -A_{2I}(\tau) & . & . & A_{II}(\tau) \end{bmatrix}$$

An element $A_{ij}(\tau)$ denotes the cumulative rate at age τ of the transition from i to j. The diagonal element $A_{ii}(\tau)$ is the cumulative rate at age τ of leaving i: $A_{ii}(\tau) = \sum_{j \neq i} A_{ij}(\tau)$. The cumulative transition rate can be a step function, with a jump at each age a transition occurs, or a continuous function. The increment of $A_{ij}(\tau)$ during the interval from τ to $\tau + d\tau$ is $dA_{ij}(\tau)$. The probability that the individual who is in i at τ will be in j at $\tau + d\tau$ is $p_{ij}(\tau, \tau + d\tau) \approx dA_{ij}(\tau)$. The probability that an individual who is in i at τ will be in i at $\tau + d\tau$ is $p_{ii}(\tau, \tau + d\tau) = 1 - \sum_{j \neq i} p_{ij}(\tau, \tau + d\tau) \approx 1 - \sum_{j \neq i} dA_{ij}(\tau)$. The matrix of transition probabilities between ages x and y, expressed in terms of the transition probabilities in small subintervals, is

$$\mathbf{P}(x, y) = \prod_{x \leq \tau < y} \mathbf{P}(\tau, \tau + d\tau) \approx \prod_{x \leq \tau < y} [\mathbf{I} - d\mathbf{A}(\tau)]$$

The equation is the solution to the Chapman-Kolmogorov equation. No assumption is made on the nature of the distribution of the transition probability (Aalen et al. 2008, p. 470). The distribution can be discrete or continuous. The product integral is a restatement of the Chapman-Kolmogorov equation.

If transition rates are continuous functions of age, then $dA_{ij}(\tau) = \mu_{ij}(\tau) d\tau$ and $d\mathbf{A}(\tau) = \boldsymbol{\mu}(\tau) d\tau$. The quantity $\mu_{ij}(\tau) d\tau$ is the probability that an individual who is in i at τ will move to j during the interval of length $d\tau$ $p_{ij}(\tau, \tau + d\tau) = \mu_{ij}(\tau) d\tau$. Since the interval is sufficiently small to ensure not more than one transition, a move from i to j implies that the individual will be in j at $\tau + d\tau$. The probability of remaining in i during the interval of length $d\tau$ is $p_{ii}(\tau, \tau + d\tau) = 1 - \sum_{j \neq i} \mu_{ij}(\tau) d\tau$. The matrix expression linking the matrix of transition probabilities during the interval from τ to $\tau + d\tau$ to the matrix of instantaneous transition rates is $\mathbf{P}(\tau, \tau + d\tau) = \mathbf{I} - \boldsymbol{\mu}(\tau) d\tau$, where $\mathbf{I}$ is the identity matrix and

$$\boldsymbol{\mu}(\tau) = \begin{bmatrix} \mu_{11}(\tau) & -\mu_{21}(\tau) & . & . & -\mu_{I1}(\tau) \\ -\mu_{12}(\tau) & \mu_{22}(\tau) & . & . & -\mu_{I2}(\tau) \\ . & . & . & & . \\ . & . & & . & . \\ -\mu_{iI}(\tau) & -\mu_{2I}(\tau) & . & . & \mu_{II}(\tau) \end{bmatrix}$$

with $\mu_{ii}(\tau) = \sum_{j \neq i} \mu_{ij}(\tau)$. If the instantaneous transition rates are continuous functions of age, $\mathbf{P}(x, y) = \prod_{x \leq \tau < y} [\mathbf{I} - \boldsymbol{\mu}(\tau) d\tau]$

In the literature, the instantaneous transition rate matrix has different configurations. The configuration used in this chapter is common in demography. The first subscript denotes the origin and the second the destination. In statistics, the off-diagonal element is the transition rate instead of minus the transition rate, and the matrix is the transpose of the matrix shown here. The reasons for choosing the configuration become clear later.

If the transition probability is a continuous function of age, a system of differential equations links transition probabilities and transition rates. The differential equations are derived from the Chapman-Kolmogorov equation. Recall that we may write

$$\mathbf{P}(x,y) = \mathbf{P}(x,\tau)\,\mathbf{P}(\tau,y)$$

Subtraction of $\mathbf{P}(\tau, y)$ from both sides of the equation and dividing by $\tau-x$ yields

$$\frac{\mathbf{P}(x,y) - \mathbf{P}(\tau,y)}{\tau - x} = \frac{[\mathbf{P}(x,\tau) - \mathbf{I}]\mathbf{P}(\tau,y)}{\tau - x}$$

and

$$\lim_{\tau \to x} \frac{\mathbf{P}(x,y) - \mathbf{P}(\tau,y)}{\tau - x} = \lim_{\tau \to x} \frac{[\mathbf{P}(x,\tau) - I]\mathbf{P}(\tau,y)}{\tau - x}$$

Since $\lim_{\tau \to x} \frac{\mathbf{P}(x,\tau) - \mathbf{I}}{\tau - x} = -\boldsymbol{\mu}(x)$, we obtain the differential equation

$$\frac{d\mathbf{P}(x)}{dx} = -\boldsymbol{\mu}(x)\mathbf{P}(x).$$

The differential equation describes continuous-time nonhomogeneous Markov processes. In physics, the equation is known as the master equation. In the social sciences, the master equation is less well known, but some important applications (under that name) exist (see, e.g. Weidlich and Haag 1983, 1988; Aoki 1996; Helbing 2010). Aoki summarises the significance of the master equation as follows: 'The master equations describe time evolution of probabilities of states of dynamic processes in terms of probability transition rates and state occupancy probabilities' (Aoki 1996, p. 116).

To solve the matrix differential equation, we may try to generalise the solution of the scalar differential equation $\frac{dp(x)}{dx} = -\mu(x)\,p(x)$. The solution, given the interval from x to y, is $p(x,y) = \exp[-\int_x^y \mu(\tau) d\tau]$, with $p(x,y)$ the probability that an individual who is alive at age x will be alive at age y and $\mu(\tau)$ the instantaneous death rate at age τ. The generalisation $\mathbf{P}(x,y) = \exp[-\int_x^y \boldsymbol{\mu}(\tau) d\tau]$ does usually not work, however. It works only if the matrices of instantaneous transition rates commute, i.e. if the matrix multiplication $\boldsymbol{\mu}(\tau)\boldsymbol{\mu}(\tau + d\tau) = \boldsymbol{\mu}(\tau + d\tau)\boldsymbol{\mu}(\tau)$ for all τ.

To solve the system of differential equations, it is replaced by a system of integral equations:

2.3 Transition Probabilities and State Occupation Probabilities

$$\mathbf{P}(x,y) = \mathbf{I} - \int_x^y \boldsymbol{\mu}(\tau)\mathbf{P}(x,\tau)\,d\tau$$

This equation is essentially a system of flow equations of the multistate model. The element $p_{ij}(x,y)$ of $\mathbf{P}(x,y)$ is:

$$p_{ij}(x,y) = p_{ij}(x,x) - \int_x^y \sum_{q \neq j} \mu_{jq}(\tau) p_{ij}(x,\tau)\,d\tau + \int_x^y \sum_{q \neq j} \mu_{qj}(\tau) p_{iq}(x,\tau)\,d\tau$$

$$p_{ij}(x,y) = p_{ij}(x,x) - \sum_{q \neq j} {}_id_{jq}(\tau, \tau + d\tau) + \sum_{q \neq j} {}_id_{qj}(\tau, \tau + d\tau)$$

$_id_{jq}(x,y)$ represents the number of moves or direct transitions from state j to state q between the ages x and y by an individual in state i at exact age x. The sum is the number of exits from state j by persons in i at x. The last term is the number of entries into state j by persons in i at x.

To derive an expression involving transition rates during the interval from x to y, we write

$$\mathbf{P}(x,y) = \mathbf{I} - \left[\int_x^y \boldsymbol{\mu}(\tau)\mathbf{P}(x,\tau)\,d\tau\right]\left[\int_x^y \mathbf{P}(x,\tau)\,d\tau\right]^{-1}\left[\int_x^y \mathbf{P}(x,\tau)\,d\tau\right]$$

$$\mathbf{P}(x,y) = \mathbf{I} - \mathbf{m}(x,y)\mathbf{L}(x,y)$$

where $\mathbf{m}(x,y)$ is the matrix of transition rates. An element $m_{ij}(x,y)$ ($j \neq i$) is the average transition rate during the interval from x to y and the diagonal element is the rate of leaving i: $m_{ii}(x,y) = \sum_{j \neq i} {}_im_{ij}(x,y)$. Schoen (1988, p. 66) shows the same matrix equation and points to the link with the flow equations commonly used in demography.

Transition probabilities serve as input in the computation of state occupation probabilities. Let $p_i(y)$ denote the probability that an individual who is alive at age y is in state i at that age and let $\mathbf{p}(y)$ denote the vector of state occupation probabilities at age y. The state probabilities at age y depend on state probabilities at an earlier age and transition probabilities, e.g. $\mathbf{p}(y) = \mathbf{P}(x,y)\mathbf{p}(x)$. This equation may be applied recursively to determine state occupancies at consecutive ages. Consider age intervals of 1 year. If the state occupation probabilities at birth are given and the transition probabilities $\mathbf{P}(x, x+1)$ are known for $0 \leq x < z-1$, with z the start of the highest, open-ended age group, then a recursive application of $\mathbf{p}(x+1) = \mathbf{P}(x,x+1)\mathbf{p}(x)$ with $0 \leq x < z-1$ produces state occupation probabilities by single years of age from birth to the highest age.

The estimation of transition probabilities from data relies on the Nelson-Aalen estimator if the waiting time distribution of a transition is not constrained and on the occurrence-exposure rate if the waiting time distribution is (piecewise) exponential. The two approaches are considered in the remainder of this section. Some packages for multistate modelling, e.g. *etm* and *mstate*, adopt the non-parametric method assuming that the multistate survival function is a step function and estimate the empirical transition matrix, while other packages, e.g. *msm* and *Biograph*, adopt the parametric method assuming that the underlying multistate process is continuous but transition rates are (piecewise) constant.

(a) Non-parametric Method

A logical estimator of $\mathbf{P}(x,y)$ is $\hat{\mathbf{P}}(x,y) = \prod_{x \leq \tau < y} [\mathbf{I} - d\hat{\mathbf{A}}(\tau)]$. Since the estimator $\hat{\mathbf{A}}(\tau)$ is a matrix of step functions with a finite number of increments in the (x,y)-interval, the product integral is the finite matrix product:

$$\hat{\mathbf{P}}(x,y) = \prod_{x \leq T_n < y} [\mathbf{I} - \Delta \hat{\mathbf{A}}(T_n)]$$

The matrix $\hat{\mathbf{P}}(x,y)$ is the *empirical transition matrix*, often denoted as the Aalen-Johansen estimator. It is a non-parametric estimator, which generalises the Kaplan-Meier estimator to Markov chains (Aalen et al. 2008, p. 122). The diagonal element is generally not equal to the Kaplan-Meier estimator. The i-th diagonal element is the probability that an individual who is in i at age x will also be in i at age y. The state may be left and re-entered during the interval. The Kaplan-Meier estimator is an estimator of the probability that an individual who is in i at age x will *remain* in i at least until age y. The state may not be left during the interval. The Kaplan-Meier estimator is $\prod_{x \leq T_n < y} \left[1 - \frac{\sum_{j \neq i} \Delta N_{ij}(T_n)}{Y_i(T_n)} \right]$.

For the covariance of the empirical transition matrix, see Aalen et al. (2008).

Consider the selection of the GLHS data on ten individuals. The Aalen-Johansen estimator of the transition probabilities are derived from the Nelson-Aalen estimator of the cumulative transition rates shown in Table 2.2. Consider the transition probability between ages 14 and 18.833. At age 14, individual 8 (ID = 180) enters his first job and enters observation. He leaves the first job at age 15.667 (see Table 2.1, JN transition). At that age, individual 3 (ID = 67) had entered observation (at age 15.167). The empirical probability of transition from J to N between ages 14 and 15.667 is $(1 - 1/2) = 0.5$. The probability that the individual is without a job at age 18.833 is 28.57 %. It is computed by the matrix multiplication:

$$[\mathbf{I} - d\mathbf{A}(15.667)] * [\mathbf{I} - d\mathbf{A}(18.167)] * [\mathbf{I} - d\mathbf{A}(18.750)] * [\mathbf{I} - d\mathbf{A}(18.833)] =$$

$$\begin{bmatrix} 0.500 & 0 \\ 0.500 & 1 \end{bmatrix} \begin{bmatrix} 1 & 1 \\ 0 & 0 \end{bmatrix} \begin{bmatrix} 0.857 & 0 \\ 0.143 & 1 \end{bmatrix} \begin{bmatrix} 0.833 & 0 \\ 0.167 & 1 \end{bmatrix} = \begin{bmatrix} 0.714 & 0.714 \\ 0.286 & 0.286 \end{bmatrix}$$

Table 2.5 shows the results. The column `etm.est` gives the probability of an occurrence before t and `etm.var` gives the variance. The probability of no occurrence is `surv`. It is the empirical survival function or Kaplan-Meier estimator of the survival function. Both the Nelson-Aalen estimator and the Kaplan-Meier estimator are *discrete* distributions with their probability mass concentrated at the observed event times. The link between the cumulative hazard estimator and the

2.3 Transition Probabilities and State Occupation Probabilities

Kaplan-Meier estimator relies on the approximation of the product integral. The product integration is the key to understanding the relation between the Nelson-Aalen and the Kaplan-Meier estimators (Aalen et al. 2008, p. 99 and p. 458). The column `delta` shows the increments of the cumulative hazard. The probability that an individual who is in state J at age 14 will be in state N at age 25 is 43.27 %. The estimate is based on all transitions before age 25, the last one at age 24.833. The probability of being in J at age 25 is the same as the probability of being in J at age 24.833, since in the sample population no transition occurred between ages 24.833 and 25. Recall that the elements of the empirical transition matrix are step functions with constant values between transition times. The probability that a 20-year-old individual who is in state J will be in N at age 25 is 41.52 %.

The `etm` function of the *etm* package computes the Aalen-Johansen estimator of the transition probability matrix of any multistate model. The entries of the Aalen-Johansen estimator are empirical probabilities. The *etm* package is used to produce the results shown in Table 2.5. The results are for a selection of the ten respondents used for illustration of the Nelson-Aalen estimator. The code is:

```
library (etm)
D<- Biograph.mvna (d.10)
tra <- attr(D$D,"param")$trans_possible
etm.0 <- etm(data=D$D,c("J","N"),tra,"cens",s=0)
```

The covariance matrix of the empirical transition matrix is derived using martingale theory (Aalen et al. 2008, pp. 124ff). The Aalen-Johansen estimator along with event counts, risk set, variance of the estimator and confidence intervals can be obtained through the `summary` function of the *etm* package:

```
summary(etm.0)$"J N"
summary(etm.0)$"N J"
```

The confidence interval is computed without transformation of the data. Transformations can be specified, however (see Beyersmann et al. 2012, p. 185).

Respondents enter observation when they start their first job. The probability of being employed at the highest age in the sample population (53) depends on the employment status at lower ages. An individual with a job at age 14 has a 37 % chance of also having a job at age 53. The percentage is the same for a person with a job at age 18. An individual with a job at age 30 has a 42 % chance of having a job at age 53. Because employment status varies with age the probability of being in a given state at a given higher age varies with age too. By varying the reference age, the changes in probabilities can be assessed. The selection of a range of reference ages is the basic idea of the landmark method. In this example, the end state is a transient state. In the landmark method, the end state is an absorbing state. In multistate life table analysis, the method of selecting different reference ages and to estimate transition probabilities conditional on states occupied at a reference age is known as the status-based life table (Willekens 1987).

Table 2.5 Aalen-Johansen estimator of transition probabilities. GLHS subsample of ten individuals

```
JN transition
      age nrisk nevent   etm.est       etm.var      surv
1  14.00000    1     0 0.0000000 0.000000000 1.0000000
2  15.16667    1     0 0.0000000 0.000000000 1.0000000
3  15.66667    2     1 0.5000000 0.125000000 0.5000000
4  17.00000    1     0 0.5000000 0.125000000 0.5000000
5  17.83333    2     0 0.5000000 0.125000000 0.5000000
6  18.16667    3     0 0.5000000 0.125000000 0.5000000
7  18.33333    4     0 0.5000000 0.125000000 0.5000000
8  18.66667    6     0 0.0000000 0.000000000 1.0000000
9  18.75000    7     1 0.1428571 0.017492711 0.8571429
10 18.83333    6     1 0.2857143 0.029154519 0.7142857
11 19.16667    5     0 0.2857143 0.029154519 0.7142857
12 19.41667    6     1 0.4047619 0.032056473 0.5952381
13 19.66667    5     0 0.4047619 0.032056473 0.5952381
14 20.91667    6     1 0.3690476 0.028351420 0.6309524
15 21.00000    6     1 0.4742063 0.028903785 0.5257937
16 21.16667    5     0 0.3556548 0.026799238 0.6443452
17 21.50000    6     0 0.2371032 0.021280425 0.7628968
18 22.41667    7     0 0.1185516 0.012347346 0.8814484
19 22.58333    8     1 0.2287326 0.020075818 0.7712674
20 23.16667    7     2 0.4490947 0.027585427 0.5509053
21 24.58333    6     1 0.5409123 0.026181931 0.4590877
22 24.83333    5     0 0.4327298 0.026119191 0.5672702
23 25.16667    6     0 0.3245474 0.023469628 0.6754526
24 26.00000    7     1 0.4210406 0.025223801 0.5789594
25 28.16667    6     0 0.3157805 0.022498163 0.6842195
26 29.75000    7     0 0.2105203 0.017385650 0.7894797
27 30.41667    8     0 0.2105203 0.017385650 0.7894797
28 30.66667    6     0 0.1052602 0.009886262 0.8947398
29 31.08333    7     0 0.1052602 0.009886262 0.8947398
30 40.25000    6     1 0.2543835 0.025396927 0.7456165
31 41.25000    5     0 0.2543835 0.025396927 0.7456165
32 41.50000    4     0 0.2543835 0.025396927 0.7456165
33 41.91667    3     0 0.2543835 0.025396927 0.7456165
34 42.75000    3     0 0.2543835 0.025396927 0.7456165
35 44.66667    2     1 0.6271917 0.075842235 0.3728083
36 52.16667    1     0 0.6271917 0.075842235 0.3728083
37 52.66667    1     0 0.6271917 0.075842235 0.3728083

NJ transition
      age nrisk nevent   etm.est       etm.var      surv
1  14.00000    0     0 0.0000000 0.000000000 1.0000000
2  15.16667    0     0 0.0000000 0.000000000 1.0000000
3  15.66667    0     0 0.0000000 0.000000000 1.0000000
4  17.00000    1     0 0.0000000 0.000000000 1.0000000
5  17.83333    1     0 0.0000000 0.000000000 1.0000000
6  18.16667    1     0 0.0000000 0.000000000 1.0000000
7  18.33333    1     0 0.0000000 0.000000000 1.0000000
8  18.66667    1     1 1.0000000 0.000000000 0.0000000
9  18.75000    0     0 0.8571429 0.017492711 0.1428571
10 18.83333    1     0 0.7142857 0.029154519 0.2857143
11 19.16667    2     0 0.7142857 0.029154519 0.2857143
12 19.41667    2     0 0.5952381 0.032056473 0.4047619
13 19.66667    3     0 0.5952381 0.032056473 0.4047619
14 20.91667    3     1 0.6309524 0.028351420 0.3690476
15 21.00000    3     0 0.5257937 0.028903785 0.4742063
16 21.16667    4     1 0.6443452 0.026799238 0.3556548
17 21.50000    3     1 0.7628968 0.021280425 0.2371032
18 22.41667    2     1 0.8814484 0.012347346 0.1185516
19 22.58333    1     0 0.7712674 0.020075818 0.2287326
20 23.16667    2     0 0.5509053 0.027585427 0.4490947
21 24.58333    4     0 0.4590877 0.026181931 0.5409123
22 24.83333    5     0 0.5672702 0.026119191 0.4327298
23 25.16667    4     1 0.6754526 0.023469628 0.3245474
24 26.00000    3     0 0.5789594 0.025223801 0.4210406
25 28.16667    4     1 0.6842195 0.022498163 0.3157805
26 29.75000    3     1 0.7894797 0.017385650 0.2105203
27 30.41667    2     0 0.7894797 0.017385650 0.2105203
28 30.66667    2     1 0.8947398 0.009886262 0.1052602
29 31.08333    1     0 0.8947398 0.009886262 0.1052602
30 40.25000    1     0 0.7456165 0.025396927 0.2543835
31 41.25000    2     0 0.7456165 0.025396927 0.2543835
32 41.50000    2     0 0.7456165 0.025396927 0.2543835
33 41.91667    1     0 0.7456165 0.025396927 0.2543835
34 42.75000    0     0 0.7456165 0.025396927 0.2543835
35 44.66667    0     0 0.3728083 0.075842235 0.6271917
36 52.16667    1     0 0.3728083 0.075842235 0.6271917
37 52.66667    0     0 0.3728083 0.075842235 0.6271917
```

2.3 Transition Probabilities and State Occupation Probabilities

The following code computes the Aalen-Johansen estimators of the transition probabilities for reference ages 18, 25, 30 and 35 (see Beyersmann et al. 2012, p. 187):

```
age. points <- c(18,25,30,35)
landmark.etm <- lapply (age.points,
    function (reference.age)
        {etm(data=D$D,
        state.names=c("J","N"),
        tra=tra,"cens",
        s=reference.age) })
```

The landmark method is also implemented in the *dynpred* package (Putter, 2011b). It is the companion package of Van Houwelingen and Putter (2011).

State occupation probabilities are derived from transition probabilities. Because all individuals are initially in J, the probability of being in state N is the transition probability JN with the youngest age as reference age (compare with Beyersmann et al. 2012, p. 190). In the subsample of ten individuals, the probability of occupying state J at age 30 is 78.95 %, and the probability of being in N is 21.05 % (Table 2.5). The 95 % confidence intervals are (0.531, 1.000) (0.7895 $\pm 1.96\sqrt{0.017}$) and (0.000, 0.469) ($0.2105 \pm 1.96\sqrt{0.017}$), respectively. The following code produces these results:

```
dd=Biograph.mvna(d.10)
etm(data=dd$D,c("J","N"),tra,"cens",s=0)
summary(etm.0)$"J N"[26, c("P","lower","upper")]
summary(etm.0)$"N J"[26, c("P","lower","upper")]
```

where dd is the data for the 10 selected individuals (*Biograph* object) and 26 is the age index associated with the age at the last transition before 30 (age 29.75).

Consider now the subsample of 201 respondents. Of the 201 respondents, 160 enter the labour market (first job) before age 20 and 41 enter after age 20. The ages at labour market entry are obtained by the code:

```
table (trunc(d3.a$start))
```

Of those who entered the labour market before age 20, 146 are in state J (91 %) and 14 in state N (9 %) at age 20. In the observation plan considered, they are under observation at age 20. Some entered observation at young ages, while others entered just before age 20. The empirical transition probabilities take into account durations under observation and durations spent in J and N. The transition probabilities condition the state occupancy on the state occupied at a reference age. A person with a job at age 14 (lowest age) has an 85.6 % chance of having a job at age 20 and 14.4 % chance of having no job. A person without a job at age 14 has a probability of 75.1 % to have a job at age 20 and 24.9 % to have no job at that age. The state probabilities at age 20 are produced by the code:

```
D=Biograph.mvna(d3.a)
tra <- Parameters(d3.a)$trans_possible
etm.0 <- etm(data=D$D,c("J","N"),tra,"cens",s=0,t=20)
```

where d3.a is the *Biograph* object with ages at transition.
To display the results for age 20, use the code:

```
summary(etm.0)$"J N"[81:84,]
summary(etm.0)$"N J"[81:84,]
```

The state probabilities at age 30 are obtained from the state probabilities at age 20 and the empirical transition probabilities between ages 20 and 30, $\hat{\mathbf{P}}(20,30)$

$$\begin{bmatrix} 0.6952 & 0.6135 \\ 0.3048 & 0.3865 \end{bmatrix} \begin{bmatrix} 0.856 \\ 0.144 \end{bmatrix} = \begin{bmatrix} 0.6835 \\ 0.3165 \end{bmatrix}.$$

The following code produces the transition matrix $\hat{\mathbf{P}}(20,30)$:

```
etm.20_30 <-
etm(data=D$D,c("J","N"),tra,"cens",s=20,t=30)
```

The product of $\hat{\mathbf{P}}(20,30)$ and $\hat{\mathbf{p}}(20)$ is:

```
t(etm.20_30$est[,,99])%*%
t(etm.0$est[,,dim(etm.0$est)[3]])[,1]
```

The state occupation probabilities at age 30 $\hat{\mathbf{p}}(30)$ can be obtained by the code:

```
etm(data=D$D,c("J","N"),tra,"cens",s=0,t=30)
```

The probability of being employed at age 30 is 68.5 % if the person is employed at the lowest age and 67.5 % if the person is not employed. Table 2.6 shows the state probabilities at selected ages. The table shows the probabilities of occupying state J (J_est) and state N (N_est) at selected ages and the 95 % confidence intervals (J_lower, J_upper) and (N_lower, N_upper) for individuals who are employed at the lowest age. The confidence intervals are computed by the summary.etm function of the *etm* package.

Table 2.6 Probabilities of being with/without a job at selected ages: non-parametric method. GLHS, 201 respondents

	age	J_lower	J_est	J_upper	N_lower	N_est	N_upper
1	15	0.827	0.926	1.000	0.000	0.074	0.173
2	20	0.786	0.856	0.926	0.074	0.144	0.214
3	25	0.641	0.707	0.774	0.226	0.293	0.359
4	30	0.618	0.684	0.749	0.251	0.316	0.382
5	40	0.624	0.699	0.774	0.226	0.301	0.376
6	50	0.600	0.688	0.775	0.225	0.312	0.400

2.3 Transition Probabilities and State Occupation Probabilities

(b) Parametric Method: Piecewise Exponential Model

If the instantaneous transition rates are constant, the distribution of the waiting time to the next transition is exponential. Assume that the instantaneous transition rates are constant in the age interval from x to y: $\mu_{ij}(\tau) = m_{ij}(x,y)$ for $x \leq \tau < y$, with $m_{ij}(x,y)$ the transition rate during the (x,y)-interval. The matrix of transition probabilities is $\mathbf{P}(x,y) = \exp[-(y-x)\mathbf{m}(x,y)]$. If transition rates are age-specific with age intervals of 1 year, then the transition probabilities between reference age x and age y are obtained by the matrix expression

$$\mathbf{P}(x,y) = \mathbf{P}(x, x+1)\,\mathbf{P}(x+1, x+2) \ldots \mathbf{P}(y-1, y)$$

with $\mathbf{P}(x, x+1) = \exp[-\mathbf{m}(x, x+1)]$.

To determine the value of $\exp[-\mathbf{m}(x,y)]$, I use the Taylor series expansion. Note that for matrix $\mathbf{A}$, $\exp(\mathbf{A})$ may be written as a Taylor series expansion:

$$\exp(\mathbf{A}) = \mathbf{I} + \mathbf{A} + \frac{1}{2!}\mathbf{A}^2 + \frac{1}{3!}\mathbf{A}^3 + \cdots$$

Hence,

$$\exp[-(y-x)\mathbf{m}(x,y)] = \mathbf{I} - (y-x)\mathbf{m}(x,y) + \frac{(y-x)^2}{2!}[\mathbf{m}(x,y)]^2$$
$$- \frac{(y-x)^3}{3!}[\mathbf{m}(x,y)]^3 + \cdots$$

(see also Schoen 1988, p. 72).

The estimator of the transition matrix is $\hat{\mathbf{P}}(x,y) = \exp[-(y-x)\hat{\mathbf{m}}(x,y)]$ with $\hat{\mathbf{m}}(x,y)$ the matrix of empirical occurrence-exposure rates in the (x,y)-interval: $\hat{m}_{ij}(x,y) = N_{ij}(x,y)/R_i(x,y)$, where $N_{ij}(x,y)$ is the observed number of moves from i to j during the interval and $R_i(x,y)$ is the exposure time in i.

In case of two states, the rate equation may be written as follows:

$$\begin{bmatrix} \hat{m}_{11}(x,y) & -\hat{m}_{21}(x,y) \\ -\hat{m}_{12}(x,y) & \hat{m}_{22}(x,y) \end{bmatrix} = \begin{bmatrix} N_{11}(x,y) & -N_{21}(x,y) \\ -N_{12}(x,y) & N_{22}(x,y) \end{bmatrix} \begin{bmatrix} R_1(x,y) & 0 \\ 0 & R_2(x,y) \end{bmatrix}^{-1}$$

where $\hat{m}_{11}(x,y) = \hat{m}_{12}(x,y)$ and $\hat{m}_{22}(x,y) = \hat{m}_{21}(x,y)$. In matrix notation: $\hat{\mathbf{m}}(x,y) = \mathbf{N}(x,y)[\mathbf{R}(x,y)]^{-1}$

Consider the example with 201 respondents. The age-specific transition rates are shown in Table 2.3. The first state is J and the second N. The JN transition rate for 18-year-old individuals is 0.0806 and the NJ transition rate is 0.3024. They are obtained by dividing the number of transitions by the exposure time in each state between ages 18 and 19. The 1-year transition probability matrix is:

$$\hat{\mathbf{P}}(18, 19) = \exp[-\hat{\mathbf{m}}(18, 19)] = \exp\left[-\begin{bmatrix} 0.0806 & -0.3024 \\ -0.0806 & 0.3024 \end{bmatrix}\right]$$

$$= \begin{bmatrix} 0.9330 & 0.2512 \\ 0.0670 & 0.7488 \end{bmatrix}$$

The probability that an individual in the sample population who on his 18th birthday has a job will be without a job on his 19th birthday is 6.7 %. The probability that an 18-year-old without a job will be with a job 1 year later is 25.1 %. Bootstrapping is used to generate confidence intervals. The mean transition probability produced by 100 bootstrap samples is 0.0665 for the JN transition, with 95 % confidence interval (0.0294, 0.1043), and 0.2583 for the NJ transition, with 95 % confidence interval (0.0000, 0.4611). The retention probabilities are 0.9335 for J, with confidence interval (0.8957, 0.9706), and 0.7417 for N, with confidence interval (0.5389, 1.0000).

The state occupation probabilities at age 30 are obtained as the product of the transition probability matrix $\hat{\mathbf{P}}(20, 30)$ and the state probabilities $\hat{\mathbf{p}}(20)$. In the subsample, 86 % is employed at age 20 and 14 % is without a job (Table 2.6). The state probabilities at age 30 are $\hat{\mathbf{p}}(30) = \hat{\mathbf{P}}(20, 30)\,\hat{\mathbf{p}}(20) = \hat{\mathbf{P}}(29, 30)\,\hat{\mathbf{P}}(28, 27) \cdots \hat{\mathbf{P}}(20, 21)\,\hat{\mathbf{p}}(20)$. It is equal to

$$\begin{bmatrix} 0.6970 & 0.6144 \\ 0.3030 & 0.3856 \end{bmatrix} \begin{bmatrix} 0.8646 \\ 0.1354 \end{bmatrix} = \begin{bmatrix} 0.6858 \\ 0.3142 \end{bmatrix}.$$

The 95 % confidence intervals of the state occupation probabilities at age 30, obtained from 100 bootstrap samples, are (0.6173, 0.7556) for J and (0.2444, 0.3827) for N. The estimates and their confidence interval are close to the figures produced by the non-parametric method (Table 2.6).

2.4 Expected Waiting Times and State Occupation Times

State occupation times, also denoted as sojourn times and exposure times, are durations of stay in a state or stage during a given period. They indicate the lengths of episodes and are expressed in days, weeks, months or years if measured for a single individual or in person-days to person-years if measured for a population. Observed sojourn times are used to determine the exposure to the risk of a transition. In this section, the focus is on *expected* sojourn times. The fundamental question is: Given a set of transition rates, what is the expected sojourn time in a state? Questions on durations of stay are omnipresent. What is the expected lifetime (life expectancy)? What is the health expectancy, i.e. how many years may a person expect to live healthy? What is the expected age at disability for those who ever become disabled? What is the expected duration of marriage at time of divorce?

2.4 Expected Waiting Times and State Occupation Times

What is the expected duration of unemployment for someone who becomes unemployed? What is the expected number of years of working life for persons who retire early? What these questions have in common is that they are about the length of periods between two reference points. The reference points may be transitions such as in the question on duration of marriage at divorce. Marriage and divorce are the two transitions. The reference point may be any point in time. When the second reference point is a transition, the expected sojourn time is equivalent to the expected waiting time to the transition.

Expected occupation times depend on transition rates between two reference ages. They also depend on the location of the observer. Suppose we want to know the number of years a person may expect to live with cardiovascular disease between ages 60 and 80. It depends on the transition rates between ages 60 and 80, including rates of death from cardiovascular disease or other causes. It also depends on the reference age because the reference age introduces dependencies on intervening transitions. The expected number of years with the disease is larger for 60-year-old individuals than for 0-year-old children because the latter category may not reach age 60.

The sojourn time between ages x and y spent in each state of the state space by state occupied at age x is $_x\mathbf{L}(x, y) = \int_x^y \mathbf{P}(x, \tau) \, d\tau$. The configuration of $_x\mathbf{L}(x, y)$ is:

$$_x\mathbf{L}(x,y) = \begin{bmatrix} _1L_1(x,y) & _2L_1(x,y) & . & . & _IL_1(x,y) \\ _1L_2(x,y) & _2L_2(x,y) & . & . & _IL_2(x,y) \\ . & . & . & . & . \\ . & . & . & . & . \\ _1L_I(x,y) & _2L_I(x,y) & . & . & _IL_I(x,y) \end{bmatrix}$$

The marginal state occupation times give the total expected sojourn time in the system by state occupied at age x (column total).

The time spent in state j between ages x and y by an individual who is in state i at exact age x is

$$_{ix}L_j(x,y) = \left[\int_x^y p_{ij}(x,t) \, dt \right]$$

and for all states of origin and states of destination: $_x\mathbf{L}(x, y) = \int_x^y \mathbf{P}(x, \tau) \, d\tau$

In the above formulation, the expected occupation time in state j is conditional on being in state i at age x. The occupation time is said to be *status-based*; it is estimated for individuals in a given state at the reference age x. The *population-based* occupation time is the expected occupation time in state j beyond age x, irrespective of the state occupied at age x. It is the sum of status-based occupation times between x and y, weighted by state probabilities at age x:

$_xL_j(x,y) = \sum_i [p_i(x) \int_x^y p_{ij}(x,\tau) d\tau] = \sum_i p_i(x) \, _{ix}L_j(x,y)$, where $p_i(x)$ is the probability that an individual is in state i at age x.

The expected state occupation times are derived from transition rates. Two approaches are considered: the non-parametric approach and the (piecewise constant) exponential model.

(a) Non-parametric Approach

Beyersmann and Putter (2014) present a non-parametric method for estimating the expected state occupation time. Divide the period between age 0 and the highest age ω in intervals. Intervals of 1 year are considered, but the method can be applied to intervals of any length. Let $p_i(x)$ denote the state occupation probability at age x. A natural estimate of the expected occupation time in i beyond age x, irrespective of the state occupied at age x, is:

$$_x\hat{L}_i(x,y) = \sum_{t=x}^{y-1} (x - (x-1))\, \hat{p}_i(x) = \sum_{t=x}^{y-1} \hat{p}_i(x)$$

The method assumes that an individual who is in state i at age x stays in i during the entire year preceding x, and an individual who leaves i between $x-1$ and x leaves at the beginning of the interval (at $x-1$). The assumption can be relaxed by reducing the length of the interval or by making alternative assumptions about ages at entry and exit. A plausible assumption is that transitions take place in the middle of the interval. That assumption is valid if the interval is sufficiently short so that at most one transition occurs during the interval. Multiple transitions during an interval (tied transitions) require an assumption about the sequence of transitions.

(b) Parametric Approach: Exponential Model

A distinction is made between expected state occupation times between two ages (closed interval) and expected state occupation times beyond a given age (open interval). The reference age may be any age at or before the start of the interval. For instance, the expected number of years in good health beyond age 65 may be computed for persons aged 65 or for persons of an age below 65, e.g. at birth or at labour market entry. The expected state occupation time may be conditioned on the state occupied (and other characteristics) at the reference age or the first age of the closed or open interval. The expected state occupation time may also be conditioned on a future transition. Consider an employment career. The age at which a person may experience a first episode without work after a period with employment is lower for those who will ever experience an episode without work than for the average population. The expected occupation time during an age interval, conditioned on a transition occurring with certainty during that interval, is less than the expected occupation time that is not conditioned on a transition occurring. For instance, the expected duration of marriage at divorce is lower for those who ever divorce than for the average married population. The latter includes those who never divorce.

The time spent in state j between ages x and y by an individual who is in state i at exact age x is $_x\mathbf{L}(x,y) = [\int_x^y \mathbf{P}(x,t)dt]$, where an element $_{ix}L_j(x,y)$ denotes the time an individual in i at age x may expect to spend in j between ages x and y. If the

2.4 Expected Waiting Times and State Occupation Times

transition rates are constant in the (x,y)-age interval (exponential model), the integration of the equation leads to

$$_xL(x,y) = \int_x^y P(x,t)dt = \int_x^y \exp[-(t-x)\mathbf{m}(x,t)]\,dt,$$

which is equal to

$$_xL(x,y) = [\mathbf{m}(x,y)]^{-1}[\mathbf{I} - \exp[-(y-x)\mathbf{m}(x,y)]],$$

provided $\mathbf{m}(x,y)$ is not singular. The expression is also shown by Namboodiri and Suchindran (1987, p. 145), Schoen (1988, p. 101) and van Imhoff (1990). If $\mathbf{m}(x,y)$ is singular, a very small value may be added to the diagonal elements of the matrix. Izmirlian et al. (2000, p. 246), who consider the case with an absorbing state (death), suggest to replace by one the zero diagonal element corresponding to the absorbing state. I choose to add a small value (10^{-8}) to the diagonal. It may be viewed as a rate of a fictitious attrition. It is too small to occur between x and y but it is large enough to make $\mathbf{m}(x,y)$ non-singular.

Taylor series expansion of $\exp[-(y-x)\mathbf{m}(x,y)]$ results in the following equivalent expression for the state occupation times (Schoen 1988, p. 73):

$$_xL(x,y) = (y-x)\left[\mathbf{I} - \frac{(y-x)}{2!}\mathbf{m}(x,y) + \frac{(y-x)^2}{3!}[\mathbf{m}(x,y)]^2 - \frac{(y-x)^3}{4!}[\mathbf{m}(x,y)]^3 + \cdots\right]$$

When the interval is short, the sojourn time may be approximated by the linear integration hypothesis, which implies the assumption of uniform distribution of events (linear model):

$$_xL(x,y) = \frac{y-x}{2}[\mathbf{I} + \mathbf{P}(x,y)]$$

The linear method is usually used in demography and actuarial science. It is often referred to as the actuarial method.

The reference age may be any age at or before the start of the interval. Consider the reference age zero. The expected time newborns may expect to spend in each state between ages x and y, by state at birth, is

$$_0L(x,y) = {_xL(x,y)}\,\mathbf{P}(0,x)$$

where $\mathbf{P}(0,x)$ represents the transition probabilities between ages 0 and x. When the reference age changes from age 0 to age x, the expected length of stay in the various states between ages x and y changes from an unconditional measure to a conditional measure. It becomes conditional on being present in the population at x. The measure is

$$_x\mathbf{L}(x,y) = {}_0\mathbf{L}(x,y)\,[\mathbf{P}(0,x)]^{-1},$$

provided the inverse of $\mathbf{P}(0,x)$ exists. The state occupation times between ages x and y, a newborn may expect, irrespective of the state occupied at birth is $_0\mathbf{L}(x,y)\mathbf{p}(0)$.

The estimation of the expected state occupation times beyond a given age requires the state occupation time beyond the highest age group. If at high ages few transitions occur, the ages are often collapsed in an open-ended age group with constant transition rates. Demographers use that approach to close the life table. Let z denote the first age of the highest open-ended age group. The sojourn time in the various states beyond age z by individuals present at z is $_z\mathbf{L}(z,\infty) = [\mathbf{m}(z,\infty)]^{-1}$, where ∞ denotes infinity.

The life expectancy at age x is the number of years an individual aged x may expect to spend in each state beyond age x, by state occupied at x or irrespective of the state occupied at x. It is $_x\mathbf{e}(x,\infty) = [\int_x^\infty \mathbf{P}(x,t)dt]$. An element $_{ix}e_j(x,\infty)$ of $_x\mathbf{e}(x,\infty)$ is the number of years an individual who is in state i at age x may expect to spend in state j beyond age x. $_x\mathbf{e}(x,\infty)$ is a matrix with the state at age x as the column variable and the state occupied beyond age x the row variable. It gives the expected remaining lifetime conditional on the state occupied at age x. In multistate demography, it is known as the *status-based life expectancy* at age x. The *population-based life expectancy* is the time an individual aged x may expect to spend in each of the states beyond age x, irrespective of the state occupied at age x. It is $_x\mathbf{e}(x,\infty)$ multiplied by the vector of state occupation probabilities at age x.

If transition rates are age-specific, i.e. piecewise constant, and the length of an age interval is 1 year, then the expected state occupation times at reference age x is

$$_x\mathbf{e}(x,\infty) = \sum_{\tau=x}^{z-1} {}_x\mathbf{L}(\tau,\tau+1) + {}_x\mathbf{L}(z,\infty)$$

with $_x\mathbf{L}(\tau,\tau+1) = [\mathbf{m}(\tau,\tau+1)]^{-1}\,[\exp[\mathbf{m}(\tau,\tau+1)] - \mathbf{I}]$ and $_z\mathbf{L}(z,\infty) = [\mathbf{m}(z,\infty)]^{-1}$.

The expected occupation time in state i depends on the rate of leaving i. If the exit rate between ages x and y is zero, an individual in i at age x will remain in i at least until age y. If a departure from i occurs during the (x,y)- interval, it will occur at an occupation time which is less than the expected occupation time. In other words, the expected occupation time, conditioned on a transition occurring, is less than the expected occupation time that is not conditioned on a transition occurring. Consider an individual in state i at age x. The expected waiting time to leaving i between x and y consists of two parts. The first is the state occupation time for stayers. It is equal to $y - x$. The probability of staying in i during the entire interval from x to y is the survival probability $_{ix}S_i(y) = \exp[-\int_x^y \mu_i(\tau)d\tau]$. The second part is the waiting time to an exit from i that occurs before y. It is denoted by $_{ix}^{oc}L_i(x,y)$. Hence, the occupation time equation is $_{ix}L_i(x,y) = (y-x)_{ix}S_i(y) + {}_{ix}^{oc}L_i(x,y)$ $[1 - {}_{ix}S_i(y)]$ and $_{ix}^{oc}Li(x,y) = \dfrac{{}_{ix}Li(x,y) - (y-x)_{ix}Si(y)}{1 - {}_{ix}Si(y)}$. It is the time an individual aged x in i spends in i on a continuous basis before leaving, provided the exit occurs before y. The occupation time equation distinguishes stayers and leavers.

2.4 Expected Waiting Times and State Occupation Times

The fraction of an interval spent in a given state if a transition occurs with certainty is frequently referred to as Chiang's 'a', after the statistician Chiang who introduced it. Chiang, who developed the measure in the context of mortality, called 'a' the fraction of the last year of life (Chiang 1968, pp. 190ff, 1984, pp. 142ff). Schoen (1988, p. 8 and p. 71) uses the concept of *mean duration at transfer* to denote the expected number of years before the transition. It is the product of Chiang's 'a' (fraction of the interval) and the length of the interval. If transitions are uniformly distributed during the interval, the survival function is linear, and 'a' is half the length of the interval. If the transition rate is constant during an interval, the waiting time to the event is exponentially distributed. Consequently, the expected time to an event that occurs with certainty is less than half the interval length. The probability that an exit from state i during the (x,y)-interval occurs during the first half of the interval, provided it occurs with certainty during the interval, is a ratio of two distribution functions: $\frac{1 - \exp\left[-\frac{y-x}{2} m_i(x, y)\right]}{1 - \exp[-(y-x) m_i(x, y)]}$.

Consider the 201 respondents and age 18. The expected occupation times in each of the states of the state space (J and N) by state on the 18th birthday is:

$$_{18}\mathbf{L}(18, 19) = \left[\begin{bmatrix} 0.0806 & -0.3024 \\ -0.0806 & 0.3024 \end{bmatrix} \right]^{-1} \left[\begin{bmatrix} 1 & 0 \\ 0 & 1 \end{bmatrix} - \begin{bmatrix} 0.9330 & 0.2512 \\ 0.0670 & 0.7488 \end{bmatrix} \right]$$

$$= \begin{bmatrix} 0.9644 & 0.1336 \\ 0.0356 & 0.8664 \end{bmatrix}$$

A person of exact age 18 with employment may expect to spend 0.036 years (less than half a month) without employment before reaching age 19. The 95 % confidence interval, produced by bootstrapping, is (0.0136, 0.0635). A person of the same age without a job may expect to be employed during 0.134 years (1.6 months) before his 19th birthday, with confidence interval (0.0323, 0.2663). A small figure (10^{-8}) has been added to the diagonal to prevent $\mathbf{m}(18,19)$ from being singular. A person aged 18 with employment, who leaves employment before age 19, may expect to leave employment after $\frac{0.9644 - 0.9330}{1 - 0.933} = 0.4687$ years or 5.6 months. The Taylor series expansion gives about the same result. A sum of four terms plus the identity matrix gives $\begin{bmatrix} 0.9644 & 0.1336 \\ 0.0356 & 0.8664 \end{bmatrix}$.

The number of years between the lowest age (14) and the highest age (54) is 40 years. Since states J and N are transient states, the total numbers of years spent in the employment career between ages 14 and 54 is 40. If a hypothetical individual starts at age 14 with a job and the employment career is governed by the occurrence-exposure rates estimated from the GLHS subsample of 201 subjects, then the expected number of years with a job is 28.66, and the number of years without a job is 11.34. The average of the 100 bootstrap samples is 28.55 and 11.45, respectively. The 95 % confidence intervals are (26.65, 30.28) and (9.72, 13.35).

2.5 Synthetic Life Histories

The methods presented in the previous sections produce state probabilities and expected occupation times that are consistent with empirical transition rates. The state probabilities and the occupation times describe the expected life history, given the data. The confidence intervals around the expected values indicate the degree of uncertainty in the data. Transition rates are differentiated by age to capture the age patterns of transitions. In this section, age-specific transition rates are considered, with age intervals of 1 year. Transition rates are piecewise constant: they vary between age groups, but they are constant within age groups. Individual life histories differ from the expected life history because of observed differences between individuals with different personal attributes, unobserved differences and chance. The chance mechanism is the subject of this section. Observed and unobserved differences are disregarded because they are beyond the scope of this chapter. Synthetic individual life histories are generated using longitudinal microsimulation (Willekens 2009; Zinn 2011, 2014; Zinn et al. 2013). The method is consistent with discrete event simulation (DEV) methods.

To explain the chance mechanism, a single transition rate will do, and to explain the basic principle of generating synthetic biographies, a single transition rate matrix is sufficient. To generate more realistic synthetic biographies, age-specific transition rates are used. Consider the 201 respondents of the GLHS sample and the observation period between labour market entry and survey date. In Sect. 2.2, the aggregate NJ transition rate was estimated at 0.096 per year (using *msm*). An individual who previously had a job (the nature of the sample) and who is currently without a job may expect to get another job in 10.4 years (1/0.096) on average. The expected waiting time during the first year is $(1/0.096)[1 - \exp(-0.096)] = 0.9534$ years. It is high because at the time the data were collected a relatively large number of respondents, in particular women, left the labour force and did not return. The probability of experiencing the event in the first year is 9.154 % $[100*(1-\exp(-0.096))]$. An individual without a job, who gets a job within 1 year, waits 0.4920 years, on average. This is a little less than 6 months. Individual waiting times are random variables; the values are distributed around these expected value. Since the transition rate is constant at 0.096, individual waiting times are exponentially distributed with a mean of 10.4 years and a variance of 108 years, assuming no competing transition intervenes in the labour market transitions. The median waiting time is 7.2 years $[\ln(2)]/0.096$.

To obtain individual waiting times that are consistent with these expected values, waiting times are drawn randomly from an exponential distribution with a hazard rate 0.096 or, alternatively, a mean waiting time of 10.4 years. A random draw is implemented in two steps. First, a random number is drawn from the standard uniform continuous distribution $U[0,1]$. Every value between zero and one is equally likely to occur. The random number drawn represents the probability that the waiting time to the transition is less than or equal to t, where t needs to be determined. Let α denote the probability. Hence, $\alpha = 1 - \exp[-0.096t]$. Suppose

2.5 Synthetic Life Histories

$\alpha = 0.54$. The value of t is derived from the inverse distribution function of the exponential distribution. It is $t = -\frac{\ln(1-\alpha)}{0.096} = -\frac{\ln(1-0.54)}{0.096} = 8.09$ years. n draws from the uniform distribution result in n individual waiting times. If n is sufficiently large, the *sample* mean is close to the expected value of 10.4 years, and the sample variance is close to 108 years. One experiment of 1,000 draws resulted in a mean waiting time of 10.11 years and a variance of 116.5 years. Another experiment resulted in a mean waiting time of 9.89 years and a variance of 87.4 years.

The transition rate estimated from data, in this example 0.096, is subject to sample variation. The rate is itself a random variable. If the number of observations is sufficiently large, the rate is a normally distributed random variable with the expected value as its mean. The 95 % confidence interval of the NJ transition rate was estimated at (0.0804, 0.1146). To incorporate the degree of uncertainty in the data in the generation of synthetic life histories, a transition rate may be drawn from a normal distribution with mean $\ln(0.096)$ and standard deviation $\sqrt{1/122} = 0.0905$. The standard deviation of the NJ transition rate was computed in Sect. 2.2 of this chapter. If the value drawn from a normal distribution is denoted by m, then the transition rate is $\exp(m)$. An alternative to drawing a transition rate from a normal distribution is to resample the data (with replacement) and to estimate the transition rate from the new sample. In this approach, the distribution of the transition rate is the distribution generated by bootstrap samples. Consider 100 bootstrap samples and 100 transition rates, one from each sample. Each of these transition rates is used to generate 1,000 individual waiting times. The collection of waiting time incorporates the effects of sample variation and the exponential distribution of waiting times. For a person without a job, the overall average waiting time to a job is 10.54 years, and the variance is 115.00 years. The NJ transition rates estimated in the bootstrap samples vary from 0.073 to 0.140, with mean rate 0.0967.

The aggregate transition rates may be used to generate employment histories. The JN transition rate is 0.0533 and the NJ transition rate is 0.0960. Recall that observations started at labour market entry (first job). Hence, N refers to being without a job, after having had at least one job. The transition rate matrix is

$$\hat{m} = \begin{bmatrix} 0.0533 & -0.0960 \\ -0.0533 & 0.0960 \end{bmatrix}.$$ Everyone starts the employment history in J. The starting time is zero, meaning that the time is measured as time elapsed since labour market entry. The employment history is simulated for 30 years (simulation stop time). The transition rates are assumed to remain constant during that period. In this example, employment histories are sequences of transitions and waiting times to transitions. They are assumed to be outcomes of a continuous-time Markov model with constant rates. The simulation runs as follows. Let t denote time. An individual starts in J at time 0. A random number is drawn from an exponential distribution with transition rate 0.0533 to determine the time to transition from J to N. One draw results in a transition at $t = 8.29$ years. To determine how long the individual stays in N, a random number is drawn from an exponential distribution with transition rate 0.096. The randomly selected time to NJ transition is 4.30 years. Hence, the individual starts a second job 12.59 years after labour market entry (8.29 + 4.30).

A new random waiting time is drawn from an exponential distribution with transition rate 0.0533 to determine the time at the second JN transition. The number is 24.00, which means that the transition would occur 36.59 years after labour market entry. The transition time exceeds the time horizon of 30 years and is not considered. When the simulation is discontinued, the individual is in state J. The function sim.msm of the *msm* package is used to generate the life history of a single individual. The code is

```
m <- array(c(0.0533,-0.0533,-0.096,0.096),
    dim=c(2,2),dimnames=list(destination=c("J","N"),
    origin=c("J","N")))
bio <- sim.msm (-t(m),mintime=0,maxtime=30,start=1)
```

where m is the transition rate matrix shown above, mintime is the starting time of the simulation, maxtime is the ending time and start is the starting state (J is state 1 and N is state 2). The object bio has two components. The first contains the state sequence and the second the transition times.

The distribution of employment histories that are consistent with the transition rates may be obtained by simulating a large number of employment histories. In this simple illustration, the transition rates are assumed not to depend on age and to remain constant during the period of 30 years. Simulation of 1,000 employment histories results in the distribution shown in Table 2.7. The most frequent trajectory is JNJ, about one third of all trajectories. The trajectories JN and J cover about one fifth each. These 3 trajectories account for 68 % of all trajectories during a period of 30 years. For each trajectory, the median ages at transition are also shown. The table is produced by the Sequences function of *Biograph*. The results of the simulation are stored in a *Biograph* object, which facilitates analysis of the simulated life histories.

Constant transition rates have been used for illustrative purposes only. Usually, age-specific transition rates are used to generate synthetic life histories. Suppose an individual enters his first job at age 21.3 (decimal year). He experiences the employment exit rate from age 21.3 onwards until (a) he enters a period without a job, (b) he experiences a competing transition, or (c) the 'observation' is censored, i.e. simulation is discontinued. In this illustration, no competing transition is considered. Hence, the waiting time to the JN transition depends on the age-specific transition rates between age 21.3 and the age at which simulation is discontinued, which in the sample of 201 respondents is 52. Age-specific transition rates are weighted by exposure time. The transition rate at age 21 is multiplied by

Table 2.7 Employment histories in virtual population, based on GLHS aggregate transition rates

	ncase	%	cum%	path	tr1	tr2	tr3	tr4
1	305	30.5	30.5	JNJ	9.12>N	19.95>J		
2	194	19.4	49.9	JN	20.35>N			
3	185	18.5	68.4	J				
4	130	13.0	81.4	JNJNJ	4.81>N	10.42>J	18.86>N	24.91>J
5	121	12.1	93.5	JNJN	6.53>N	13.28>J	25.83>N	

2.5 Synthetic Life Histories

the duration of exposure, which is 0.7 years (22.0–21.3). The transition rates at age 22 and higher are multiplied by one. The sum of the age-specific transition rates beyond age 21 is the cumulative transition rate, computed at age 21. The waiting time to the JN transition is determined by a random draw from an exponential waiting time distribution associated with the cumulative transition rate computed at age at labour market entry. The age at the JN transition is the current age plus the waiting time to the JN transition. Suppose a waiting time of 3.4 years is drawn. The individual will enter a period without a job at age 24.4. If the waiting time is such that the age at transition exceeds the highest age in the *observation* scheme, then the *observation* is censored at the highest age.

If the number of states exceeds two, the destination state must be determined in addition to the time to transition. A multinomial distribution is used. The distribution is derived from the origin-destination-specific transition rates. If $m_{ij}(x,y)$ is the (i,j)-transition rate between ages x and y, then the probability of selecting state j, conditional on leaving i, is $_iq_j(x,y) = \frac{m_{ij}(x,y)}{\sum_{j \neq i} m_{ij}(x,y)}$, with $\sum_{ji} q_j(x,y) = 1$. The probability is an event probability, not a transition probability. The probabilities are used to partition the interval between the minimum probability (0) and the maximum probability (1): $\{0, \ _iq_1, \ _iq_1 + _iq_2, \ _iq_1 + _iq_2 + _iq_3 \ldots, 1\}$. A random number is drawn from a standard uniform distribution, and the interval that corresponds to its value determines the destination state. The method is implemented in the *msm* package.

The method of estimating time to transition and destination state consists of two steps. The first uses the exit rate from the current state, i say, to determine the time to transition (exit from i). The exit rate is taken from the diagonal of the transition rate matrix. The second step is to determine the destination, conditional on leaving the current state. This method was suggested by Wolf (1986). An alternative but equivalent method relies on the destination-specific transition rates. Consider an individual in state i at age x. For each possible destination j random waiting times are drawn from exponential distributions with parameters the cumulative (i,j)-transition rates between x and the highest age: $A_{ij}(x, \omega) = \int_x^\omega \mu_{ij}(\tau) d\tau$. If transition rates are piecewise constant (age-specific), the cumulative hazard is piecewise linear. The smallest random waiting time determines the destination. The two methods rely on the theory of competing risks and assume that the waiting times corresponding to the distinct destinations are independent. Zinn (2011, pp. 177ff) shows that the two methods give similar results. Notice that the two methods are also consistent with discrete event simulation (DEVS), although only the second method stores randomly drawn waiting times in event queues before selecting the shortest waiting time. The *LifePaths* (Statistics Canada[2]) and *MicMac* microsimulation models (Gampe et al. 2009) use event queues. The *msm* package uses exit rates and conditional destination probabilities.

For illustrative purposes, the transition rates in Table 2.3 are used to generate synthetic employment histories for 2010 individuals, 10 for each observation in the

---
[2] http://www.statcan.gc.ca/microsimulation/lifepaths/lifepaths-eng.htm

GLHS subsample of 201 respondents. For each individual in the GLHS sample, 10 employment histories are simulated to reduce the Monte Carlo variation. The employment career is simulated between a low age and a high age. The ages are determined by individual observation periods in the GLHS subsample of 201 respondents. For instance, individual 1 enters the labour market at age 17 and is 52 at interview. In the virtual population, ten individuals enter the labour market at age 17 and are interviewed at age 52. Individual 4 is 22 at labour market entry and 31 at interview. The ages of labour market entry and interview of that respondent are imposed on ten individuals in the virtual population. The simulated employment histories cover the same age intervals as the observed employment histories. Differences between simulated and observed employment trajectories are due to sample variation affecting the estimated transition rates and Monte Carlo variation in the simulation. Table 2.8 shows the main employment trajectories in the

Table 2.8 Employment histories in observed population and virtual population, based on age-specific GLHS transition rates

```
A. Observed trajectories: males and females combined
    ncase    %    cum%   case      tr1           tr2           tr3           tr4
 1    67  33.33  33.33     J
 2    54  26.87  60.20   JNJ  21.71>N  26.17>J
 3    44  21.89  82.09    JN  24.88>N
 4    16   7.96  90.05  JNJNJ 20.83>J  23.96>J  25.62>N  29.62>J
 5    10   4.98  95.02  JNJNJ 20.12>N  21.21>J  29.62>N

B. Simulated trajectories: males and females combined
    ncase    %    cum%  case      tr1           tr2           tr3           tr4
 1   627  31.19  31.19     J
 2   531  26.42  57.61   JNJ  22.99>N  27.33>J
 3   294  14.63  72.24    JN  27.2>N
 4   245  12.19  84.43  JNJN  21.21>N  24.3>J   30.31>N
 5   218  10.85  95.27  NJNJ  20.66>N  22.31>J  26.92>N  32.43>J

C. Observed trajectories: males
    ncase    %    cum%      case      tr1          tr2          tr3          tr4          tr5          tr6
 1    52  49.06  49.06        J
 2    41  38.68  87.74      JNJ  21.92>N  25.33>J
 3     6   5.66  93.40    JNJNJ  18.42>N  20.17>J  22.71>N  24.04>J
 4     3   2.83  96.23       JN  27.5>N
 5     3   2.83  99.06  JNJNJNJ  18.17>N  19.67>J   21.5>N  22.08>J  33.17>N  35.75>J

D. Simulated trajectories: males
    ncase    %    cum%     case      tr1          tr2          tr3          tr4          tr5          tr6
 1   518  48.87  48.87       J
 2   314  29.62  78.49     JNJ  21.5>N   24.93>J
 3   131  12.36  90.85   JNJNJ  20.54>N  22.54>J  26.81>N  28.85>J
 4    35   3.30  94.15    JNJN  21.3>N   23.37>J  34.4>N
 5    23   2.17  96.32 JNJNJNJ  20.4>N   21.65>J  22.52>N  23.85>J  28.4>N   30.62>J

E. Observed trajectories: females
    ncase    %    cum%     case      tr1          tr2          tr3          tr4          tr5          tr6
 1    41  43.16  43.16      JN  24.67>N
 2    15  15.79  58.95       J
 3    13  13.68  72.63     JNJ  21.5>N   29.58>J
 4    10  10.53  83.16    JNJN  20.12>N  21.21>J  29.62>N
 5    10  10.53  93.68   JNJNJ  23.21>N  26.29>J  27.62>N  32.25>J
 6     5   5.26  98.95  JNJNJN  18.5>N   19.67>J  27.17>N  28.42>J  32.58>N
 7     1   1.05 100.00 JNJNJNJ  21.92>N  22.08>J  33.83>N  35.08>J  39.83>N  40.17>J

F. Simulated trajectories: females
    ncase    %    cum%    case      tr1           tr2           tr3           tr4
 1   337  35.47  35.47      JN  25.32>N
 2   183  19.26  54.74    JNJN  21.13>N  25.5>J   30.11>N
 3   174  18.32  73.05     JNJ  24.43>N  31.99>J
 4   139  14.63  87.68       J
 5    62   6.53  94.21   JNJNJ  20.91>N  24.31>J  28.8>N   37.05>J
```

observed and the simulated population. For a given trajectory, the number of simulated trajectories should be about 10 times the observed trajectories because 10 simulations were performed for each observation. The table also shows the median ages at transition. The results differ considerably because in the GLHS, which was organised in 1981, women and men report very different employment histories, and the transition rates are not differentiated by sex. If the transition rates are estimated separately for males and females and employment trajectories are produced for the two sexes separately, the simulated trajectories are much closer to the observations (Table 2.8). Among females, JN is the most frequent trajectory, whereas it is quite rare among males. For both men and women, the model accurately estimates the proportion of persons employed continuously throughout the observation period. For women, it underestimates permanent withdrawal from the labour market after a single employment episode and overestimates re-entry. That may be due to a cohort effect with younger cohorts more likely to re-enter the job market after a period of absence. The sample size is too small to estimate age-specific transition rates by sex and birth cohort.

2.6 Conclusion

Life histories are operationalised as state and event sequences. Synthetic life histories describe sequences that would result if individual life courses are governed by transition rates estimated from life history data. Transition rates link real and synthetic life histories. If transition rates are accurate, synthetic biographies mimic observed life paths. Life history data are generally incomplete. They do not cover the entire life span. By combining data from similar individuals, the transition rates may cover the entire life span. The estimation of transition rates is crucial. In this chapter, two estimation methods are described. The first is non-parametric and the second is parametric, or more appropriate, partial parametric. The non-parametric approach is common in biostatistics. The Nelson-Aalen estimator of transition rates is distribution-free; it does not rely on an assumption that the data are drawn from an underlying probability distribution. The partial parametric method is common in demography, epidemiology and actuarial science. The occurrence-exposure rate computed for an age interval assumes that the transition rate is constant within the interval. Occurrence-exposure rates vary freely between intervals. The two methods converge when the interval gets infinitesimally small.

Transition rates are used to generate synthetic biographies. Synthetic biographies describe life histories in terms of state occupation probabilities and expected state occupation times. Life expectancies, healthy life expectancies and active life expectancies are examples of state occupation times. Life histories generated by the most likely transition rates, given the data, are expected life histories. They apply to a population. Few individuals have a life path that coincides with the expected life history. Microsimulation is used to determine the distribution of individual life histories around expected life histories. The method presented in this chapter involves drawing individual waiting times to transitions from piecewise exponential waiting time distributions. Sequences of waiting times are obtained by joining randomly drawn waiting times. The method, which is referred to as longitudinal microsimulation, is described in the chapter. The added value of synthetic individual life paths is the information they provide on the distribution of (1) state and event sequences and (2) state occupation times around expected values. Synthetic individual biographies describe life paths in a virtual population. The virtual population closely resembles the real population if (1) transition rates are accurately estimated and (2) the observation plan applied to the real population is also applied to the virtual population, i.e. simulated life segments fully coincide with observed life segments.

The variation of individual life histories indicates uncertainties in the data and uncertainties associated with drawing random numbers from probability distributions. The uncertainties translate into uncertainties in transition rates, transition and state probabilities and expected state occupation times. Uncertainties in transition rates can be measured assuming that transition rates or transformations of transition rates are normally distributed (asymptotic theory). The distributions of probabilities and occupation times are more complicated and cannot always be expressed analytically. In the chapter, bootstrapping is used to estimate the uncertainties in transition probabilities, state probabilities and occupation times. If the cohort biography (expected life path) is computed for each bootstrap sample, the distribution of cohort biographies can be determined. By combining bootstrapping and longitudinal microsimulation, synthetic individual biographies can be produced that incorporate uncertainties in the data and uncertainties introduced by the microsimulation (Monte Carlo variation). The latter results from drawing random numbers from probability distributions. The precision of the method of computing synthetic biographies from real data is measured by comparing summary statistics of virtual and real populations.

The methods described in this chapter are implemented in *Biograph* and other packages discussed in this book. The packages have in common that they adopt a counting process point of view (Aalen et al. 2008).

Chapter 3
The Biograph Object

3.1 Introduction

A *Biograph* object is a data frame of individual life history data. All information on the life history of a person is stored in a single record. That data format is known as wide format. The wide format differs from the long format, in which information on an episode or a transition is contained in a separate record. The structure of the data frame is described in Sect. 3.2 of this chapter. In a *Biograph* object, life history data are organised chronologically starting with the first reported state of the life course and the first transition. That data structure is consistent with the life course as a sequence of events and a sequence of states. Converting raw data from surveys, registers or follow-up studies into a *Biograph* object can be cumbersome. Most surveys are not organised from a life history perspective but from a life domain perspective. In Sect. 3.3, I describe how to convert the GLHS data into a *Biograph* object. The GLHS data structure is only one of the many possible data structures. It is not possible to develop a single conversion method for all known data structures. More on how to create a *Biograph* object and several examples may be found in Annex A. Data analysis may require some operations on the data before the analysis can start. In multistate modelling, that may involve the removal from the data of transitions to the same state (intrastate transitions). In the GLHS data, job changes are intrastate transitions. Other operations may change the observation window. *Biograph* includes functions to change the observation window. One function selects transitions between two time points (calendar time) or between two ages. Another function delineates an observation window by two events or by an event and the survey date. These operations change the structure of the data. Data restructuring is the subject of Sect. 3.4. In Sect. 3.5 of this chapter, I review formats of life history data and list functions that may be used to convert one data format into another. A description of life histories includes information on states occupied during the period of observation, on transitions between states and on the dates of transition. Different ways exist to report dates. Most people use calendar dates, but dates may also be measured as time elapsed since a reference date or a reference event. The Century Month Code (CMC), used in the GLHS, measures dates as the number of months elapsed since 1 January 1900. Other surveys may express dates differently. Section 3.6 covers different date formats and R functions, including *Biograph* functions, for converting one date format into another.

It takes time and effort to create a *Biograph* object. It is a good investment, however, because *Biograph* offers access to packages in CRAN for survival analysis, sequence analysis and competing risks and multistate modelling. The packages include *survival*, *Epi*, *TraMineR*, *mstate*, *msm*, *mvna* and *etm*. *Biograph* includes functions that convert a *Biograph* object into objects required by these packages: survival object, Lexis object (*Epi*), state-sequence object (*TraMineR*), msdata object (*mstate*) and data frames for *mvna*, *etm* and *msm*. The data structures of the objects required by these packages as input are documented in this chapter.

3.2 Description of a *Biograph* Object

A *Biograph* object is a data frame with one record for each subject. A record stores data on personal attributes, the sequence of states occupied during the period of observation and the reported transitions between states. The data structure is a wide format, as opposed to the long format with one record for each episode or transition. Table 3.1 shows a selection of the GLHS survey data, used by Blossfeld and Rohwer (2002). The data were briefly discussed in Chap. 1. The data are collected retrospectively and cover the period from birth to survey date. The 201 individuals experience 600 job episodes and 382 episodes without a job.

Consider subject 1. He is a male born in March 1929 (CMC 351). The birth cohort is 1929–1931. He enters the first job in March 1946 (CMC 555) at age 17. Information on that first job episode ends at the beginning of November 1981 (CMC 983), which is the survey date. Blossfeld and Rohwer assume that the transition occurs at the beginning of a month and that the survey takes place at the end of the month. If the month of censoring is given and not the calendar date, *Biograph* assumes that censoring occurs at the beginning of the month. Therefore, 1 month is added to the censoring month given by Blossfeld and Rohwer: CMC 982 becomes CMC 983 (see Sect. 3.6).

Table 3.1 *Biograph* object: GLHS data

	ID	born	start	end	sex	edu	marriage	LMentry	cohort	path	Tr1	Tr2	Tr3	Tr4	Tr5	Tr6	Tr7
1	1	351	351	983	Male	17	679	555	1929-31	NJ	555	NA	NA	NA	NA	NA	NA
2	2	357	357	983	Female	10	762	593	1929-31	NJJJN	593	639	673	893	NA	NA	NA
3	3	473	473	983	Female	11	870	688	1939-41	NJJJJJN	688	700	730	742	817	829	NA
4	4	604	604	983	Female	13	872	872	1949-51	NJN	872	927	NA	NA	NA	NA	NA
5	5	377	377	983	Male	11	701	583	1929-31	NJJJ	583	651	788	NA	NA	NA	NA
6	6	492	492	983	Male	11	781	691	1939-41	NJNJNJNJ	691	717	728	754	771	847	859
7	7	476	476	983	Female	9	748	652	1939-41	NJJJJN	652	705	730	736	751	NA	NA
8	8	609	609	983	Male	11	881	838	1949-51	NJJJ	838	844	892	NA	NA	NA	NA
9	9	377	377	983	Male	12	690	591	1929-31	NJJJJ	591	602	634	643	NA	NA	NA
10	10	382	382	983	Male	11	824	580	1929-31	NJJNJ	580	701	843	862	NA	NA	NA

3.2 Description of a *Biograph* Object

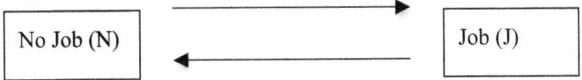

Fig. 3.1 Labour market data: state space and transitions. GLHS

Subject 2 is a female. She enters observation at birth (CMC 357). The observation is censored at CMC 983 at age 52. She enters the first job at the beginning of month 593 (CMC) at age 19 and starts a new job at the beginning of month 639 at age 23. The third job episode starts at the beginning of month 673 at age 26. It ends at the end of month 892 and is followed by a period without a job, starting at the beginning of month 893. The observation is censored at survey date at the beginning of month 983, when the respondent is aged 44. At time of interview the respondent has no job.

When multiple events occur during the same month, it is assumed that the events occur at the same time, i.e. at the beginning of the month.[1]

Blossfeld and Rohwer study the 600 job episodes. *Biograph* considers the full employment career that includes 600 job spells and 382 spells without a job. It addresses the complete sequence of both states and events that characterise the employment domain of the life course. Figure 3.1 shows the state space and the possible transitions.

The data include the subject identification number (ID), date of birth, start and end of observation (observation period or observation window), covariates and information on states occupied during the observation period: the state sequence and the dates of transitions. In *Biograph*, a state is denoted by a single character. A state sequence is a character string; it is the successive states occupied during the observation period. The dates are ordered chronologically, with the date at the first transition displayed first, followed by the date at the second transition, etc. The ordering is consistent with the state sequence. The number of states occupied during the observation period is equal to the length of the character string denoting the state sequence.

In R, objects may have attributes attached to it. A *Biograph* object has three attributes. The first is the format of the dates, in this case CMC. The second attribute is the format of the date of birth, in this case also CMC. The third attribute consists of parameters that characterise the data. Object attributes will be explained later in this chapter.

---

[1] Some packages for (multistate) survival analysis in R do not permit multiple events in the same time unit.

In the *Biograph* object a record contains the following variables (columns):

ID: identification number of respondent. ID is a numeric value. The values do not need to be sequential, but they need to be numeric. Character variables are not allowed.

born: date of birth of respondent. The date may be in CMC or another date format. The date format is one of the attributes of the *Biograph* object.

start: onset of observation

end: end of observation

Four covariates: sex (sex), highest educational attainment before entry into the labour market (edu), date (CMC) of marriage (marriage) and date (CMC) of entry into the labour market

path: sequence of states occupied during the observation period. The variable path must be a character variable. Each state is represented by a single character.

Tr*: transition dates in CMC. The maximum number of transitions is determined by the data. In this subsample, it is 12.

The variable path (for life path) is a character variable representing the sequence of states occupied during the observation period. The path should be a character variable; otherwise, *Biograph* gives an error message and stops. You should check that the variables are of the required type, using the str(GLHS) command. The variables pres and NOJ are omitted since these variables are associated with job episodes and not with persons.

The length of the string path gives the number of states an individual occupies during the period of observation. The number of states the i-th individual occupies is nchar(GLHS$path[i]). The respondent occupying the largest number of states in the observation period is produced by the code:

```
GLHS[nchar(GLHS$path)==max(nchar(GLHS$path)),]
```

It is the person with ID 194. The number of covariates may vary between data sets. *Biograph* determines the number of covariates from the position of the variable path in the data frame. In the data record, path always follows the covariates. The column number that contains the variable path is identified by the function locpath:

```
locpat <- locpath (GLHS)
```

It is column 10. In locpath, the position of path is identified by the following code:

```
which(GLHS[1,]==GLHS[1,"path"],arr.ind=TRUE)[2]
```

3.3 How to Create a *Biograph* Object?

The code shows why the name of the state sequence must be 'path' and why path should be a character variable for the method to work. Any other variable name will not work.

A *Biograph* object has three attributes attached to it. The first is the date format. Possible date formats are CMC, year, age and calendar date. A calendar date is a character string accepted by the as.Date function of base R. In the GLHS data, the format is CMC. The attribute is defined by the code:

```
attr(GLHS,"format.date") <- "CMC"
```

The second attribute is the date of birth format. The attribute is defined by the code:

```
attr(GLHS,"format.born") <- "CMC"
```

The third attribute is a set of parameters that characterise the data. The function Parameters extracts the parameters from the data. The following code defines the attribute:

```
attr(GLHS,"param")   <- Parameters (GLHS)
```

The function Parameters is a function of the *Biograph* package. It derives from the *Biograph* object (data set) a set of parameters that characterise the data, such as sample size, state space, numbers of transitions, etc. The function also determines the transitions that are included in the data. The function is documented in Chap. 4.

3.3 How to Create a *Biograph* Object?

In this section, I describe how to convert the GLHS data published by Blossfeld and Rohwer (2002) into a *Biograph* object. The programme create.GLHS.r converts the published data into a *Biograph* object. The programme is not part of the *Biograph* package, but it is distributed with the package. It is located in the documentation folder of the package source.

The published data file is an episode file. The filename is rrdat. The data are conveniently included in the *Biograph* package. The data object rrdat can be retrieved by typing data(rrdat) after loading the *Biograph* package. The data file can also be downloaded from the designated website http://oldsite.soziologie-blossfeld.de/eha/tda/ using the following code, provided the computer is connected to the Internet:

```
url.tda <- "http://oldsite.soziologie-
 Blossfeld.de/eha/tda/cf_files/Data/RRDAT.1"
rrdat.1 <- as.matrix (read.table(file=url.tda),header=FALSE)
colnames(rrdat.1) <- c("ID","NOJ","TS","TF","SEX","TI","TB","TE",
   "TM","PRES","PRES1","EDU")
rownames(rrdat.1) <-c(1:nrow(rrdat.1))
rrdat <- data.frame(rrdat.1)
```

Table 3.2 GLHS input data for Blossfeld and Rohwer's TDA programme (rrdat)

(1)	(2)	(3)	(4)	(5)	(6)	(7)	(8)	(9)	(10)	(11)	(12)
1	1	555	982	1	982	351	555	679	34	−1	17
2	1	593	638	2	982	357	593	762	22	46	10
2	2	639	672	2	982	357	593	762	46	46	10
2	3	673	892	2		357	593	762	46	−1	10
Variable	Name	Description									
1	ID	Identification number of subject									
2	NOJ	Serial number of the job episode									
3	TS	Starting time of the job episode									
4	TF	Ending time of the job episode									
5	SEX	Sex (1 male; 2 females)									
6	TI	Date of interview (CMC)									
7	TB	Date of birth (CMC)									
8	T1	Date of entry into the labour market (CMC) (denoted by TE)									
9	TM	Date of marriage (CMC) [0 if not married]									
10	PRES	Prestige score of current job, i.e. of job episode in current record of data file									
11	PRESN	Prestige score of the next job (if missing, −1)									
12	EDU	Highest educational attainment before entry into labour market									

A selection of the GLHS survey data is presented in Table 3.2. The data contain the date of birth and 5 covariates: sex, date of marriage, prestige score of the current job, prestige score of the next job and level of education. Observation starts at birth (TB) and ends at the date of interview (TI). A job episode is identified by a serial number (NOJ) and is characterised by the starting date of the episode (TS) and the ending date (TF). The starting date of the first job episode is the date of entry into the labour market. Dates are given in Century Month Code (CMC).

The *Biograph* object is prepared in five steps. The first is the specification of the state space and the possible transitions. The state space consists of two states: no job (N) and job (J). Everyone starts in state N. In this simple case, three transitions are possible: from no job to job (NJ), from job to no job (JN) and from a job to another job (JJ). In other state spaces, some transitions may not be possible. If the state space consists of marital statuses, for instance, the transition from married to never married is not feasible. The second step is the selection of covariates. The third step is the specification of the observation window for each subject. It requires the dates at start and end of observation. In the fourth step, the state sequence is determined and the dates at transition are recorded. In the fifth and final step, all data are stored in a data frame, three data attributes are attached to the data frame. The first attribute is the format of the transition dates, the second the format of the dates of birth and the third a set of parameters that characterise the data. The parameters include the transition matrix, i.e. the matrix of possible and relevant transitions.

3.4 Data Restructuring   59

The `reshape` function is used to convert the long format to a wide format. When creating the wide format, the attributes of episodes (NOJ, PRES and PRESN) are omitted and a new covariate (birth cohort) is defined.

The Blossfeld-Rohwer data are limited to job episodes, with information on the starting month and ending month of a job episode. The authors assume that job episodes start at the beginning of a month and end at the end of a month. In *Biograph*, the end of an episode is not considered explicitly because the end of an episode is the beginning of a new episode. Episodes are assumed to start at the beginning of the month. From the data on job episodes, the start dates and end dates of episodes without a job are extracted.

Three attributes are added to the data set. The first is the format of the transition dates:

```
attr(GLHS,"format.date") <- "CMC"
```

The second is the format of the birth dates:

```
attr(GLHS,"format.born") <- "CMC"
```

The third is the set of parameters:

```
attr(GLHS,"param") <- Parameters (GLHS)
```

The parameters include the matrix of feasible transitions that some packages require (`Parameters(GLHS)$tmat`).

In Chap. 8, the creation of a Biograph object is described using the data from the Netherlands Family and Fertility Survey (NLOG98). Annex A illustrates the creation of a `Biograph` object using other data than the GLHS and the NLOG98. The data include hypothetical data and real data. The first hypothetical data set carries information on three subjects, the second on 22 subjects. The third example of how to prepare a *Biograph* object uses data from the Survey of Health, Ageing and Retirement in Europe (SHARE). The SHARE survey is modelled after the US Health and Retirement Survey (HRS). The fourth example uses data from the National Family Health Survey of India, which is one of many Demographic and Health Surveys (DHS) organised in Third World countries and countries in transition. The fifth example uses medical data included in the *mstate* package for multistate modelling in R, developed by Putter and colleagues at Leiden University Medical Center. The data cover 2,279 leukaemia patients who had a bone marrow transplant. The final example uses simulated life history data.

3.4 Data Restructuring

In applied research, an analysis is often performed on a subset of a (sample) population or part of an observation period. First, I consider a selection of a subset of data. Data restructuring is considered next. Suppose we want to restrict the analysis of GLHS data to a subset of the sample population, e.g. women born in 1939–1941.

To select the subset of the sample population, the `subset` function of base R is used:

```
GLHS.c1 <- subset
    (GLHS,GLHS$sex=="Female"&GLHS$cohort=="1939-41")
```

or `GLHS[GLHS$sex=="Female"&GLHS$cohort=="1929-31",]`.

The use of the `subset` function removes the attributes. They need to be added to the `GLHS.c1` object.

Biograph includes three functions to select subsets of data. The first function, `Remove.intrastate`, selects transitions to destination states that differ from the origin states and removes transitions to the same state. In the GLHS data, many transitions are from one job to another job. In multistate event history analysis, these transitions are referred to as intrastate moves as opposed to interstate moves. Some packages for multistate survival analysis require that the intrastate transitions are removed, e.g. the *mvna* and the *mstate* packages. The second and third functions, `ChangeObservationWindow.e` and `ChangeObservationWindow.t`, redefine the observation window. These functions are presented now.

(a) *Remove intrastate transitions*.

To function `Remove.intrastate` removes intrastate transitions from the data set:

```
GLHS.0 <- Remove.intrastate (Bdata=GLHS)
```

The object `GLHS.0` is the data with intrastate transitions removed and the attributes of the *Biograph* object are updated. The attribute changes because intrastate transitions are no longer possible. Table 3.3 shows the first records of the new data.

(b) *Change observation window*.

Two functions change the observation window. The first function, `ChangeObservationWindow.e`, selects observations between two transitions or a transition and the survey date. The second function, `ChangeObservationWindow.t`, selects observations between two time points or two ages. The (age at) survey date may be one of these points. Before these functions are called, the function `Parameters` needs to be invoked (see further).

The function `ChangeObservationWindow.e` defines an observation window from entry into a given state of the state space (entry state) to entry into another

Table 3.3 *Biograph* object: GLHS data with intrastate transitions removed

	ID	born	start	end	sex	edu	marriage	LMentry	cohort	path	Tr1	Tr2	Tr3	Tr4	Tr5	Tr6	Tr7
1	1	351	351	983	Male	17	679	555	1929-31	NJ	555	NA	NA	NA	NA	NA	NA
2	2	357	357	983	Female	10	762	593	1929-31	NJN	593	893	NA	NA	NA	NA	NA
3	3	473	473	983	Female	11	870	688	1939-41	NJN	688	829	NA	NA	NA	NA	NA
4	4	604	604	983	Female	13	872	872	1949-51	NJN	872	927	NA	NA	NA	NA	NA
5	5	377	377	983	Male	11	701	583	1929-31	NJ	583	NA	NA	NA	NA	NA	NA
6	6	492	492	983	Male	11	781	691	1939-41	NJNJNJNJ	691	717	728	754	771	847	859
7	7	476	476	983	Female	9	748	652	1939-41	NJN	652	751	NA	NA	NA	NA	NA
8	8	609	609	983	Male	11	881	838	1949-51	NJ	838	NA	NA	NA	NA	NA	NA
9	9	377	377	983	Male	12	690	591	1929-31	NJ	591	NA	NA	NA	NA	NA	NA
10	10	382	382	983	Male	11	824	580	1929-31	NJNJ	580	843	862	NA	NA	NA	NA

3.4 Data Restructuring

given state (exit state). In the original GLHS data, the observation window extends from birth to survey date. All state occupancies and transitions since birth are considered. Suppose we want to start observation at labour market entry and end observation at survey date. The segment of life before labour market entry needs to be removed from the data. The new data set that results consists of observations that start at labour market entry. In calling the function ChangeObservationWindow.e, the entry state should be specified. The exit state is set equal to NA if observation ends at survey date. The following code results in an observation window that starts at labour market entry and ends at survey date:

```
entry <- "J"
exit  <- NA
GLHS.y2 <- ChangeObservationWindow.e
    (Bdata=GLHS,entrystate=entry,exitstate=exit)
```

Table 3.4 shows selected result.

If you want to limit the observation from birth to labour market entry, use:

```
entrystate <- "N"
exitstate  <- "J"
GLHS.y3 <- ChangeObservationWindow.e
    (Bdata=GLHS,entrystate,exitstate)
```

Table 3.5 shows selected results.

The function ChangeObservationWindow.t defines an observation window as the period between two points in time or between two ages. Suppose we wish to study the GLHS observations recorded between CMC 600 and CMC 800. The starting time of observation is 600 and the ending time 800. The time interval is given in the time scale used in the *Biograph* object.

If the dates are given in CMC, the interval must also be given in CMC. Events that occur later than CMC 800 are omitted. The code is:

```
GLHS.y4 <- ChangeObservationWindow.t
    (Bdata=GLHS,
    starttime=600,
    endtime=800,
    covs.dates=c("marriage","LMentry"))
```

Since the covariates include date variables (date of marriage and date of labour market entry), these dates need to be considered too. Table 3.6 shows a selection of the observations recorded between CMC 600 and CMC 800.

Table 3.4 *Biograph* object: GLHS data with observation window starting at labour market entry

	ID	born	start	end	sex	edu	marriage	LMentry	cohort	path	Tr1	Tr2	Tr3	Tr4	Tr5	Tr6
1	1	351	555	983	Male	17	679	555	1929-31	J	NA	NA	NA	NA	NA	NA
2	2	357	593	983	Female	10	762	593	1929-31	JJJN	639	673	893	NA	NA	NA
3	3	473	688	983	Female	11	870	688	1939-41	JJJJJN	700	730	742	817	829	NA
4	4	604	872	983	Female	13	872	872	1949-51	JN	927	NA	NA	NA	NA	NA
5	5	377	583	983	Male	11	701	583	1929-31	JJJ	651	788	NA	NA	NA	NA
6	6	492	691	983	Male	11	781	691	1939-41	JNJNJNJ	717	728	754	771	847	859
7	7	476	652	983	Female	9	748	652	1939-41	JJJJN	705	730	736	751	NA	NA
8	8	609	838	983	Male	11	881	838	1949-51	JJJ	844	892	NA	NA	NA	NA
9	9	377	591	983	Male	12	690	591	1929-31	JJJJ	602	634	643	NA	NA	NA
10	10	382	580	983	Male	11	824	580	1929-31	JJNJ	701	843	862	NA	NA	NA

Table 3.5 *Biograph* object: GLHS data with observation window starting at birth and ending at labour market entry

```
   ID born start end     sex edu marriage LMentry cohort path Tr1 Tr2 Tr3 Tr4 Tr5 Tr6 Tr7 Tr8
1   1  351  351 555   Males  17      679     555 1929-31   NJ 555  NA  NA  NA  NA  NA  NA  NA
4   2  357  357 593 Females  10      762     593 1929-31   NJ 593  NA  NA  NA  NA  NA  NA  NA
9   3  473  473 688 Females  11      870     688 1939-41   NJ 688  NA  NA  NA  NA  NA  NA  NA
10  4  604  604 872 Females  13      872     872 1949-51   NJ 872  NA  NA  NA  NA  NA  NA  NA
13  5  377  377 583   Males  11      701     583 1929-31   NJ 583  NA  NA  NA  NA  NA  NA  NA
17  6  492  492 691   Males  11      781     691 1939-41   NJ 691  NA  NA  NA  NA  NA  NA  NA
21  7  476  476 652 Females   9      748     652 1939-41   NJ 652  NA  NA  NA  NA  NA  NA  NA
24  8  609  609 838   Males  11      881     838 1949-51   NJ 838  NA  NA  NA  NA  NA  NA  NA
28  9  377  377 591   Males  12      690     591 1929-31   NJ 591  NA  NA  NA  NA  NA  NA  NA
31 10  382  382 580   Males  11      824     580 1929-31   NJ 580  NA  NA  NA  NA  NA  NA  NA
```

Table 3.6 *Biograph* object: GLHS observations from CMC 600 to CMC 800

```
   ID born start end    sex edu marriage LMentry cohort    path Tr1 Tr2 Tr3 Tr4 Tr5
1   1  351   600 800   Male  17      679     555 1929-31      J  NA  NA  NA  NA  NA
2   2  357   600 800 Female  10      762     593 1929-31    JJJ 639 673  NA  NA  NA
3   3  473   600 800 Female  11      870     688 1939-41  NJJJJ 688 700 730 742  NA
4   4  604   604 800 Female  13      872     872 1949-51      N  NA  NA  NA  NA  NA
5   5  377   600 800   Male  11      701     583 1929-31    JJJ 651 788  NA  NA  NA
6   6  492   600 800   Male  11      781     691 1939-41 NJNJNJ 691 717 728 754 771
7   7  476   600 800 Female   9      748     652 1939-41 NJJJJN 652 705 730 736 751
8   8  609   609 800   Male  11      881     838 1949-51      N  NA  NA  NA  NA  NA
9   9  377   600 800   Male  12      690     591 1929-31   JJJJ 602 634 643  NA  NA
10 10  382   600 800   Male  11      824     580 1929-31     JJ 701  NA  NA  NA  NA
```

A similar procedure can be used to define an observation window between two ages. First, convert the CMCs in the *Biograph* object to ages (for a description of the function, see below):

```
GLHS.a <- date.b(Bdata=GLHS,
                 format.in="CMC",
                 selectday=1,
                 format.out="age",
                 covs=c("marriage","LMentry"))
```

The function ChangeObservationWindow.t can be used with the new data set. To select observations between ages 20 and 40, use:

```
GLHS.y5 <- ChangeObservationWindow.t
              (Bdata=GLHS.a,
               starttime=20,
               endtime=40,
               covs.dates=c("marriage","LMentry"))
```

3.5 Other Data Formats

The *Biograph* data format has one row per subject. It is one of several data formats used in R packages for the analysis of transition data, state sequences and event sequences. *Biograph* has a number of functions that convert a *Biograph* object into a data frame that can be accessed by other packages. Packages sometimes require not only a particular input data structure but also specific column labels. *Biograph* takes care of that too. Before the conversion functions are presented, I briefly review data structures.

Three data types may be associated with life histories that are represented by sequences of states and transitions between states: status data, event data and episode data. In economics, episodes are generally referred to as spells. *Status data* are common for repeated measurements such as panel surveys. For each measurement or observation, the time in a given time scale (e.g. age or calendar time) and the state occupied are recorded. If at two consecutive points in time different states are recorded, a transition has occurred. No information is usually available on the date of the transition. Status data are interval-censored data: the time interval in which the transition occurs is known, but the precise date is not. The origin state is the prior state; the destination state is the current state. *Event data* show for each event or transition the (exact) date, the origin state and the destination state. *Episode data* are closely related to event data. They show for each episode the state occupied, date at start of episode, date at end of episode (stop) and the reason for ending. A status (0–1) variable is used to denote whether the end of an episode is due to the transition of interest (1) or an event unrelated to the transition being studied (censoring) (0). This data structure is referred to as the counting process data structure. The format was proposed by Andersen and Gill (1982). It is used in the *survival* package (Therneau 1999, 2014; Lumley 2004) and other packages for survival analysis. The format allows for left truncation and right censoring. The period between start and end defines the time period exposed to the risk of experiencing the transition.

The distinction between status data and event data is mirrored in the description of life histories. Life histories are described as state sequences or event sequences. *Biograph* uses both types of life history data but emphasises state sequence.

The description of life histories follows one of two data formats: a wide format with one record per subject and a long format with one record for each episode or transition. In the latter format, data on an individual are distributed over several records, one for each transition or episode. The wide format is common in social sciences and health sciences. For example, the Demographic and Health Surveys uses the wide format. *TraMineR*, an R package for describing and visualising state and event sequences, uses the wide format (Gabadinho et al. 2011). The long format is common in event history analysis because it is considered to be more flexible. Blossfeld and Rohwer (2002) use the long format to present episode data. In their terminology, the wide format is known as person file and the long format as episode file. For further discussion on the structure of episode data, see Alter and Gutmann (1999).

Gabadinho et al. (2012) distinguish the same three data types, but they also consider additional data formats. For instance, the wide format includes a data format in which successive states are given in consecutive columns (the state-sequence (STS) format), a format in which successive states are listed together with the duration in the state (the state-permanence-sequence (SPS) format), and the format in which successive states are listed without the duration (the distinct-state-sequence (DSS) format). The sequence of states occupied may be displayed in an extended format or a compressed format. In the extended format, the state occupied is recorded every year (or other time unit) and the state sequence is a vector of length equal to the number of ages that are covered by the observation window. In the compressed format a state sequence is represented by (i) a sequence of letters or combination of letters (words) or (ii) a sequence of numerical codes. The codes are separated by a separation character. Gabadinho et al. also consider the long format, covering the episode format and the event format. In the episode format, which is referred to as SPELL format, there is one line for each spell (episode), and a spell is characterised by the state occupied, a starting date and an ending date. In the event format, referred to as vertical time-stamped-event (TSE) format, there is one record for each transition and a transition is characterised by the transition number and the time at which the transition occurs.

Now I consider three data structures in more detail: person data (wide format), episode data (long format) and event data (long format).

(a) *Person data (wide format)*

The *Biograph* object has data in a wide format (person file). A single record contains all data of an individual. The number of records equals the sample size. A state is denoted by a single character and the state sequence is a character string (the path variable).

TraMineR (Gabadinho et al. 2012) uses the data format with one record per subject (wide format). In the extended format, state sequences are given as vectors of states. The data set is a matrix with subject ID as the row variable and age as the column variable. Table 3.7 shows a selection of GLHS data (subjects 1–10 and ages 15–25 and 40–45) in the extended format. The states are out of a job (N), in a job (J) and censored (+). The same table can be obtained from the object produced by the Occup function of *Biograph* (see next chapter). The code to generate the data is Occup(GLHS)$st_age_1[1:10,c(16:26,41:46)]. The object may be used as input to *TraMineR*.

The extended format can be converted to a compressed format by the seqconc function of the *TraMineR* package:

```
library (TraMineR)
DTraMineR <- seqconc (occup$st_age_1,sep="-")
```

In the compressed format a sequence is represented as a character string. The states are represented by words or numerical codes separated by a specific separation character. In *TraMineR* the default separator is '−'. The separator can be omitted provided a state is represented by a single character or digit:

```
DTraMineR2 <- seqconc (occup$st_age_1,sep="")
```

Table 3.8 shows a selection of the data in the compressed format. Note that each string has 54 characters, which is the number of ages from 0 to 53. The number of characters is nchar(DtraMineR2[1]).

The function seqdef of the *TraMineR* package converts DTraMineR in a sequence object, a pivotal object in the *TraMineR* package (see further).

(b) *Episode data (long format)*

Blossfeld and Rohwer (2002) use the long format to present episode data. Several packages in CRAN use the long format, e.g. *survival*, *eha*, *mvna*, *etm*,

3.5 Other Data Formats 65

Table 3.7 GLHS data in *TraMineR* extended format: states occupied at birthdays

```
      age
ID    15   16   17   18   19   20   21   22   23   24   25   40   41   42   43   44   45
 1   "N"  "N"  "N"  "J"  "J"  "J"  "J"  "J"  "J"  "J"  "J"  "J"  "J"  "J"  "J"  "J"  "J"
 2   "N"  "N"  "N"  "N"  "N"  "J"  "J"  "J"  "J"  "J"  "J"  "J"  "J"  "J"  "J"  "J"  "N"
 3   "N"  "N"  "N"  "J"  "J"  "J"  "J"  "J"  "J"  "J"  "J"  "N"  "N"  "N"  "+"  "+"  "+"
 4   "N"  "N"  "N"  "N"  "N"  "N"  "N"  "N"  "J"  "J"  "J"  "+"  "+"  "+"  "+"  "+"  "+"
 5   "N"  "N"  "N"  "J"  "J"  "J"  "J"  "J"  "J"  "J"  "J"  "J"  "J"  "J"  "J"  "J"  "J"
 6   "N"  "N"  "J"  "J"  "N"  "J"  "J"  "N"  "N"  "J"  "J"  "J"  "+"  "+"  "+"  "+"  "+"
 7   "J"  "J"  "J"  "J"  "J"  "J"  "J"  "J"  "N"  "N"  "N"  "N"  "N"  "N"  "+"  "+"  "+"
 8   "N"  "N"  "N"  "N"  "N"  "J"  "J"  "J"  "J"  "J"  "J"  "+"  "+"  "+"  "+"  "+"  "+"
 9   "N"  "N"  "N"  "J"  "J"  "J"  "J"  "J"  "J"  "J"  "J"  "J"  "J"  "J"  "J"  "J"  "J"
10   "N"  "N"  "J"  "J"  "J"  "J"  "J"  "J"  "J"  "J"  "J"  "N"  "J"  "J"  "J"  "J"  "J"
```

Table 3.8 GLHS data in *TraMineR* compressed format

```
[1]   "NNNNNNNNNNNNNNNNNNNJJJJJJJJJJJJJJJJJJJJJJJJJJJJJJJ+"
[2]   "NNNNNNNNNNNNNNNNNNNNJJJJJJJJJJJJJJJJJJJJJJJJNNNNNNNN+"
[3]   "NNNNNNNNNNNNNNNNNNNJJJJJJJJJJNNNNNNNNNNNN++++++++++"
[4]   "NNNNNNNNNNNNNNNNNNNNNNNJJJJNNNNNN++++++++++++++++++++"
[5]   "NNNNNNNNNNNNNNNNNNNNJJJJJJJJJJJJJJJJJJJJJJJJJJJJJJJ+++"
[6]   "NNNNNNNNNNNNNNNNNNNJJNJJNNJJJJJJJNJJJJJJJJJJ+++++++++++++"
[7]   "NNNNNNNNNNNNNNNNJJJJJJJJJNNNNNNNNNNNNNNNNNNNN++++++++++++"
[8]   "NNNNNNNNNNNNNNNNNNNJJJJJJJJJJJJ++++++++++++++++++++++"
[9]   "NNNNNNNNNNNNNNNNNNNNJJJJJJJJJJJJJJJJJJJJJJJJJJJJJJJJJJ+++"
```

Epi and *mstate*. The *survival* and *eha* packages use the same long format. The other packages use different long formats. In the long format used by the first two packages, the data are in a data frame with a row for each episode and at least the following columns:

Tstart: starting date of episode
Tstop: ending date of episode
Event: indicator variable, indicating whether the episode ends in the event of interest (1) or censoring (0)

If all episodes start at the same date (e.g. 0), the Tstart column may be omitted. In that case, the Tstop variable is replaced by a variable labelled time. The data format is known as the counting process data format, which was proposed by Andersen and Gill (1982). The Surv function of the *survival* package converts data in a counting process format to a survival object. The same Surv function is used in the *eha* package. Note that the presence or absence of Tstart implies different time scales. If Tstart and Tstop are given, the time scale measures time in calendar time, CMC, days since 1 January 1970 or another exogenous time scale. If time is used, the time scale measures time since entry in the current state. The variable time is equal to Tstop − Tstart. In the context of multistate modelling, Putter et al. (2007) refer to the first time scale as the *clock forward* approach and to the second as the *clock reset* approach.

Table 3.9 shows the GLHS data in episode format, as required by the *survival* package. There is one record for every episode. The number of records is therefore equal to the number of episodes. In the GLHS data, the subsample has a total of

Table 3.9 GLHS data in episode format

```
   ID OR  DES  Tstart Tstop status trans sex pres edu marriage NOJ  TE  cohort  born
1   1 N    J     351   555    1     1    1   0   17    679     0  555 1929-31  351
2   1 J    cens  555   983    0     2    1   0   17    679     0  555 1929-31  351
3   2 N    J     357   593    1     1    2   0   10    762     0  593 1929-31  357
4   2 J    J     593   639    1     3    2   0   10    762     0  593 1929-31  357
5   2 J    J     639   673    1     3    2   0   10    762     0  593 1929-31  357
6   2 J    N     673   893    1     2    2   0   10    762     0  593 1929-31  357
7   2 N    cens  893   983    0     1    2   0   10    762     0  593 1929-31  357
8   3 N    J     473   688    1     1    2   0   11    870     0  688 1939-41  473
9   3 J    J     688   700    1     3    2   0   11    870     0  688 1939-41  473
10  3 J    J     700   730    1     3    2   0   11    870     0  688 1939-41  473
11  3 J    J     730   742    1     3    2   0   11    870     0  688 1939-41  473
12  3 J    J     742   817    1     3    2   0   11    870     0  688 1939-41  473
13  3 J    N     817   829    1     2    2   0   11    870     0  688 1939-41  473
14  3 N    cens  829   983    0     1    2   0   11    870     0  688 1939-41  473
```

982 episodes, 600 job spells and 382 episodes without a job. The state occupied during the episode is given in the OR (origin) column. The starting date of the episode is given by Tstart and the ending date by Tstop. An episode may end because the subject experiences a transition to a new episode or an unrelated transition, or the observation is terminated. The status variable denotes whether the ending of an episode is caused by an event (transition of interest) (status=1) or censoring (status=0). If status is equal to one, the destination state is given in the DES (destination) column. The variable trans denotes the transition number. These numbers are contained in the object Parameters(GLHS) $tmat, produced by the Parameters function of *Biograph*. The NJ transition has number 1, the JN transition 2 and the JJ transition 3. The transition number is followed by the covariates and the date of birth (column 'born').

The data in the long format are produced by the code:

```
Dlong <- Biograph.long (Bdata=GLHS)
```

The results are stored in object Dlong, which consists of two components. The first, Dlong$Devent, has event data (see Section c). The second, Dlong $Depisode, has episode data. The component Dlong$Depisode is a data frame with 982 rows. The Biograph.long function uses the reshape function from the *stats* package because of its speed. The reshape function generates an event file and Biograph.long converts the event file into an episode file.

Some packages, including *mvna* and *mstate*, require that intrastate transitions are omitted. In that case, a transition from J to J is not possible. The function Remove. intrastate removes intrastate transitions.

An object of class Lexis is the main data object of the *Epi* package. It represents follow-up data in multiple time scales, such as calendar time, age and time since a reference event (e.g. labour market entry). In this book, two time scales are considered: calendar time and age. The data format is a long format with one record for each episode. The Lexis object is a data frame with a variable for each time scale and four variables with reserved names starting with lex:

3.5 Other Data Formats

`per`	calendar time at start of episode
`age`	age at start of episode
`lex.dur`	length of the episode (duration of follow-up)
`lex.Cst`	state occupied during the episode, also referred to as current state and entry state. It is the state in which the follow-up takes place
`lex.Xst`	exit status (eXit state), i.e. the state taken up after a transition out of lex.Cst. It is also referred to as destination state
`lex.id`	Subject identification number

The arguments `per`, `age` and `lex.dur` define the start and length of the episode in two time scales (calendar time and age). Only two of the three elements need to be given. They should be numeric. The third element is imputed. The arguments `lex.Cst` and `lex.Xst` define the state at entry and the state at exit. They are character variables. The Lexis object may contain other variables, e.g. covariates. The function `Biograph.Lexis` converts a *Biograph* object into a Lexis object:

```
Dlexis <- Biograph.Lexis (Bdata=GLHS,
                  Dlong=Dlong$Depisode)
```

The function relies on the `Lexis` function of the *Epi* package to convert the data. If the argument `Dlong` is missing, it is computed. The `Lexis` function converts the arguments `lex.Cst` and `lex.Xst` from character variables to factors. The function produces a Lexis object with the six variables listed above and with covariates and other data copied from the *Biograph* object GLHS. For details on the Lexis object, see Plummer and Carstensen (2011).

Table 3.10 shows the Lexis object for the first four respondents in the GLHS subsample. The required variables are shown and one variable (status) is added.

Table 3.10 Lexis object: GLHS data

	lex.id	per	age	lex.dur	lex.Cst	lex.Xst	status
1	1	1929.162	0.00000	17.0000000	N	J	1
2	1	1946.162	17.00000	35.6712329	J	J	0
3	2	1929.666	0.00000	19.6630137	N	J	1
4	2	1949.329	19.66301	3.8328767	J	J	1
5	2	1953.162	23.49589	2.8383562	J	J	1
6	2	1956.000	26.33425	18.3287671	J	N	1
7	2	1974.329	44.66301	7.5041096	N	N	0
8	3	1939.329	0.00000	17.9178082	N	J	1
9	3	1957.247	17.91781	1.0000000	J	J	1
10	3	1958.247	18.91781	2.5020585	J	J	1
11	3	1960.749	21.41987	0.9993113	J	J	1
12	3	1961.748	22.41918	6.2520548	J	J	1
13	3	1968.000	28.67123	1.0000000	J	N	1
14	3	1969.000	29.67123	12.8328767	N	N	0
15	4	1950.247	0.00000	22.3353919	N	J	1
16	4	1972.582	22.33539	4.5796766	J	N	1
17	4	1977.162	26.91507	4.6712329	N	N	0

The first column is the subject identification number, the second the calendar date at the start of an episode, the third the age at the start, the fourth the duration of the episode (in years), the fifth the entry state or state occupied during the episode, the sixth the exit state or destination state and the last column the status at exit (1 in case of a transition and 0 if the observation is censored). The table is produced by the following code:

```
Dlexis[1:17,c(6,1,2,3,4,5,12)]
```

The Lexis object for a single episode, e.g. the episode between birth and job entry, may be obtained directly from a *Biograph* object in three steps. First, the dates in the *Biograph* object are converted to calendar years:

```
yr<- date_b (Bdata=GLHS,
        format.in="CMC",
        selectday=1,
        format.out="year",
        covs=c("marriage","LMentry"))
```

Second, a transition is selected. The following function selects the transition NJ. Respondents that did not experience the NJ transition are removed from the data (KEEP=FALSE). If KEEP=TRUE, the records pertaining to respondents who do not experience the NJ transition are not removed, but the dates of the NJ transition are set equal to NA.

```
jn <- TransitionAB (Bdata=yr,
        transition="NJ",keep=FALSE)
```

The data frame `jn` has 201 rows because every respondent enters the labour market once. The function `table(trunc(jn$year))` gives the number of respondents by year of the first job entry. The respondents who do not enter the labour market at time of censoring are removed in the `jn` object, i.e. the cases are not kept. In this example no respondent is removed because all respondents enter the labour market before survey date. The third step is required only if some respondents do not experience the transition. In that step, respondents who do not experience the transition at time of censoring are removed from the `yr` object:

```
yr2 <- subset (yr,yr$ID%in%jn$id)
```

The following code produces the Lexis object:

```
Lcoh <- Lexis(
        id = yr2$ID,
        entry = list( per=yr2$start ),
        exit  = list( per=jn$year, age=jn$year-yr2$born
),
        exit.status = rep(1,nrow(yr2)),
        data=yr2,
        merge=TRUE)
```

The result is shown in Table 5.1 in Chap. 5. This completes the presentation of the Lexis object.

The package *mvna* uses as input a data.frame of the form

3.5 Other Data Formats

```
data.frame(id,from,to,time) or
data.frame(id,from,to,entry,exit) with
```

id	subject identification number
from	the state from where the transition occurs (state occupied during the episode)
to	the state to which a transition occurs (direction of transition at the end of the episode)
either time	time when a transition occurs, measured as time elapsed since start of episode (time when current episode, which starts at time 0, ends)
or entry	entry time in state/episode
exit	exit time from state/episode

The function Biograph.mvna converts data from the *Biograph* format to the *mvna* format:

```
Dmvna <- Biograph.mvna (Bdata=GLHS)
```

The mvna package does not accept intrastate transitions, i.e. transitions to the same state (e.g. from job to job). It requires a transition matrix that indicates that intrastate transitions are absent. The Biograph.mvna function performs four operations on data in *Biograph* format. First, it checks whether intrastate transitions are present, which is the case when at least one diagonal element of the transition matrix is not NA (missing values). If that is the case, then it calls the Remove.intrastate function to remove the intrastate moves. Second, it calls the Parameters function to determine the parameters associated with the *Biograph* object with intrastate transitions removed. The *mvna* package requires the transition matrix Parameters(Remove.intrastate(GLHS))$tmat. Third, it calls the Biograph.long function to create an object having the data in the long format. Fourth, it adds to the data frame the variables entry and exit and it changes the variable name of the subject identification numbers from ID to id.

The function Biograph.mvna creates an object with three components. The first component is Dmvna$D, which is a data frame with the variables id, from, to, entry and exit. That data frame is used by the *mvna* package. The second component is Dmvna$D.cov, which is the same data frame augmented by the covariates and some other information. The third component, Dmvna$cens, is the code for censored observations. The function adds the 'format.date', 'format.born' and 'param' attributes to the components Dmvna$D and Dmvna$Dcov.

The object Dmvna$D has columns with the labels id (for ID), from (for OR), to (for DES), entry (for Tstart) and exit (for Tstop). The time scale, which in the original data is calendar time in CMC, is changed to age. Since the CMC at birth is included as a covariate in Dmvna$D.cov (variable born), age can easily be converted back to calendar time. The reason for using age is that the cumulative

Table 3.11 GLHS data in *mvna* format

	id	from	to	Tstart	Tstop	status	trans	born	entry	exit
1.2	1	N	J	351	555	1	2	351	0.00000	17.00000
1.15	1	J	cens	555	983	0	1	351	17.00000	52.67124
2.2	2	N	J	357	593	1	2	357	0.00000	19.66302
2.3	2	J	N	593	893	1	1	357	19.66302	44.66302
2.15	2	N	cens	893	983	0	2	357	44.66302	52.16713
3.2	3	N	J	473	688	1	2	473	0.00000	17.91781
3.3	3	J	N	688	829	1	1	473	17.91781	29.67123
3.15	3	N	cens	829	983	0	2	473	29.67123	42.50411
4.2	4	N	J	604	872	1	2	604	0.00000	22.33539
4.3	4	J	N	872	927	1	1	604	22.33539	26.91506
4.15	4	N	cens	927	983	0	2	604	26.91506	31.58630

hazard is shown for different ages. A selection of data from the GLHS data frame, with the variables from, to, entry and exit, is shown in Table 3.11.

The *mstate* package requires data in a particular long format, the 'msdata' format. In this format, each subject has a number of rows equal to the number of transitions for which he is at risk (Putter et al. 2007); transitions to the same state are not allowed. In other words, the package requires one record for each *potential* transition. Since a censored observation could have resulted in any of the possible destinations, one record is added for every possible destination. For instance, if a person has a job and the observation is censored, then there is only one transition that could occur but did not because of censoring: the JN transition. The JJ transition cannot occur because transitions to the same state are not allowed. The consideration of each potential transition is rooted in the theory of competing risks in which every possible destination is considered. This data structure allows flexible model specification, as will be demonstrated later in this book.

An object of class 'msdata' is a data frame with at least the following variables:

id	subject identification
from	the state from where the transition occurs (starting state)
to	the state to which a transition occurs (receiving state or destination state)
trans	the transition number
Tstart	the starting time in the state from where the transition occurs (origin state)
Tstop	the ending time in the state from where the transition occurs
status	status variable, with 1 indicating an event (transition) and 0 censoring

The 'msdata' class of objects requires an attribute that contains the transition numbers. It is the 'trans' attribute, referring to the transition matrix of possible transitions (similar to the tmat object produced by the Parameters function).

The Biograph.mstate function produces a data frame in the 'msdata' format (object of class 'msdata') from a data frame in the *Biograph* format.

3.5 Other Data Formats

It performs three operations. First, it checks to determine whether the intrastate transitions are removed. If they are not yet removed, it calls the Remove.intrastate function to remove the intrastate moves. Using the Parameters function, it defines the transition matrix, i.e. the matrix that shows the feasible transitions and the number of each transition (matrix tmat). In this case the NJ transition is transition 1 and the JN transition is transition 2. In the new transition matrix, intrastate transitions are absent. Second, it calls the Biograph.long function to create an object having the data in the long format. Third, it determines for a subject in a given state all possible transitions (destinations; competing risks) and specifies one record for each possible destination. The Dmstate object is of class 'msdata' and carries the 'format.date', 'format.born' and 'param' attributes. The 'param' attribute includes the matrix of feasible transitions tmat, which is used by the *mstate* package: attr(Dmstate,"param") $tmat.

Table 3.12 shows the GLHS data in the format required by *mstate*. It is produced by the following code (covariates are omitted):

```
Dmstate <- Biograph.mstate (Bdata=GLHS)
```

The object produced contains also several covariates (not shown): the date of birth in CMC, the year of birth (decimal year), sex, education, date of marriage (CMC), date of labour market entry (CMC) and birth cohort.

Consider the first respondent in Table 3.12. The observation was censored while he was employed (J). Hence, there is one possible hypothetical transition: JN. The possible transition did not occur before the end of the observation (status = 0). Respondent 2 was out of a job (N) when the observation was censored. Here the one possible hypothetical transition is NJ, since J is the only possible destination of a transition out of N.

Other packages have also utilities to convert data formats. The *Epi* package includes the function msdata.Lexis that converts a data frame of the class Lexis (wide format) into a long data frame required by *mstate*. The function emt.Lexis produces data in the format required by the *etm* package. The function msprep of the *mstate* package converts data in a wide format to the long format. The function can be applied only in the absence of transitions to previous states. Multistate models in which back transitions do not occur or are not allowed are known as

Table 3.12 GLHS data in msdata format for *mstate* package

	ID	OR	DES	Tstart	Tstop	status	trans	born	OD	Episode	Tstarta	Tstopa	from	to
1.2	1	N	J	351	555	1	1	351	NJ	1	0.00000	17.00000	1	2
1.15	1	J	N	555	983	0	2	351	cens	2	17.00000	52.66667	2	1
2.2	2	N	J	357	593	1	1	357	NJ	1	0.00000	19.66667	1	2
2.3	2	J	N	593	893	1	2	357	JN	2	19.66667	44.66667	2	1
2.15	2	N	J	893	983	0	1	357	cens	3	44.66667	52.16667	1	2
3.2	3	N	J	473	688	1	1	473	NJ	1	0.00000	17.91667	1	2
3.3	3	J	N	688	829	1	2	473	JN	2	17.91667	29.66667	2	1
3.15	3	N	J	829	983	0	1	473	cens	3	29.66667	42.50000	1	2
4.2	4	N	J	604	872	1	1	604	NJ	1	0.00000	22.33333	1	2
4.3	4	J	N	872	927	1	2	604	JN	2	22.33333	26.91667	2	1

irreversible Markov chains and progressive multistate models (Meira-Machados and Roca-Pardinas 2012).

(c) *Event data (long format)*

The reshape function in the *stats* package of R reshapes a data frame between wide format with repeated measurements in separate columns of the same record and long format with the repeated measurements in separate records. The function is:

```
zx <- reshape (GLHS,
    idvar="ID",
    varying=list((locpath(GLHS)+1):(ncol(GLHS))),
    v.names="date",
    direction="long")
```

The zx object has for each subject 12 records, one for each of the maximum number of transitions. The number of records in the zx object is 2,412 (=201*12). If a transition does not occur and the date is not applicable (NA), then the 'date' column shows NA. The redundant records can be removed as follows:

```
zx2 <- zx[!is.na(zx$date),]
```

The zx2 object has 781 records.

Respondents may experience more than one transition. The Reshape function lists the first transition first. It adds the second, third and subsequent transitions at the end of the object. This implies that zx is sorted by the line number of the transition and not by subject ID. To get the data sorted by subject ID, use:

```
Dlong.reshape <- zx2[order(zx2$ID),].
```

The reshape function creates 'time' and 'date' columns. The 'time' column shows the line numbers of transitions experienced by the individual with a given ID and the 'date' column shows the dates of the transitions. The reshape function does not give the state of origin and the state of destination of a transition. The

```
Dlong.reshape$OD <- substr(Dlong.reshape$path,
            Dlong.reshape$time,
            Dlong.reshape$time+1)
```

following command gives the origin and destination:

The result of these steps is shown in Table 3.13.

To complete the construction of the event data structure, the date format of transitions and birth dates and the transition matrix are added as attributes (note that *mstate* needs the transition matrix tmat):

```
attr(Dlong.reshape,"format.date") <-
            attr(GLHS,"format.date")
attr(Dlong.reshape,"format.born") <-
            attr(GLHS,"format.born")
attr(Dlong.reshape,"trans") <-
attr(Remove.intrastate(GLHS),"param")$tmat
```

3.5 Other Data Formats

Table 3.13 GLHS data in long format, produced by reshape function of *stats* package

	ID	born	start	end	sex	edu	marriage	LMentry	cohort	path	time	date	OD
1.1	1	351	351	983	Male	17	679	555	1929-31	NJ	1	555	NJ
2.1	2	357	357	983	Female	10	762	593	1929-31	NJJJN	1	593	NJ
2.2	2	357	357	983	Female	10	762	593	1929-31	NJJJN	2	639	JJ
2.3	2	357	357	983	Female	10	762	593	1929-31	NJJJN	3	673	JJ
2.4	2	357	357	983	Female	10	762	593	1929-31	NJJJN	4	893	JN
3.1	3	473	473	983	Female	11	870	688	1939-41	NJJJJN	1	688	NJ
3.2	3	473	473	983	Female	11	870	688	1939-41	NJJJJN	2	700	JJ
3.3	3	473	473	983	Female	11	870	688	1939-41	NJJJJN	3	730	JJ
3.4	3	473	473	983	Female	11	870	688	1939-41	NJJJJN	4	742	JJ
3.5	3	473	473	983	Female	11	870	688	1939-41	NJJJJN	5	817	JJ
3.6	3	473	473	983	Female	11	870	688	1939-41	NJJJJN	6	829	JN
4.1	4	604	604	983	Female	13	872	872	1949-51	NJN	1	872	NJ

Table 3.14 GLHS data in *msm* format

	ID	born	path	time	age	OR	DES	trans	firstobs	stateN	state
1.1	1	351	NJ	1	0.00000	#	N	NA	1	N	1
1.2	1	351	NJ	2	17.00000	N	J	NA	1	J	2
1.14	1	351	NJ	3	52.66667	J	cens	NA	1	J	2
2.1	2	357	NJJJN	1	0.00000	#	N	NA	1	N	1
2.2	2	357	NJJJN	2	19.66667	N	J	NA	1	J	2
2.3	2	357	NJJJN	3	23.50000	J	J	NA	1	J	2
2.4	2	357	NJJJN	4	26.33333	J	J	NA	1	J	2
2.5	2	357	NJJJN	5	44.66667	J	N	NA	1	N	1
2.14	2	357	NJJJN	6	52.16667	N	cens	NA	1	N	1
3.1	3	473	NJJJJN	1	0.00000	#	N	NA	1	N	1

The *msm* package requires event data and a long format. For each transition, the date and the destination state are required. Entry into observation and censoring are treated in the same way as events. The function Biograph.msm produces a data object for the *msm* package. The conversion is time consuming. The long format is stored in the data frame Dmsm. To create input data for *msm* from data in the *Biograph* format, use the utility Biograph.msm:

```
Dmsm <- Biograph.msm (Bdata=GLHS)
```

Table 3.14 shows part of the data in the object Dmsm, created by the above statement (the covariates are omitted). The variables are:

ID	identification number
born	CMC at birth
path	state sequence
time	event (including entry in the first state)
date	date of transition (in CMC code)
age	age at transition
OR	origin state
DES	destination state (state occupied after the transition)
trans	transition number
firstobs	dummy denoting the first transition (first transition = 1)

`stateN`   state occupied after the transition (except for censoring, in which case state denotes the state occupied at time of censoring)

`state`   state occupied after the transition(number) (see `stateN`)

At entry into observation, the state of entry is denoted as a destination state. The origin state is not applicable and is denoted by #. For instance, respondent with ID 1 enters observation at CMC 352. The state of entry is N. Note that the state associated with the CMC at censoring is the state occupied at time of censoring.

3.6 A Note on Dates

In the GLHS, transition dates are given in CMC, i.e. months elapsed since 1 January 1900. The same practice is adopted in the Demographic and Health Surveys. Other surveys and follow-up studies express dates as days elapsed since a reference date. Reference dates vary. For instance, the Framingham Heart Study (FHS), which is a longitudinal study that started in 1948–1950 and is widely used in epidemiology, and the US Health and Retirement Survey (HRS) count the number of days since 1 January 1960. The date is often referred to as SAS dates because that practice is adopted in the SAS data analytic software. Some studies use age or time elapsed since a reference event other than birth. Calendar dates are used too to express the date at transition. It is sometimes useful to switch between date formats. For instance, calendar dates can easily be interpreted, much easier than CMC or days elapsed since 1 January 1960, but they are not very suitable for computations. In the study of the life course, the time to event is often measured by the age of the individual. Another useful date measure is the decimal year. It is the calendar year of a transition augmented by the fraction of the year. For instance, a transition that occurs on 5 March 2012 occurs at time 2012.175 and a transition on 10 October 2012 occurs at time 2012.773. For an overview of different date representations, conversion methods and applications, see Willekens (2013b).

Biograph includes several functions to convert dates in one format to dates in another format. They are presented in this section. First, a few general comments on dates and a selection of conversion methods are provided.

The most common representation of dates is the character representations (day/month/year) and (month/day/year). Dates are also expressed in number of days, weeks or months since a reference date. For instance, in R dates are represented as the number of days since 1 January 1970, with negative values for earlier dates (R reference manual, version 3.0.0 (2013-04-03), p. 120). They are printed following the rules of the current Gregorian calendar. Although the date should be an integer, this is not enforced in the internal representation. To convert a date given as a character string into number of days since the reference date

3.6 A Note on Dates

(1 January 1970), consider 9 October 2008. The as.Date function of base R converts character data to dates.

```
Mydate <- as.Date ("2008-10-09")
Refdate <- as.Date ("1970-01-01")
days <- Mydate - Refdate
```

The number of days between 1 January 1970 and 9 October 2008 is 14,161.

In event history analysis, the reference date is often 1 January 1900. Suppose an event occurs on 4 May 1988. The number of days since the reference date is:

$$\text{mdy.date}(5,4,1988) - \text{mdy.date}(1,1,1900) = 32265$$

Authors use different methods to convert the number of days to years. Some take a year to be 365.25 days (e.g. Kalbfleisch and Prentice 2002). The Framingham Heart Study (FHS) expresses the dates of the exams in number of days since 1 January 1960. If SAS dates are used, for a person born on 1 January 1960, the value is 0, and for a person born on 11 July 1955, the value is $-1,635$, and for a person born on 12 November 1962, it is 1,046. These figures can be converted into exact number of years since the beginning of the twentieth century:

$$EY = 1960 + DATE/365.25$$

where DATE is the date of the event in days since 1 January 1960 and EY is the date of the event in exact years (Mamun 2003). For instance, if the DATE of an event is -460, the event occurs in 1958 and more specifically at 1958.741.

Mamun (2003) uses a different method to determine the exact number of years since the reference date, which he takes to be 1 January 1900:

$$EY = YEAR + (MONTH - 1)/12 + (DAY - 1)/(30.437 * 12)$$

For instance, 4 May 1988 is 88.3415 years since the beginning of the twentieth century:

$$88 + (5 - 1)/12 + (4 - 1)/(30.437 * 12) = 88.34154702$$

The date in exact years may be converted back in year, month and day of occurrence, using the following formula (where TRUNC means truncation):

$$YEAR = TRUNC(EY)$$
$$MONTH = TRUNC[(EY - YEAR) * 12] + 1$$
$$DAY = TRUNC[(EY - YEAR - (MONTH - 1)/12) * 30.437 * 12] + 1$$

For instance, 88.3415470 is:

$$\text{YEAR} = \text{TRUNC}[88.3415470] = 88$$
$$\text{MONTH} = \text{TRUNC}[(88.3415470 - 88) * 12] + 1 = 5 \text{ (MAY)}$$
$$\text{DAY} = \text{ROUND}[(88.34154702 - 88 - (5-1)/12) * 30.437 * 12] + 1 = 4$$

The conversion is not always perfect because it does not account for the different numbers of days in a month and the changing number of days in the month of February.

Dates are often expressed in months since a reference date. For instance, the Century Month Code (CMC), used in several studies in demography and health, represents the date as the number of months since 1 January 1900 (see, e.g. Blossfeld and Rohwer 2002). The approach is adopted in the Demographic and Health Surveys and several other surveys. The dates in exact years may be converted into dates in CMC:

$$\text{DATECMC} = (\text{EY} - 1900) * 12$$

Consider 4 May 1988. The date in CMC is 88.34154702 * 12 = 1,060.098564. The month is CMC 1060 and the day is ROUND[0.098564 * 30.437] + 1 = 4.

The CMC measures the months elapsed since 1 January 1900. For instance, CMC 555 is March 1946 and CMC 1100 is August 1991. The CMC is generally an integer number but may be a real number. If the date is known precisely (day, month and year), the CMC is a real number. If the date is known approximately (month), the CMC is an integer number. If CMC is an integer, the transition is assumed to take place at the beginning of the month. If the CMC is an integer value (e.g. if dates are measured in months as in many demographic surveys), *Biograph* assumes that the onset of observation, censoring and the events occur at the beginning of a month. That is important since surveys may assume that events occur at the beginning of a month, but that censoring occurs at the end of a month (e.g. the GLHS data distributed by Blossfeld and Rohwer (2002) and Blossfeld et al. (2007)).

From the Century Month Codes, the years of the transitions can be obtained. The year is 1900+(CMC−1)/12, since January 1900 is month 1. The result is a real value, which is often used as such. In several applications, the real number is converted into year and month. For instance, a transition that occurs at CMC 1100 occurs in the year 1900+trunc((1,100−1)/12) = 1991. The month is (CMC−12*trunc((CMC−1)/12)) = 8.

3.6 A Note on Dates

The *Biograph* functions that convert dates in one format to dates in a different format are:

Function	Conversion
cmc_as_year	cmc to decimal year
cmc_as_age	cmc to age
cmc_as_Date	cmc to date of class Date
Date_as_year	date of class Date to decimal year
Date_as_cmc	date of class Date to cmc
Date_as_age	date of class Date to age
year_as_Date	decimal year to date of class Date
year_as_cmc	decimal year to cmc
year_as_age	decimal year to age
age_as_Date	age to date of class Date
age_as_year	age to decimal year

For possible date formats, you are referred to the R *Date* package.

For instance, the following code converts the marriage dates in CMC to calendar dates (dates of class Date); it is assumed that marriages occur at the beginning of the month:

```
z <- cmc_as_Date (
        GLHS$marriage,
        selectday=1,
        format.out="%Y-%m-%d")
```

If `selectday`=15, the event is assumed to occur in the middle of the month. To convert CMC to decimal year, use:

```
z <- cmc_as_year (GLHS$marriage,selectday=1)
```

The marriage date of the first respondent is CMC 679 or 1956.497 or 1 July 1956.

The age at marriage is obtained by converting CMC to age:

```
z <- cmc_as_age (GLHS$marriage,
                born=GLHS$born,
                format.born="CMC")
```

Object z has two components. The first gives the date in decimal year and the second gives the age. The first respondent marries at age 27 (z$age[1]).

Biograph has a generic function that integrates the different functions listed above. It is the `date_convert` function. The function requires the input and output formats of the dates. For instance, the following function converts 01/01/2011 to 1 January 2011:

```
b <- date_convert(d='01/01/2011',
            format.in='%m/%d/%Y',
            format.out='day-month-year')
```

To determine the age on 01/01/2011 of a person born on 20 September 1980, use the function:

```
bb<- date_convert("01/01/2011",
         format.in="%d/%m/%Y",
         format.out="age",
         born="20/9/1980",
         format.born="$d/$m/$Y")
```

The age is 30 years and the fraction of the year is 0.2814. The object bb has four components. The first is the age in seconds; the second is the age in days; the third is the age in years, months and days; and the fourth is the age in decimal year.

The function date_b converts an entire *Biograph* object. The following code produces calendar dates in the format day/month/year:

```
GLHSb <- date_b(GLHS,
         format.in="CMC",
         selectday=1,
         format.out="%d%b%Y",
         covs=c("marriage","LMentry"))
```

Table 3.15 shows transition dates for a random sample of ten respondents. It is a selection of rows and columns of GLHSb. It is produced using the following code:

```
GLHSb[GLHSb$ID%in%sample(GLHSb$ID,10,replace=FALSE),
     c(1:4,7,8,10,11:12)]
```

The function date_b uses the function cmc_as_Date that converts CMC format to an object of class 'Date'. Note that the functions CMC.years and CMC.ages in the first release of *Biograph* (January 2011) have been replaced in *Biograph 2.0* by the more general date_b function.

3.7 Conclusion

The *Biograph* object is a data frame of individual life histories. The object has one record for each individual in the sample. Events are ordered chronologically. The object contains the input data for the *Biograph* package and keeps information on essential characteristics of the data. The characteristics are stored in attributes of the object. When the data are in *Biograph* format, all functions of the package can easily be applied. In addition, the data can be easily converted into another format

Table 3.15 Calendar dates of transitions in GLHS

```
ID      born      start     end       marriage  LMentry   path       Tr1       Tr2
3    3  01May1939 01May1939 01Nov1981 01Jun1972 01Apr1957 NJJJJJN    01Apr1957 01Apr1958
9    9  01May1931 01May1931 01Nov1981 01Jun1957 01Mar1949 NJJJJ      01Mar1949 01Feb1950
12   12 01May1939 01May1939 01Nov1981 01Sep1967 01May1954 NJJJJ      01May1954 01Mar1967
28   28 01May1931 01May1931 01Nov1981 01Apr1960 01Apr1954 NJJJJ      01Apr1954 01Aug1955
43   44 01Apr1949 01Apr1949 01Nov1981 01Jan1974 01Oct1966 NJJJJNJJJ  01Oct1966 01Feb1967
72   75 01Jun1931 01Jun1931 01Nov1981      <NA> 01Aug1945 NJJ        01Aug1945 01Aug1971
90   94 01Nov1949 01Nov1949 01Nov1981 01Oct1971 01Nov1970 NJ         01Nov1970      <NA>
146  151 01Feb1951 01Feb1951 01Nov1981      <NA> 01May1968 NJ         01May1968      <NA>
163  169 01Sep1951 01Sep1951 01Nov1981 01Jul1973 01Apr1968 NJJJ       01Apr1968 01Jul1978
174  180 01Aug1940 01Aug1940 01Nov1981 01Mar1966 01Aug1954 NJNJNJ     01Aug1954 01Apr1956
```

3.7 Conclusion

and subsets of data can be selected. *Biograph* includes conversion utilities and functions that select subsets of data.

The preparation of a *Biograph* object involves (a) defining events as transitions between states of a state space and (b) ordering events chronologically. Since in most data collections, data on events are not organised chronologically but by domain of life, the data restructuring may take time. After the transitions are properly identified, the *Biograph* utility Sequences.ind.0 orders dates of transition chronologically and determines the state sequence. In Annex A, a utility is used to convert several data sets into a *Biograph* object.

Chapter 4
Exploratory Data Analysis

4.1 Introduction

Biograph contains several functions for exploratory transition data analysis. In this chapter I describe the functions and the objects they generate. The following functions are covered:

(a) Parameters derives from a *Biograph* object several characteristics of the data, such as the sample size, state space, absorbing states and transition matrix.
(b) AgeTrans finds the ages at transition. Age is exact up to the time unit used in the analysis (e.g. month) and is given in decimal form.
(c) YearTrans finds the calendar years of transitions. The calendar year indicates the *decimal year*, which gives the year and the fraction of the year.
(d) SamplePath shows, for a selection of subjects, the state sequence recorded during the period of observation.
(e) OverviewEpisodes displays summary information on episodes.
(f) OverviewTransitions displays summary information on transitions, e.g. the number of transitions by state of origin and state of destination and the mean ages at transition.
(g) Sequences counts the different state sequences experienced by subjects in the sample.
(h) Occup identifies for every age the states occupied at that age by subjects in the sample. It also identifies state occupation times (durations of stay) in each state by age. It determines that information for each subject in the sample and for groups of subjects you select.
(i) Trans counts transitions by age, state of origin and state of destination.
(j) RateTable produces the main output table of the *Biograph* package, namely, Stable, which is a data frame with the necessary data (occurrences and exposure times) for computation of age-specific transition rates by age,

origin and destination. It also produces an object with the censored cases by age and state occupied at time of censoring.

Results of the computations are stored in objects: variables and data frames. The objects are returned to the programme calling the function.

This chapter consists of six sections. In the first section I present functions that extract from the observations general characteristics of the (sample) population. They include the sample size, the state space, the total number of episodes and transitions, etc. I also discuss ways to extract information from the data using functions of R Base. Finally, I present a function to extract information on a particular transition between two states. Functions that provide detailed information on episodes and transitions are covered in Sect. 4.2. Open episodes are distinguished from closed episodes. Functions that extract individual sample paths from the data and produce frequency tables of empirical state sequences are presented in Sect. 4.3. In the next section, I present functions that determine state occupancies and exposure times by age. State occupancy refers to the state an individual of a given age occupies (micro). It also refers to the distribution of the population of that age between the states (macro). These functions are generic. They produce information for a selected individual, for a selected group of individuals in the population or for the entire (sample) population. The possibility to extract information for selected individuals is particularly useful for identifying outliers. Groups of individuals may be formed on the basis of any characteristic or combination of characteristics included in the data. In Sect. 4.5, covariates are used to differentiate individuals in a population and to create groups. No new functions are introduced in this section, but I show how generic functions can be applied to subsets of the (sample) population in order make comparisons. Section 4.6 is the conclusion of the exploratory analysis.

4.2 The Multistate System and Its Measurement

The function Parameters explores the *Biograph* object and extracts information on the multistate system being described by the data: (1) number of observations (sample size), (2) state space, (3) possible transitions, (4) age groups, (5) states of origin and destination, (6) covariates, etc. The function returns a list or parameters for use in tabulations and computations. Parameters is invoked by the following command:

```
param <- Parameters (GLHS)
```

The object returned by Parameters contains the following components:

1. nsample: sample size.

4.2 The Multistate System and Its Measurement

2. numstates: number of states in the state space (produced by the StateSpace function called by Parameters).
3. namstates: state labels. The state space is determined by the StateSpace function. States are identified by a single character. The labels are stored in a character vector.
4. absorbstates: character vector of absorbing states. They are determined as states that are not left during the observation period. In the absence of absorbing states, it is NULL.
5. iagelow: lowest age in the (sample) population.
6. iagehigh: highest age in the (sample) population.
7. namage: labels for the single years of age from the lowest age (iagelow) to the highest age (iagehigh).
8. nage: number of age groups.
9. maxtrans: maximum number of transitions experienced by an individual during the observation period. It is determined by the number of dates of transitions in the *Biograph* data frame. It is the maximum number of states occupied by a subject minus one: max(nchar(GLHS$path))-1.
10. ntrans: total number of transitions.
11. trans_possible: transition matrix with elements 'true' indicating that the transition from i to j is feasible transition and 'false' indicating that the transition is not possible.
12. tmat: transition matrix indicating for each possible transition the transition number from 1 to n, where n is the number of possible (i,j) transitions.
13. transitions: different representations of transitions.
14. nntrans: transition matrix with, for each possible transition, the transition count.
15. locpat: column of the *Biograph* object that contains the state sequence (*path*).
16. ncovariates: number of covariates that the *Biograph* object contains.
17. covariates: character vector of covariate names.
18. format.date: format of the dates in the *Biograph* object.
19. format.born: format of date of birth in the *Biograph* object.

Parameters: invokes other functions that are part of *Biograph*:

(a) string_nb: removes blanks in the character variable *string*.
(b) stringf: converts a character string (*string*) into a vector of characters (*str_char*). The number of characters in the string is the length of the vector.
(c) StateSpace: uses GLHS$path to determine the number of states (numstates) and the state labels (namstates).

The StateSpace function determines the state space from the individual state sequences in the path column of the *Biograph* object. The function generates a character vector with as elements the different states identified in the state sequence (path column) of the *Biograph* object. The vector represents the state space. In the GLHS data, the number of states is 2 and the names of the states are 'N' and 'J'.

The first element of the vector is the state encountered first in the data. The second element is the state encountered next. The data determine the sequence of elements of the state space vector. To determine the state space used in the GLHS data, invoke the StateSpace function:

```
statespace <- StateSpace (GLHS)
```

The function produces an object with two components. The first (statespace $namstates) is a character vector with the state labels. It is {'N','J'}. The second (statespace$absorbstates) is a character vector with absorbing states. In the absence of absorbing states, NULL is returned.

For tabulation purposes a different order of states may be desired. StateSpace may be used to change the order of states in the state space. For instance, if you wish the sequence to be 'J' and 'N' rather than 'N' and 'J', use:

```
StateSpace (GLHS,newnamstates=c("J","N"))
```

The object namstates is now changed.

In the GLHS data, the age variable iagelow is 0 and iagehigh is 53. The number of age groups is 54, and the labels are 0, 1, 2, ..., 53. The value of maxtrans is 12. To determine the ID of the individual(s) with the maximum number of states occupied during the observation period, use the code:

```
GLHS$ID [nchar(GLHS$path)== max(nchar(GLHS$path))]
```

The associated record number is:

```
which (nchar(GLHS$path)== max(nchar(GLHS$path))
```

It is individual in line 188 (with ID 194).

The number of possible transitions is 3. The possible transitions are NJ, JN and JJ. Two transition matrices indicate the possible transitions. The first, param $trans_possible, is a matrix of logical values that are TRUE if the transition is possible and FALSE otherwise. In some statistical packages for estimating multistate models, e.g. *mvna* and *mstate*, this matrix is referred to as the transition matrix and is used to distinguish transitions that are possible from transitions that are not possible. The second, param$tmat, shows the transition numbers:

```
         To
From   N  J
   N  NA  1
   J   2  3
```

The count of transitions is param$nntrans:

4.2 The Multistate System and Its Measurement

```
           Destination
   Origin  N    J
   N       0   323
   J     181   277
```

The object param$transitions shows for each transition the state of origin and the state of destination, in character and numerical format:

```
   Trans OR DES ORN DESN
1    1    1   2   N    J
2    2    2   1   J    N
3    3    2   2   J    J
```

The *Biograph* object stores the dates of the transitions in the columns starting at locpat+1, where locpat<- locpath (GLHS). To display the dates, use the command GLHS[,(locpat+1):ncol(GLHS)].

The function AgeTrans obtains the ages at transition from the dates at transition and the dates of birth. It also determines the ages at entry into observation and the ages at exit. It is called by the following command:

```
agetrans <- AgeTrans (Bdata=GLHS)
```

It returns the following objects:

(a) agetrans$ages: object with for each subject, the ages at transition. The ID of the subject is also given.
(b) agetrans$ageentry: for each subject, age at entry into observation.
(c) agetrans$agecens: for each subject, age at censoring.
(d) agetrans$st_entry: for each subject, state at time of entry into observation.
(e) agetrans$st_censoring: for each subject, state at end of observation (censoring).

Consider subjects with ID 3 and 208. Their ages at transition are given by

```
agetrans$ages[rownames(agetrans$ages)%in% c(3,208),]
```

The ages at entry and at censoring and the states at entry and at censoring may be obtained in the same way for any individual. The following code generates a frequency table of ages at censoring. The ages are from the lowest age (iagelow) to the highest age (iagehigh) in the data.

```
namage <- c(param$iagelow:param$iagehigh)
censored_by_age <- table(cut(agetrans$agecens,
                    breaks=namage,
                    include.lowest=TRUE,
                    right=FALSE))
```

Age is a continuous variable. To transform age into an interval variable, i.e. to generate age intervals, the cut function of R Base may be used. The intervals are defined by the breaks argument, which gives a set of breakpoints. Unless specified otherwise, intervals are closed on the right and open on the left except for the lowest interval. It means that the lowest value is excluded from the interval and the highest value is included. The interval is denoted by (a,b], where a and b are the lowest and highest values, respectively. If include.lowest is TRUE, then the lowest value is included and the highest excluded. The interval is [a,b). In demography, age intervals usually include the lowest age and exclude the highest age. For instance, the age group 20–25 includes individuals aged 20 and excludes individuals aged 25. The censored cases by age and sex are obtained using the code:

```
table(cut(agetrans$agecens,
            breaks=namage,
            include.lowest=TRUE,
            right=FALSE),
            GLHS$sex)
```

The frequency table of ages at entry into observation (agetrans$ageentry) may be obtained in a similar way. To tabulate states at censoring by sex, use table(agetrans$st_censoring,GLHS$sex).

The age profile of the first transition, irrespective of the type of transition, is agetrans$ages[,1], that of the second transition is agetrans$ages[,2], etc. The mean ages at transition are produced by the command:

```
zmean <-
   apply(agetrans$ages,2,function(x) mean(x,na.rm=T))
```

The mean age at censoring (survey date) is mean(agetrans$agecens). It is 41.4 years.

The function YearTrans determines the calendar years in which transitions occur and expresses the dates at transition in decimal years. It is invoked by the following command:

```
yeartrans <- YearTrans (GLHS)
```

The difference between two calendar years (real values; in decimal form) gives the length in years of the episode between two transitions. The function returns the

4.2 The Multistate System and Its Measurement

object `yeartrans`. It gives for each respondent in the sample population the calendar years at transition.

Note that the frequency table of `agetrans$ages` by `yeartrans` gives the number of transitions by age and calendar year. That information can be displayed in a Lexis diagram (see further) and used for age-period-cohort analysis. The following statement tabulates the number of transitions by age and calendar year:

```
table(trunc(agetrans$ages),
      trunc(yeartrans[,5:ncol(yeartrans)]))
```

To tabulate the number of transitions by 5-year age groups and periods of 5 years, use:

```
a1 <- cut(agetrans$ages,breaks=seq(0,55,by=5))
b1 <- cut(yeartrans[,5:ncol(yeartrans)],
          breaks=seq(1943,1983,by=5))
z <- table (a1,b1)
```

The first year with a transition is 1943 and the last year 1983. The total number of transitions (`sum(z)`) is 781, which is the sum of z and also the sum of the transitions by origin and destination. Note that the table shows the total number of transitions by age group and calendar period. To get the first transition only, convert the vectors `a1` and `b1` to matrices

```
locpat <- locpath(GLHS)
a1mat <- matrix(a1,c(nsample,ncol(GLHS)-locpat))
b1mat <- matrix(b1,c(nsample,ncol(GLHS)-locpat))
```

and use `table(a1mat[,1],b1mat[,1])`.

Transitions may also be grouped by birth cohort. The years of birth of subjects are `trunc(data.frame(yeartrans)$born)`. Let us define a birth cohort as consisting of subjects born during a period of 5 years, e.g. during the period 1950–1954 or 1985–1989. These births cohorts are defined by the code:

```
bb <- trunc(data.frame(yeartrans)$born)
c1 <- cut(bb,breaks=seq(5*trunc(min(bb)/5),
          5*trunc(max(bb)/5+1),by=5))
```

The three-dimensional table that shows the number of first transitions by age group, calendar period and birth cohort is produced by the code:

```
table(a1mat[,1],b1mat[,1],c1)
```

The *survival* package has a `tcut` function, which is similar to the `cut` function of R Base used here:

```
require (survival)
z <- tcut(agetrans$agecens,
       breaks=c(namage,60),
       labels=namage)
```

z is an object containing the value of `agetrans$agecens` and with three attributes:

- `attr(,"cutpoints")` the cutpoints
- `attr(,"labels")` the labels of the intervals
- `attr(,"class")` the class 'tcut'

The number of censored cases by age is obtained by `table(trunc(z))`. It is

```
29 30 31 32 39 40 41 42 49 50 51 52
 2 25 27 17  1 22 17 15  2 36 25 12
```

with in the first row the age (age interval) and in the second row the number of censored cases in that interval.

Note that the table is the same as the one obtained by the following code:

```
table(cut(agetrans$agecens,breaks=namage))
```

If a value of `agetrans$agecens` is equal to the lowest value of the interval, `tcut` excludes that value from that interval and includes it in the previous interval.

Age profiles of transition are obtained using the `TransitionAB` function. The function extracts information on a given transition from the data. The transition is denoted by the state of origin and the state of destination. A state is represented by the character in `namstates`. Consider entry into first job, which is the transition from state N to state J. The following command extracts information on first job entry:

```
z <- TransitionAB (GLHS,"NJ")
```

The information is obtained in two steps. In the first step, the position of the given transition in the event sequence is determined for each subject. The event sequence is given by the string variable `GLHS$path`. In the case of first job entry, it is trivial since it is always the second position in the character string `GLHS$path`. In the second step, the date of the transition of interest is selected from the GLHS object.

The object z has eight components. The first, `z$case`, is the transition. The second, `z$n`, is the number of individuals experiencing the transition. The third, z$id, is the vector of identification numbers of the individuals experiencing the transition. The fourth, z$pos, is the position of the transition in GLHS$path. The remaining components give for each transition the date of the transition (z$date), the age (z$age) and calendar year (z$year) of the transition and the birth cohort (z$cohort) of the respondent experiencing the transition.

The command

```
zJN <- TransitionAB (GLHS,"JN")
```

extracts information on the first JN transition, i.e. on the first job exit followed by a period out of employment. Subsequent JN transitions are disregarded.

The following code gives the numbers of NJ transitions by age, calendar year and birth cohort:

```
table(trunc(z$age),trunc(z$year),trunc(z$cohort))
```

To tabulate the number of transitions by 5-year age group and birth cohort in periods of 5 years, use the code:

```
a1 <- cut(z$age,breaks=seq(0,55,by=5))
table (a1,c1)
```

4.3 Episodes and Transitions

The functions OverviewEpisodes and OverviewTransitions provide summary information on episodes and transitions and stores the information in data frames. The information produced by OverviewEpisodes includes number of episodes, types of episodes and mean lengths of episodes. Summary information on transitions includes possible transitions, number of transitions by origin and destination and mean ages of transitions.

The functions are invoked by the following commands:

```
seq.ind <- Sequences.ind (GLHS$path,namstates)
overviewE <- OverviewEpisodes(
            Bdata=GLHS,
            seq.ind=seq.ind)
overviewT <- OverviewTransitions (
            Bdata=GLHS,
            seq.ind=seq.ind,
            agetrans=agetrans)
```

The function `OverviewEpisodes` produces an object with five components:

(a) `overviewE$n`: number of observations (sample size)
(b) `overviewE$ne`: number of episodes
(c) `overviewE$nt`: number of transitions
(d) `overviewE$types`: types of episodes: open and closed intervals
(e) `overviewE$sojourn`: total state occupation time in each state (in time units used in the data; in this case months)

Table 4.1 shows `overviewE$types`. The number of job episodes is 600, and the number of episodes without a job is 382. The GLHS subsample has 580 closed episodes, 122 episodes without a job (N) and 458 job episodes (J). At the start of observation (at birth), all respondents are out of job (see episode type LOpen). LOpen episodes are relatively long because few transitions occur at young ages. At survey, 59 are out of a job and 142 have a job (episode type ROpen).

Table 4.2 shows `overviewE$sojourn`. All the 201 respondents combined spend 40,762 months with a job and 59,208 months without a job. Closed episodes represent less than one third of the total observation time.

The function `OverviewTransitions` produces an object with two components:

(a) `Ttrans`: the number of transitions of each type
(b) `meanage`: mean ages at transition by type

The first component contains the total number of transitions by origin and destination. It also gives the number of censored cases by state at time of censoring. The object is shown in Table 4.3.

The mean ages at transition, `overviewT$meanage`, are shown in Table 4.4.

Table 4.1 Types of episodes. GLHS

Episode	LROpen	LOpen	ROpen	Closed	Total
N	0	201	59	122	382
J	0	0	142	458	600
Total	0	201	201	580	982

Table 4.2 State occupation times by type of episode. GLHS

Episode	LROpen	LOpen	ROpen	Closed	Total
N	0	43958	10571	4679	59208
J	0	0	18194	22568	40762
Total	0	43958	28765	27247	99970

4.4 State and Event Sequences: Individual and Aggregate

Table 4.3 Transitions and censoring, by state of origin and destination. GLHS

```
           Destination
Origin    N    J  Total  Censored  TOTAL
N         0  323   323         59    382
J       181  277   458        142    600
Total   181  600   781        201    982
```

Table 4.4 Mean ages at transition and censoring. GLHS

```
          Destination
Origin     N      J    censored
N        NaN   20.61      41.38
J      24.02   26.11      40.06
```

Note that the mean age at all transitions from N to J is higher than the mean age at first entry in the labour market, i.e. the first NJ transition. The mean age at labour market entry is given by the commands:

```
z <- TransitionAB (GLHS,"NJ")
mean (z$age, rm.na=TRUE)
```

The mean age at entry is 18.7 years.

The rate of job exit is the number of job episodes during the period of observation that are not right censored (458) divided by the total time spent with a job (40,762). It is $458/40{,}762 = 0.0112$. That rate is equal to the parameter of the exponential transition rate model without covariates, as expected (Blossfeld and Rohwer 2002, p. 92). The rate calculated by dividing the number of transitions by the exposure time is an occurrence-exposure rate. It is an estimator of the transition rate of the population.

4.4 State and Event Sequences: Individual and Aggregate

A particularly useful function is SamplePath. It produces sample paths for selected subjects. Subjects are selected by their ID. The IDs of the selected subjects are stored in a vector. The vector may contain a few subjects but may also include all subjects under observation. The function SamplePath checks whether the IDs selected are included in the data and removes IDs that are not recognised. For instance, the following command requests the employment careers of subjects with ID 1, 30 and 208 (GLHS data):

```
        samplepaths <- SamplePath
                (Bdata=GLHS,subjectsID=c(1,30,208))
```

where subjectsID is a set of subject IDs. The object samplepaths is a list object with as elements the employment careers of the selected individuals. Box 4.1 shows the employment careers of respondents with IDs 1 (samplepaths [[1]]), 30 (samplepaths[[2]]) and 208 (samplepaths[[3]]).

The function Sequences.ind produces, for each subject, the sequence of states occupied during the period of observation. The state sequences can be used in other functions. The states are given in numeric variables and not in character variables. The numeric value is determined from the character variable GLHS $path. The function is called by:

```
        ist <- Sequences.ind (path=GLHS$path)
```

The state sequences for a selection of subjects are shown in Table 4.5. The subjects with ID 1, 10, 70 and 208 are selected. The list is produced by the statement:

```
        z <- ist[GLHS$ID %in% c(1,10,70,208),]
```

The object z presents states by number rather than by label. Hence the sequence of states that makes up the observed segment of the life course is denoted by characters in the object GLHS$path and by numbers in object ist. The number indicates the position of the state in the state space. Pattern matching (grep command) is used to derive that number from the state space.

State N is coded one and state J 2. The coding may be reversed, using the namstatesnew argument of the function:

```
        ist2 <- Sequences.ind (path=GLHS$path,
                                namstatesnew=c("J","N"))
```

Box 4.1: Sample Paths for Selected Subjects. GLHS

```
ID  1
$born
[1] "Subject ID = 1  Date of birth 351 (01Mar29)"

$start_end
  Start  Start2  Stop   Stop2
1   351  01Mar29  983  01Nov81

$path
  Episode State EntryDate1 EntryDate2 EntryAge Durat OR DE
1       1     N       351    01Mar29     0.00   204  0  1
2       2     J       555    01Mar46    17.00   428  1  2
3       3  Cens       983    01Nov81    52.67    NA  2  0

ID  30
$born
[1] "Subject ID = 30  Date of birth 364 (01Apr30)"

$start_end
  Start  Start2  Stop   Stop2
1   357  01Sep29  983  01Nov81

$path
  Episode State EntryDate1 EntryDate2 EntryAge Durat OR DE
1       1     N       364    01Apr30     0.00   169  0  1
2       2     J       533    01May44    14.08   144  1  2
3       3     N       677    01May56    26.08   306  2  1
4       4  Cens       983    01Nov81    51.59    NA  1  0

Continued
ID 208
$born
[1] "Subject ID = 208  Date of birth 485 (01May40)"

$start_end
  Start  Start2  Stop   Stop2
1   473  01May39  983  01Nov81

$path
  Episode State EntryDate1 EntryDate2 EntryAge Durat OR DE
1       1     N       485    01May40     0.00   230  0  1
2       2     J       715    01Jul59    19.17    22  1  2
3       3     N       737    01May61    21.00     6  2  1
4       4     J       743    01Nov61    21.50    13  1  2
5       5     N       756    01Dec62    22.58   227  2  1
6       6  Cens       983    01Nov81    41.50    NA  1  0
```

Table 4.5 Selected individual state sequences. GLHS

```
         Transition
ID       1  2  3  4  5  6  7  8  9  10 11 12 13
  1      1  2  0  0  0  0  0  0  0   0  0  0  0
 10      1  2  2  1  2  0  0  0  0   0  0  0  0
 70      1  2  2  0  0  0  0  0  0   0  0  0  0
208      1  2  1  2  1  0  0  0  0   0  0  0  0
```

Table 4.6 Most frequent state and event sequences. GLHS

	ncase	%	cum%	M_age_entry	M_age_exit	ns	case	tr1	tr2	tr3	tr4	tr5
1	23	11.44	11.44		0	40.58	3	NJN	18.58>J	24.42>N			
2	19	9.45	20.90		0	49.92	3	NJJ	18>J	24.92>J			
3	17	8.46	29.35		0	40.17	4	NJNJ	18.58>J	22.5>N	27.25>J		
4	16	7.96	37.31		0	36.96	2	NJ	19.75>J				
5	16	7.96	45.27		0	41.71	4	NJJJ	17.38>J	21.54>J	27.33>J		
6	11	5.47	50.75		0	40.67	4	NJJN	18.17>J	21.08>J	25.08>N		
7	10	4.98	55.72		0	41.79	5	NJJJJ	18.25>J	23.54>J	32.58>J	36.71>J	
8	9	4.48	60.20		0	40.25	6	NJNJNJ	17.83>J	21.08>N	23.67>J	24.92>N	29.83>J
9	8	3.98	64.18		0	50.75	5	NJNJJ	16.62>J	20.75>N	22.92>J	39.67>J	
10	8	3.98	68.16		0	45.50	6	NJNJJJ	17.54>J	20.75>N	22.04>J	26.58>J	30.25>J
11	8	3.98	72.14		0	41.42	5	NJNJN	17.54>J	20.71>N	21.21>J	26.88>N	
12	6	2.99	75.12		0	51.25	5	NJJJN	17.62>J	20.62>J	23.46>J	32.67>N	

The function Sequences determines and orders individual sequences in the sample population. The command

```
seq <- Sequences(GLHS,mean_median="median")
```

returns a frequency table of state sequences. The object seq has two components. The first is the choice of mean or median. The second contains the table of sequences. Table 4.6 shows the 12 most frequent sequences: seq$sequences [1:12,]. The number of different sequences is nrow(seq), and the number of subjects included in the sequence table is sum(seq$ncase). The 201 individuals included in the subsample experience 48 different pathways. The most prevalent sequence is NJN. Among the 201 respondents, 23 (11.4 %) experience the NJN sequence and 19 (9.4 %) experience the trajectory NJJ. The persons who experience the sequence NJN enter the labour market at a median age of 18.6 and leave their first job at a median age of 24.4. They are interviewed (censored) at a median age of 40.6. The following command lists the 23 respondents.

```
z<- subset(GLHS,GLHS$path=="NJN")
```

Of the 23 respondents, 21 are females and 2 are males. All women who left the job are married, and the age at leaving the job is related to the age at marriage.

For each sequence recorded in the sample, the following information is given:

(a) ncase is the number of respondents with the indicated state sequence.
(b) % is the proportion of the state sequence in the sample.
(c) cum% is the cumulative proportion.

(d) `M_age_entry` is the mean age at entry into observation.
(e) `M_age_exit` is the mean age at end of observation (interview).
(f) `ns` is the number of states (episodes) in the state sequence.
(g) `case` is the state sequence (character variable).
(h) `tr*` is the median ages at transition (or mean age, depending on the function argument).

4.5 State Occupancies, Transitions and State Occupation Times

Biograph contains four functions to display state occupancies, transitions and state occupation times for selected individuals, groups of individuals and the entire sample. The functions are `state_age`, `state_time`, `Occup` and `Trans`. The `state_age` function displays, for a selected individual or each of a group of individuals, the state occupied at a given age and the transitions during two consecutive ages. For instance,

```
state_age (GLHS,20,208)
```

shows that individual with ID 208 is in state J at exact age 20. The following code displays the states occupied at birthdays between ages 20 and 25:

```
state_age (GLHS,20:25,208)
```

The states individuals 33 and 208 occupy at birthdays between 20 and 25 are given by the code

```
state_age (GLHS,20:24,c(33,208))
```

The function `state_age` produces an object with three components. The first shows the state labels. A '−' indicates that the individual is not under observation yet, and a '+' indicates that the observation has ended. The second component shows the state occupied at the given age or the states occupied at the selected ages. The third component shows the number of individuals in each state at consecutive ages.

The function `state_time` displays the states selected individuals occupy at each age (from the lowest to the highest age). For instance,

```
state_time(GLHS,33)
```

shows the states individual 33 occupies at each age between birth and age 53. The states occupied by individuals 33 and 208 are obtained by

```
ss <- state_time(GLHS,c(33,208))
```

The function `state_time` produces object `ss` with four components:

(a) `ss$state`: states occupied at consecutive birthdays between the lowest age and the highest age
(b) `ss$state.n`: the number of selected individuals in each state at consecutive birthdays
(c) `ss$sjt_age_1`: the number of years (or time units) the selected individuals spend in each state between consecutive birthdays
(d) `as$tjst`: for each age, the number of years (or time units) the selected individuals spends in each state

The function `Occup` produces detailed information on (a) state occupancies by age and (b) state occupation times by age and state. The function is called by the following command:

$$\text{occup <- Occup (Bdata=GLHS)}$$

The function calls the function `state_time`, which determines for given individuals state occupation times at all ages. The function `state_time` calls `AgeTrans` and `state_age`. The latter determines, for each individual under observation, the state occupied at each consecutive birthday. `Occup` returns an object, `occup` say, with the following components:

(a) `occup$state_occup`: state occupancies, number of subjects by age and state occupied. Censored cases are listed too. Age is the exact age, and, consequently, the state occupancies are the states on birthdays (and more precise, on 0:00 a.m.).
(b) `occup$st_age_1`: for each subject the states occupied at consecutive birthdays. For instance, the states occupied by the 10th subject between the minimum and the maximum ages (0 and 53) are given by `occup$st_age_1 [10,]`. It shows the state occupied at each consecutive birthday. This data format is also used by the *TraMineR* package, where it is referred to as the 'extended format of state sequence data'.
(c) `occup$sjt_age_1`: for each subject and each age, the number of years in each of the states. Consider subject 10. The number of years spent in the different states during each single year of age between 0 and 53 is `occup $sjt_age_1[10,,]`. 'Censored' is treated as a fictitious state.
(d) `occup$tsjt`: total number of years spent in each state between two consecutive ages, by all subjects combined.

The object `occup` is of class 'occup.S'. The `Occup` function attaches the class to the object.

An individual, who makes a transition at his or her birthday, is allocated to the next age, and the state occupied on his birthday is the origin state (because the transition occurs later than midnight at 0:00 a.m.). For instance, an individual who leaves a job in the month of his 23rd birthday is considered to be 23 years at the time of leaving the job. This procedure is standard in demographic analysis. A different

4.5 State Occupancies, Transitions and State Occupation Times

result is obtained when the R function *cut* is applied. In R the default interval between a and b is defined as (a,b], which comprises the values of x that are larger than a and smaller or equal to b: $\{x \mid a < x \leq b\}$. The code `table(cut(ages,1:highest_age))` allocates transitions at birthday (or in the month that has the birthday) incorrectly to the age in the previous year. Consider the following code:

```
GLHS.a<- date_b (GLHS,
                 format.in='CMC',
                 selectday=1,
                 format.out="age")
ages <- GLHS.a$end
highest_age=54
table(cut(ages,1:highest_age))
```

The number of respondents with observations censored at age 29 in completed years, i.e. between ages 29 and 30, is 5 (which is (29,30]). Two persons are aged 29 at the time of interview, and 3 have the interview on their 30th birthday.

To close the interval on the left and open on the right ([29,30)), the following code should be used:

```
table(cut(ages,1:highest_age,include.lowest=TRUE,
                             right=FALSE))
```

The following code shows the state occupation times by state and age for the subject with identification number 188:

```
print (round(occup$sjt_age_1[GLHS$ID==188,,],3))
```

For this application, the transitions to the same state have been removed. Individual 188 is a female, born in CMC 500 and experiences five transitions between the states N and J, at CMC 705, 817, 834, 844 and 964. The observation is censored at CMC 983.

Table 4.7 shows, for ID 188, the observed state occupation times in the different states. The table shows the individual contribution to the transitions and, more importantly, to the state occupation times. The state occupation times are key figures in the estimation of transition rates. The option to investigate the individual contributions to transitions and state occupation times in the estimation of transition rates is considered one of the major strengths of *Biograph*. Note that the individual contributes to both closed episodes and open episodes. The person enters the first job at age $(705-500)/12=17.08$ and leaves employment at age $(817-500)/12=26.42$. She gets a new job at age $(834-500)/12=27.83$, which she leaves at age $(844-500)/12=28.67$ years. The last job is entered at age $(964-500)/12=38.67$, and she still has that job when the observation ends at age $(983-500)/12=40.25$ years. Note that the function `cmc_as_age` may be used to get the age and calendar year at labour market entry, e.g. `cmc_as_age(705,500,"cmc")`.

Table 4.7 Individual state occupation times by age. Respondent with ID 188. GLHS

```
      state
Age         N         J Censored Total
  0   1.000  0.000      0.00       0
  1   1.000  0.000      0.00       0
  2   1.000  0.000      0.00       0
  3   1.000  0.000      0.00       0
  4   1.000  0.000      0.00       0
  5   1.000  0.000      0.00       0
  6   1.000  0.000      0.00       0
  7   1.000  0.000      0.00       0
  8   1.000  0.000      0.00       0
  9   1.000  0.000      0.00       0
 10   1.000  0.000      0.00       0
 11   1.000  0.000      0.00       0
 12   1.000  0.000      0.00       0
 13   1.000  0.000      0.00       0
 14   1.000  0.000      0.00       0
 15   1.000  0.000      0.00       0
 16   1.000  0.000      0.00       0
 17   0.083  0.917      0.00       0
 18   0.000  1.000      0.00       0
 19   0.000  1.000      0.00       0
 20   0.000  1.000      0.00       0
 21   0.000  1.000      0.00       0
 22   0.000  1.000      0.00       0
 23   0.000  1.000      0.00       0
 24   0.000  1.000      0.00       0
 25   0.000  1.000      0.00       0
 26   0.583  0.417      0.00       0
 27   0.833  0.167      0.00       0
 28   0.333  0.667      0.00       0
 29   1.000  0.000      0.00       0
 30   1.000  0.000      0.00       0
 31   1.000  0.000      0.00       0
 32   1.000  0.000      0.00       0
 33   1.000  0.000      0.00       0
 34   1.000  0.000      0.00       0
 35   1.000  0.000      0.00       0
 36   1.000  0.000      0.00       0
 37   1.000  0.000      0.00       0
 38   0.667  0.333      0.00       0
 39   0.000  1.000      0.00       0
 40   0.000  0.250      0.75       0
 41   0.000  0.000      1.00       0
 42   0.000  0.000      1.00       0
 43   0.000  0.000      1.00       0
 44   0.000  0.000      1.00       0
 45   0.000  0.000      1.00       0
 46   0.000  0.000      1.00       0
 47   0.000  0.000      1.00       0
 48   0.000  0.000      1.00       0
 49   0.000  0.000      1.00       0
 50   0.000  0.000      1.00       0
 51   0.000  0.000      1.00       0
 52   0.000  0.000      1.00       0
 53   0.000  0.000      1.00       0
```

4.5 State Occupancies, Transitions and State Occupation Times

Table 4.8 Observed aggregate state occupation times at selected ages. GLHS

	state			
Age	N	J	Censored	Total
0	201.00	0.00	0.00	201
30	57.58	127.75	15.67	201
40	36.25	83.17	81.58	201
50	17.92	37.25	145.83	201

The following command may be used to create an object with the state occupation times for selected ages:

```
z <- occup$tsjt[match(ageprint,param$namage),]
```

where `ageprint` is the vector of the ages to be printed and `namage` is the vector with age labels, e.g.

```
ageprint <- c(0,30,40,50)
```

An alternative is to get the age labels from the rownames. The following command selects the ages 0, 30, 40 and 50 from `occup$tsjt`.

```
z <- occup$tsjt[rownames(occup$tsjt) %in% c(0,30,40,50),]
```

The results are shown in Table 4.8.

The object `occup$tsjt` shows for all subjects combined the time spent in each of the states between two consecutive ages. The time shown in the column 'censored' is the number of years lost to observation due to censoring at ages below or at the age indicated. The total time (in months) subjects are observed in each state is `round(apply(occup$tsjt,2,sum),2)`:

```
      N          J     Censored     Total
4934.00    3396.83     2523.17  10854.00
```

The total state occupation time is 201*54 = 10,854 years, with 53 the highest age in completed years (age 0 ... 53). The total number of years of observation is 4,934 + 3,396.83 = 8,330.83 years or 99,970 months. It is the same as the number of months computed by `OverviewEpisodes`.

The number of respondents by state occupied at consecutive ages is presented in Fig. 4.1. The data are contained in object `occup$state_occup`. For instance, at their 32nd birthday, 45 persons are out of job and 102 have a job. Information on 54 persons is missing because they are below 32 at the time of survey. The graph is produced by the function `plot.occup.S`, which plots an object of class 'occup.S':

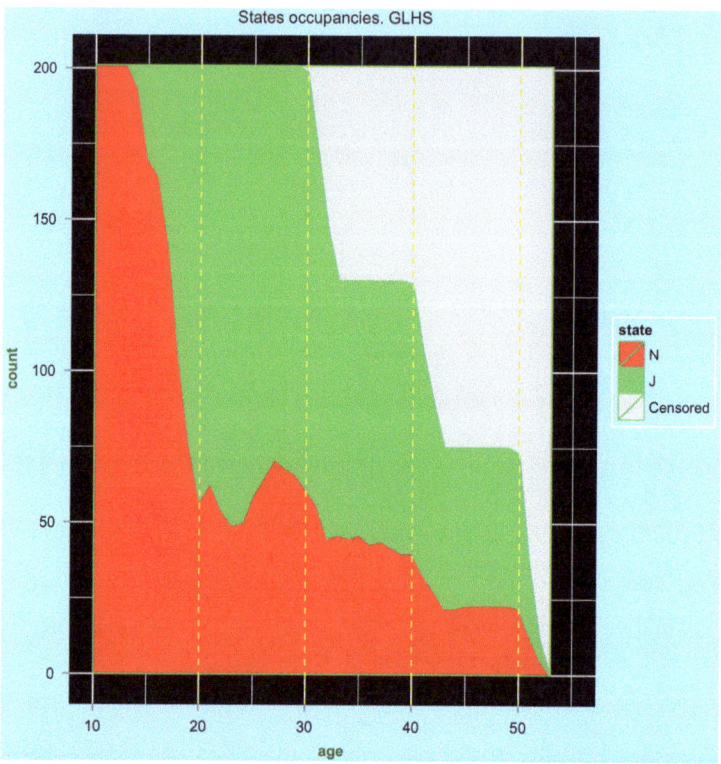

Fig. 4.1 State occupancies by age. GLHS

```
z<- plot (x=occup$state_occup,
    namstates.desired=c("N","J","Censored"),
    colours=c("red","green","lightgrey"),
    title="States occupancies. GLHS",
    area=TRUE,
    xmin=10,
    xmax=55)
```

Note that class(occup$state_occup) is 'occup.S'.

The function Trans produces data on transitions by origin, destination and age. For example,

```
trans <- Trans(Bdata=GLHS)
```

Trans creates the following objects:

(a) trans$Ttrans: matrix showing number of transitions by origin and destination and censored cases.

4.5 State Occupancies, Transitions and State Occupation Times

Table 4.9 Number of transitions by origin and destination and mean ages. GLHS

```
a. Number of transitions
        Destination
Origin    N    J Total Censored
    N     0  323   323       59
    J   181  277   458      142
 Total  181  600   781      201

b. Mean ages
        Destination
Origin    N       J censored
    N   NaN   20.61    41.38
    J 24.02   26.11    40.07
```

Table 4.10 Number of transitions at selected ages. GLHS

```
, , origin = N

     destination
Age  N J censored
 25  0 3       0
 26  0 8       0

, , origin = J

     destination
Age   N  J censored
 25  11 10       0
 26  14 11       0
```

(b) `trans$meanage`: mean ages at transition.
(c) `trans$trans`: for each age the number of transitions by origin and destination.
(d) `trans$trans_during_interval`: for each subject and each age interval, the number of transitions during that interval. This component can be used to investigate multiple transitions.

The objects `trans$Ttrans` and `trans$meanage` are shown in Table 4.9.
The number of transitions the sample population experiences at selected ages is produced by

`trans$trans[rownames(trans$trans) %in%ageselect,,]`

and is shown in Table 4.10 for `ageselect=c(25,26)`.
To display the age-specific transitions by origin and destination, use:

```
aperm(trans$trans[rownames(trans$trans)
           %in%ageselect,,],c(3,2,1))
```

Table 4.11 Data for calculation of transition rate, selected ages. GLHS

```
,  ,  State = N

       Case
Age    Occup       PY  Leaving  N  J  Censored
 0      201  201.00         0   0  0         0
25       58   62.00         3   0  3         0
40       41   36.25         9   0  4         5
50       22   17.92        11   0  1        10

,  ,  State = J

       Case
Age    Occup       PY  Leaving  N  J  Censored
 0        0    0.00         0   0   0        0
25      143  139.00        21  11  10        0
40       88   83.17        22   1   3       18
50       51   37.25        28   2   0       26
```

The function RateTable is a particularly useful function in the process of estimating transition rates. The object combines information on transitions and durations of exposure. That information is needed for the estimation of the transition rates. In addition, it keeps for tabulation purposes the state occupancies and the mean ages at transition. For example,

```
ratetable <- RateTable (GLHS,occup,trans)
```

RateTable returns two data frames:

(a) ratetable$Stable
(b) ratetable$censored_by_age

The first, ratetable$Stable, is an object in the format of a table with the state occupancies by age, exposure times by age and state and transitions by age and by origin and destination. Table 4.11 shows the information for the ages 0, 25, 40 and 50. It is produced by the following command:

```
ratetable$Stable[rownames(ratetable$Stable)
              %in% c(0,25,40,50),,]
```

ratetable$Stable is an array with three dimensions: the first is age, the second is state occupied at birthday and the third is a set of measures that pertain to persons of the indicated age in the indicated state at the last birthday: number of subjects occupying that state at that birthday, state occupation time in that state between the last and next birthday, number leaving that state between the two birthdays and destination. The object `Stable` is used for further data processing, e.g. for the calculation of transition rates in the multistate life table.

For each state `ratetable$Stable` shows:

(a) Number of subjects in that state at exact ages. For instance, in the GLHS, at exact age 25, 58 respondents are out of a job and 143 have a job. The total is 201 (sample size). Note that, if an individual makes a transition at his or her birthday, then the state occupied at the birthday is the origin state (see description of `occup$state_occup`).
(b) Total state occupation time during the period of observation spent in each of the states between two consecutive ages, by all subjects combined. The 201 respondents together spent 62.00 years out of job between the 25th and 26th birthday and 139.00 years with a job. The same information, but arranged differently, is also shown in the output file `tsjt.out` (see below).
(c) Direct transitions by state of origin, state of destination and age. For instance, 3 respondents without a job got a job between ages 25 and 26; 11 persons with a job left the job to be out of a job and 10 moved to another job. No observation was censored at age 26. Note that an individual, who makes a transition at his or her birthday, is allocated to the correct age.

The second object returned by `RateTable` is `ratetable $censored_by_age`. It is the number of subjects censored by age and state occupancies at censoring. The information is used for microsimulation with censoring. Note the difference with `agetrans$agecens`. The latter gives for each individual in the sample population the age at censoring.

4.6 Covariates

The methods described above may be extended to exploratory transition data analysis with covariates. The simplest approach is to split the data set based on values of a covariate or sets of covariates and use *Biograph* functions for each subset separately. By way of illustration, consider state sequences recorded in the GLHS and suppose we want to determine whether the employment career of the younger cohort differs from that of the older cohort. To split the data set, use the `split` function of **R Base**. The following command splits the GLHS data in two data sets, one for each cohort:

```
GLHS.cohort <-
        split(GLHS,as.factor(GLHS$cohort))
```

The object `GLHS.cohort` is an object of type 'list' with three components: a data frame with the records for individuals born before in the 1929–1931 period, a

Table 4.12 State and event sequences, by birth cohort. GLHS

```
a. Born in 1929-31
    ncase      %   cum% M_age_exit  ns   case        tr1        tr2        tr3        tr4    tr5
1      10  13.33  13.33     50.83    3    NJJ   16.33>J    30.79>J
2       8  10.67  24.00     50.58    3    NJN   18.29>J    23.58>N
3       6   8.00  32.00     50.75    2     NJ   16.96>J
4       6   8.00  40.00     51.29    4   NJJJ   18.75>J    23.38>J       31>J
5       6   8.00  48.00     50.92    5  NJNJJ   15.46>J       21>N    28.67>J    41.5>J
6       5   6.67  54.67     51.83    5  NJJJN   18.33>J    21.75>J    24.25>J    35.5>N
7       4   5.33  60.00     51.17    5  NJJJJ   19.21>J    25.04>J    33.38>J    44.96>J
8       4   5.33  65.33     51.88    6 NJNJJJ   17.54>J    25.33>N    26.58>J    38.5>J   46>J
9       3   4.00  69.33     51.42    4   NJJN      17>J    21.5>J     24.67>N
10      3   4.00  73.33     50.83    5  NJJNJ   16.5>J     26.58>J    34.33>N    35.33>J

Born in 1939-41
    ncase      %   cum% M_age_exit  ns   case        tr1        tr2        tr3        tr4    tr5
1       7  12.73  12.73     41.00    4   NJNJ   18.92>J    20.42>N    27.08>J
2       5   9.09  21.82     41.58    4   NJJJ   17.17>J    19.5>J        25>J
3       5   9.09  30.91     41.25    6 NJNJNJ   17.08>J    23.17>N    25.17>J       26>N 33.25>J
4       4   7.27  38.18     41.42    3    NJN   19.29>J    24.62>N
5       3   5.45  43.64     41.08    5  NJJJJ   16.5>J     27.83>J    34.25>J    36.83>J
6       3   5.45  49.09     42.67    4   NJJN   19.17>J    22.17>J    25.33>N
7       3   5.45  54.55     41.33    5  NJNJN   17.67>J    19.83>N    20.92>J    25.5>N
8       2   3.64  58.18     41.92    2     NJ   19.62>J
9       2   3.64  61.82     40.33    3    NJJ   22.71>J       24>J

Born in 1949-51
    ncase      %   cum% M_age_exit  ns   case        tr1        tr2        tr3        tr4    tr5
1      11  15.49  15.49     31.25    3    NJN   18.17>J    26.83>N
2       8  11.27  26.76     31.12    2     NJ   22.29>J
3       8  11.27  38.03     32.00    4   NJNJ   18.5>J     23.83>N    27.12>J
4       7   9.86  47.89     31.00    3    NJJ   18.42>J    22.67>J
5       5   7.04  54.93     30.58    4   NJJJ   17.58>J    20.42>J    27.17>J
6       5   7.04  61.97     31.67    4   NJJN   18.17>J    19.25>J    21.75>N
7       4   5.63  67.61     31.42    6 NJNJNJ   18.08>J    20.25>N    22.42>J    24.75>N   29>J
8       3   4.23  71.83     32.42    5  NJJJJ   20.67>J    20.92>J    25.5>J     27.92>J
9       3   4.23  76.06     31.33    6 NJJNJJ      17>J    21.33>J    25.92>N    26.83>J 28.42>J
```

data frame with the records for individuals born in 1930–1941 and a data frame for individuals born in 1949–1951. To display the three components, use `str(GLHS.cohort)`. The component `GLHS.cohort$"1949-51"`, or alternatively `GLHS.cohort[[3]]`, contains the data for the respondents born in 1949–1951. Among the 201 respondents, 75 were born in the period 1939–1941, 55 in the period 1939–1941 and 71 were born in 1949–1951. To list the first ten records of the first data frame, use

```
GLHS.cohort$"1929-31"[1:10,]
```

or

```
GLHS.cohort[[1]][1:10,]
```

The state sequences by birth cohort are obtained by the following commands:

```
seq.c1 <- Sequences (GLHS.cohort[[1]])$sequences
seq.c2 <- Sequences (GLHS.cohort[[2]])$sequences
seq.c3 <- Sequences (GLHS.cohort[[3]])$sequences
```

4.6 Covariates

Table 4.12 shows the most prevalent pathways for the three cohorts. The sequence NJN accounts for 11 % of the employment trajectories in the oldest cohort, 7 % in the middle cohort and 15 % in the youngest cohort. The ages at transition are median ages.

To illustrate the use of covariates further, consider the age profile at entry into the labour market. One way of plotting the age profiles is by covariate. Consider the first cohort:

```
z <- subset(GLHS,GLHS$cohort=="1929-31")
attr(z,"format.date") <- attr(GLHS,"format.date")
attr(z,"format.born") <- attr(GLHS,"format.born")
attr(z,"param") <- attr(GLHS,"param")
z.c1 <- TransitionAB(Bdata=z,
          transition="NJ",keep=FALSE)
```

and similarly for the second and third cohort. The ages at labour market entry are given in z.c1$age.

An alternative is to use a Trellis plot, i.e. a panel of graphic displays. Figure 4.2 shows the age distribution at labour market entry by birth cohort and sex. It is a density plot produced by the following commands:

```
library (lattice)
z <- TransitionAB(GLHS,"NJ")
zzz <- as.data.frame(cbind (ID=GLHS$ID,
         cohort=GLHS$cohort,
         sex=GLHS$sex,
         Entry=z$age))
zzz$cohort <- factor(zzz$cohort,
    labels=c("1929-31","1939-41","1949-51"))
zzz$sex <- factor(zzz$sex,
    labels =c("Males","Females"))

densityplot (~Entry|sex,data=zzz,
    plot.points="rug",
    main="Age at labour market entry",
    sub= paste("Total number of entries with known covariates is ",
    length(na.omit(zzz$Entry)),sep=""),
    xlab="Age",
    scale=list(x=list(alternating=FALSE)),
    groups=cohort,
    ref=TRUE,
    auto.key=TRUE)
```

Figure 4.2 shows that women born in 1939 or later enter the labour market later than women born in 1929–1931. Men enter later if they are born in 1949–1951. The distribution of the age at labour market entry is wider for the oldest cohort.

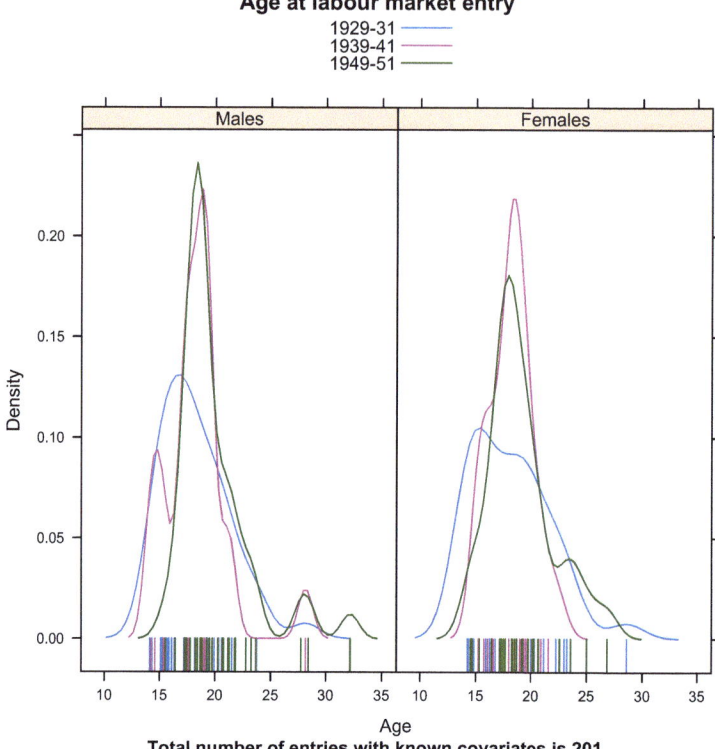

Fig. 4.2 Trellis plot of age distribution at labour market entry, by birth cohort and sex. GLHS

The figure reveals that the age profile of labour market entry for the 1939–1941 birth cohort is a mixture of two age profiles.

4.7 Conclusion

Data analysis starts by getting acquainted with the data. It involves looking at the data, the computation of summary measures, the identification of patterns and peculiarities such as outliers and the display of data for visual inspection. The tools presented in this chapter offer summary measures but also a detailed look at the data. The measures and tabulations that are produced for the sample population may also be produced for a subset of that population and even for each member separately. The purpose of a detailed look at life history data is to get a feeling for the data before embarking on statistical analysis. For instance, what is the share of open episodes, i.e. censored observations? What are the most frequent transitions and event sequences? Is a transition soon followed by another transition? The answers to these questions provide information that is useful for describing the

4.7 Conclusion

life paths of the sample population and at the same time support further statistical analysis. For instance, a detailed account of open and closed episodes helps the construction and understanding of the likelihood function in survival models. The purpose of a full documentation of the computation of event counts and state occupation times is to promote understanding of the method underlying the estimation of transition rates. The object Stable has all the necessary information to estimate age-specific transition rates by origin and destination. It is therefore considered one of the most useful objects produced by the *Biograph* package. Visualisation of the data and life histories is the subject of the next chapter.

Chapter 5
Visualisation of Life Histories

5.1 Introduction

Data visualisation is the graphic presentation of data to reveal complex information at a glance (Steele and Iliinsky 2010). The challenge is to map data to a visual display that reveals the range of values of variables and relations between variables. Visualisation of data can be an effective introduction to formal statistical modelling. Ages at marriage may be displayed as points in a scatter plot to assess the distribution of ages and to identify outliers. The marriage duration of a person may be displayed as a line connecting age at marriage and current age or age at marriage dissolution. The end point may be marked if the marriage has been dissolved and not marked if the marriage is intact at the end of the observation period. Visualisation of life histories poses particular challenges. The first is conceptual. The life history is a multistage process of development in which stages create a basis for subsequent stages. In this book the life course is conceptualised as sequences of states and sequences of events. In each domain of life, a state and event sequence can be identified. A second challenge is embedding. The life course is embedded in a historical context, and the visualisation should reveal how developmental processes vary in time. That requires at least two time scales: age and calendar time. The Lexis diagram, named after the demographer Wilhelm Lexis (1837–1914), meets that challenge. Each line in a Lexis diagram represents the follow-up of a single individual from entry to exit on two time scales: age and calendar time. The Lexis diagram is widely used and has inspired improved visualisations of life histories. Some of that research is reviewed in the brief historical note in Sect. 5.1. A third challenge is to reveal significant information at a glance. The graph should convey essential information and highlight the unexpected.

One of the great strengths of R is the graphics capabilities. In this chapter, I use two general-purpose and two special-purpose graphics packages to display life history data. The general-purpose packages are *lattice* and *ggplot2*. *Lattice*, developed by Sarkar (2008, 2014), is designed to combine multiple plots in a page. It is modelled on the Trellis graphic originally developed by Cleveland (1993) and written in S. The *ggplot2* package, developed by Wickham (2009, 2010, 2014), starts from the grammar of graphics (Wilkinson 2005, 2012) to compose graphics using a set of independent components and multiple layers. Section 5.1 contains a brief description of the grammar of graphics, which is implemented in *ggplot2*. The special-purpose packages are *Epi* and *TraMineR*. *Epi*, developed by Carstensen (2013), presents state sequences and event sequences in Lexis diagrams. *TraMineR*, developed by Gabadinho et al. (2011, 2012) and maintained by Ritschard (2014), includes several functions for the visualisation of state sequences. In Sect. 5.2 *ggplot2* functions are illustrated using GLHS data. The Lexis diagram is covered in Sect. 5.3. The visualisation of state distributions and state sequences is the subject of Sect. 5.4.

5.2 Points of Departure

In this book, the life course is approached as a sequence of states and sequence of transitions between states. Visualisation of the life course means visualisation of sequences highlighting transition dates (or ages) and sojourn times. The study of a single transition or a single episode is a first step. A scatter diagram of individual ages at transition by one or several covariates may reveal significant differences and may function as a guide for more formal analysis. Outliers are easily identified. The simplest visual representation of multiple transitions is the event chart. Each individual is represented by a single horizontal line, and transitions are denoted by various symbols placed along the line. The x-axis denotes the time scale, and subject ID is shown along the y-axis. Time can be calendar time or time elapsed since a reference event, e.g. birth or entry in a study. The event chart was introduced by Goldman (1992). Lee et al. (2000) review and discuss developments. They distinguish three basic formats of event charts: (a) calendar event chart, which displays calendar dates of transitions along the x-axis; (b) interval event chart, which displays times elapsed since a reference event along the x-axis; and (c) Goldman event chart, which shows the interval date along the x-axis and the calendar date along the y-axis. One of the extensions they consider is using different colours to represent episodes of life. The authors developed `event.chart`, which is a function of the *Hmisc* package in CRAN to display different types of event charts. For an application of event charts in the analysis of event sequences in longitudinal studies, using the *Hmisc* package, see Dubin and O'Malley (2010). For the methods, see Dubin et al. (2001).

Pleasant et al. (1996) developed *LifeLines* and later *LifeFlow* and *EventFlow* to visualise individual life histories.[1] Horizontal lines represent different domains of life. Medical conditions may be represented by one line and employment history by

---

[1] http://www.cs.umd.edu/hcil/members/cplaisant/

5.2 Points of Departure

another. Icons indicate events. Line colour and thickness illustrate relationships or the significance of events.

In 1996, Francis and Fuller (1996) discussed the usefulness of exploratory visualisation of event histories as a precursor to more formal statistical modelling and reviewed a number of visualisation methods. They selected the Lexis diagram as the main graphical method for displaying life histories. The Lexis diagram represents events and episodes in two time scales: age (individual time) and calendar time. Calendar time is shown on the x-axis and age on the y-axis. The authors extend the Lexis diagram, which displays for each individual a single lifeline or life history, to a Lexis pencil displaying multiple life histories. The multiple histories may relate to domains of life, partners or household members. Different colours are used to denote the stages of life in a lifeline. Lifelines of different domains of life are displayed side by side resembling a pencil. Francis and Fuller note that the Goldman event chart is essentially a Lexis diagram with axes reversed.

The grammar of graphics (Wilkinson 2005) is a systematic approach to statistical graphics. It describes the mapping of data to objects displayed in a graphic and the aesthetic attributes of the objects. The aesthetic attributes or aesthetics are visual properties that affect the way observations are displayed. To represent data, numerical values should be translated into positions in a coordinate system, shapes, sizes and colours. Aesthetic mapping (aes) is the mapping of data to positions, shapes, sizes and colours. For instance, to highlight changes in age at marriage over time, ages at marriage of members of a population may be represented by points in an age-time coordinate system (e.g. Lexis diagram). Points, lines, histograms and bar charts are geometric objects (geom) used to display the data. To determine whether the changes in marriage age differ between males and females, the point may be replaced by a circle if the subject is a male and a triangle when it is a female. Colours may be used to distinguish levels of education. To distinguish between first- and higher-order marriages, the data set may be split, and separate plots may be shown in two panels for easy comparison.

The grammar of graphics is implemented in *ggplot2* (Wickham 2009). Wickham makes a distinction between the information content of a plot and its beauty. The information content is controlled by: (1) the geometric object used to display observations (points, lines, histogram) and (2) the position of observations in the plot and the shape, size and colour of the geometric object. The beauty is determined by non-data-related elements, such as title, axis labels, background, grid lines, legend, etc. In *ggplot2* position, shape, size and colour are referred to as *aesthetics*. Geometric objects, denoted by *geom*, and the aesthetics control the information content of a plot. The appearance of non-data-related elements are controlled by the *theme system* of *ggplot2*. The range of geoms, aesthetics and themes make *ggplot2* a flexible plotting system. A plot may consist of multiple *layers*. Each layer may come from a different data set and have a different geometric object and aesthetic mapping (Wickham 2009, pp. 42ff, 2010). For instance, a histogram may be placed on a scatter plot. In addition, data may be split into subsets, and a panel of similar graphs may be used to display the subsets.

The display of subsets of data in panels is referred to as *faceting*. The plotting system enables the user to specify many details of a plot. There is no need to specify all the details because aesthetics have a default. In addition, *ggplot2* includes a function for quick plots: the `qplot` function. These different components of *ggplot2* are briefly described in this section. For details, the reader is referred to Wickham (2009) and the *ggplot2* website (http://ggplot2.org/).

The data and the mapping of data to aesthetics are specified the `ggplot` function. The data mapping is done in the `aes` argument. The mapping of data to aesthetics is controlled by scales. It determines how numerical values in the data are mapped to positions, shapes, sizes and colours. For instance, the position on the x-axis may be determined by the value of a variable or the log of the value. Discrete variables may be represented by different shapes. A continuous variable may be converted to an interval variable represented by different colours or may not be converted and represented by a colour gradient, obtained by linear interpolation of colours. Every aesthetic has a default scale. For instance, if we select colours to distinguish levels of education, default colours are selected unless a scale function is used to overwrite the default (in this case the scale function is `scale_colour_manual`). A scale function starts with `scale_`, followed by the name of the aesthetic and the name of the scale (for details, see Wickham 2009, pp. 93ff and the scale section of the *ggplot2* website http://had.co.nz/ggplot2/). Scales that control the position of an observation in the plot, i.e. the position on the x- and y-axes, are called a position scale. Shape scales control the shape of the mapping of numerical values to shapes. Scales that control the mapping of values to colour are colour scales. The colour scale may be defined manually by specifying the colours by name or hexadecimal number and using the `scale_colour_manual` function. An alternative is to select colours from a palette. Common colour palettes are rainbow, which is part of Base R, or the ColorBrewer palette provided by the RColorBrewer package in CRAN.

5.3 Basic Graphics with *ggplot2*

In this section, I uses the *ggplot2* package. The package needs to be installed, including packages it needs: *reshape*, *plyr*, *proto*, *digest*, *RColorBrewer* and *colorspace*. Suppose we want to determine whether men and women of different birth cohorts enter the labour market at different ages. The IDs of the subjects are shown on the x-axis, and the age at labour market entry is shown on the y-axis. Cohorts are represented by colours and sexes by shapes. The function `TransitionAB` may be used to select the ages at labour market entry (NJ transition) from the *Biograph* object. The ages at labour market entry are also included in the GLHS data (GLHS$LMentry; age in CMC). The scatter plot is shown in Fig. 5.1. It is produced by the `qplot` (*q*uick plot) function of the *ggplot2* package. The code is:

5.3 Basic Graphics with *ggplot2*

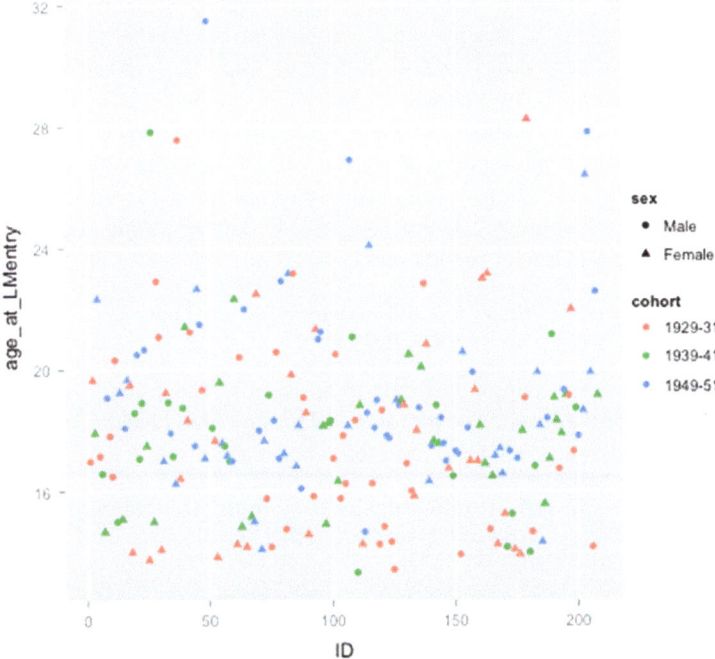

Fig. 5.1 Scatter plot of ages at labour market entry, by birth cohort and sex. GLHS

```
z <- TransitionAB (Bdata=GLHS,"NJ")
GLHS$age_at_LMentry <- z$age
qplot(ID,
      age_at_LMentry,
      data=GLHS,
      colour=cohort,
      shape=sex)
```

The youngest age at labour market entry is 13 years and the highest is 31 years. Visual inspection of the scatter plot does not reveal a significant effect of birth cohort and sex. To display the number of labour market entries by cohort and sex, use table(GLHS$cohort,GLHS$sex).

Instead of using the quick plot facility, the plot may be constructed layer by layer. A layer has five components. The first is the data, in this case age at labour market entry. The second is the set of aesthetic mappings, which describe how variables in the data are mapped to aesthetic properties of the layer: position in the coordinate system, shape, size and colour. The position is determined by the x-axis and the y-axis. In this case, subject identification number ID is displayed on the x-axis and age at labour market entry (LMentry) is displayed on the y-axis. In other words, x-position is mapped to ID and y-position to age at labour market entry. The aes function of *ggplot2* describes the mapping of data to aesthetics. The third component is the geometric used to draw the layer. In ggplot2 point, line, histogram and bar chart are geometric objects. A geometric object describes the type of object used to display the data. The object is denoted by geom. The geometric object to display points is geom_point, and the object to display a bar chart is geom_bar. In principle, histograms are for continuous variables and bars for discrete variables (Wickham 2009, p. 14). The following code produces a scatter plot of ages at labour market entry:

```
p <- ggplot (GLHS,aes(x=ID,y=z$age))
pp <- p + geom_point ()
```

The first line is the mapping of data to aesthetics. The second line specifies a layer and displays the result. The plot is saved as a graphic object (pp). To display Fig. 5.1, we need to add colour to represent cohort and a shape to represent sex:

```
p <- ggplot (GLHS,aes(x=ID,y=age_at_LMentry,
         colour=cohort,shape=sex))
p + gcom_point ()
```

The plot uses the default mappings of data into aesthetic. The default can be overwritten by specifying the aesthetic in the layer. The following code replaces the default colours by dark red, dark green and purple:

```
colours=c("1929-31"="darkred",
         "1939-41"="darkgreen","1949-51"="purple")
p + geom_point (aes(colour=cohort))
            +scale_colour_manual(values=colours)
```

To see whether gender differences by cohort vary with education, two education levels are derived from years of education. The first level is lower secondary education or less (years of education less than or equal to 11). The second level is middle school or higher. The following code produces two scatter diagrams of ages at labour market entry by birth cohort and sex, one for subjects with lower secondary education or less and one for subjects with middle school or higher. The first plot is produced by the quick plot function qplot, the second by constructing the plot layer by layer using the ggplot function. The quick plot is produced by the code:

```
GLHS.e <- GLHS
GLHS.e$edu2<- factor (ifelse (GLHS$edu<=11,1,2),
              labels=c("-LowerSec","Middle+"))
qplot(ID,age_at_LMentry,
      data=GLHS.e,
      colour=cohort,
      shape=sex,
      facets=edu2~.)
```

5.3 Basic Graphics with *ggplot2*

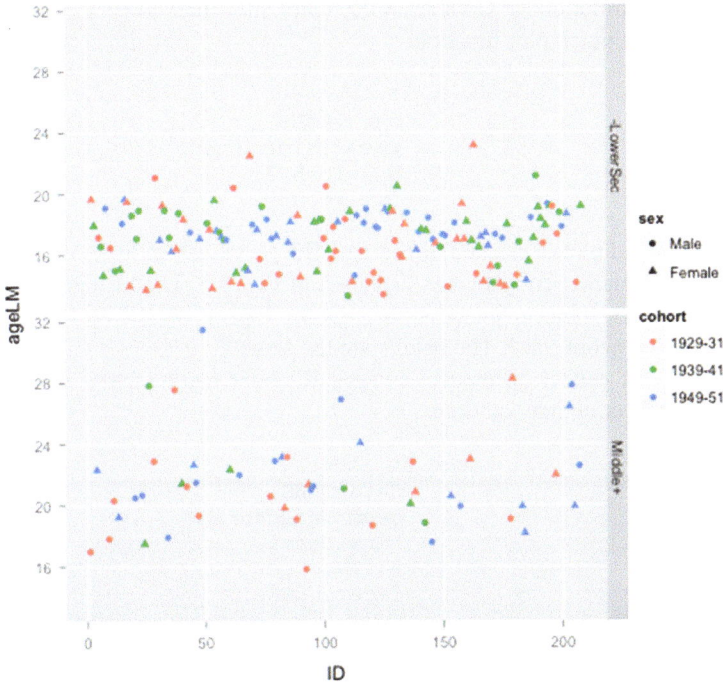

Fig. 5.2 Scatter plot of ages at labour market entry by cohort, sex and level of education. GLHS

Figure 5.2 shows the result.

The function uses faceting, which is the splitting of data into subsets and displaying the same graph for each subset.

The same plot may be produced using the ggplot function:

```
p <- ggplot (GLHS.e,
    aes(x=ID,y=age_at_LMentry,colour=cohort,shape=sex))
p + geom_point() + facet_grid(edu2~.)
```

Two types of faceting are provided in *ggplot2*: facet_grid and facet_wrap. The first produces a two-dimensional grid of panels, defined by two variables. In this case one variable (edu2) is used. The dot denotes the absence of a column variable. The second type of faceting produces a one-dimensional ribbon of panels that is wrapped into two dimensions:

```
        p + geom_point() + facet_wrap(~edu2,nrow=2)
```

The plot is not shown.

The age distribution at labour market entry may be shown in a histogram, produced by the quick plot function:

```
qplot(age_at_LMentry,
        data=GLHS,
        geom="histogram",
        binwidth=1,
        fill=cohort)
```

The command plots a stacked histogram. The plot is not shown. A histogram of ages at labour market entry by sex is shown in Fig. 5.3. The histogram is one of several geometric objects included in *ggplot2*. The geom 'histogram' may be replaced by the geom 'bar'. The results are the same.

To assess the gender differences in ages at labour market entry by cohort, the technique of faceting may be used.

```
qplot(age_at_LMentry,
        data=GLHS,
        geom="histogram",
        binwidth=1,
        fill=cohort,
        facets=sex~.)
```

The same figure may be produced using the `facet_grid` function:

```
qplot(age_at_LMentry,
        data=GLHS,geom="histogram",
        binwidth=1)
   + facet_grid(sex~.)
```

An alternative approach is to use the `ggplot` function, mapping the position on the x-axis to age at labour market entry and the filling of stacked values to cohort:

```
p2 <- ggplot (GLHS.e,
             aes(x=age_at_LMentry,fill=cohort))
p2 + geom_bar() + facet_grid(sex~.)
```

The histogram has one position aesthetic (x-axis) and a fill aesthetic. The following code plots the age at labour market entry by cohort, sex and level of education (Fig. 5.3):

```
p2 + geom_bar() + facet_grid(edu2~sex)
```

The previous two plots show information on the 201 respondents in the subsample of the GLHS. We now consider the 600 job spells and 382 episodes without a job experienced by the respondents, a total of 982 episodes. Suppose we want to compare J and N episodes and open and closed episodes. Of the job spells, 458 are closed episodes and 142 are open. Of the 382 N episodes, 122 are closed, 201 start at onset of observation and 59 are terminated at survey (censoring). Let us display

5.3 Basic Graphics with *ggplot2*

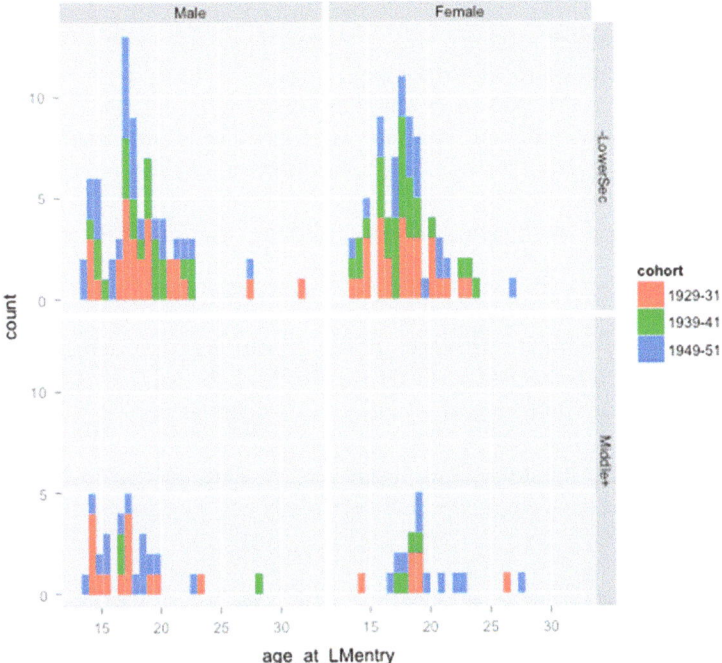

Fig. 5.3 Bar charts of age distribution at labour market entry, by sex, level of education and birth cohort. Facet grid of GLHS data

the 982 episodes, using colours and shapes to distinguish between N and J episodes and open and closed intervals. Using the theme system of *ggplot*, a few elements are added to make the visual appearance of the plot more complete and attractive for publication.

The beauty of a plot is determined by non-data-related elements, such as title, axis labels, axis tick labels, legend labels, legend key labels, grid lines, background colour and fonts in parts of the plot. The appearance of non-data-related elements is controlled by the *theme system* (Wickham 2009, Chap. 8). Themes do not affect the geoms and the aes function that maps data to aesthetics. The information content of a plot is controlled by the geom and the mapping of data in aesthetics. The beauty of the plot is controlled by the theme system. The theme system was rewritten in version 0.9.2 of *ggplot2* released in September 2012.

The theme system can be changed locally for a single plot or globally for all future plots. In earlier versions of *ggplot2*, the function opts would update elements of the theme locally, and the function theme_update updates the elements globally (Wickham 2009, p. 146). The function opts is deprecated, and its tasks are incorporated in the theme function. The functions theme_xx have also been deprecated (with xx blank, line, text, segment and rect). The function theme_update may be used to modify a small number of elements of the current theme. The function theme modifies a theme setting, and the function theme_set completely overwrites a theme. The command theme_get() displays the current setting of the themes.

A theme controls the appearance of a single item on the plot. The title, the legend name and the x-axis label are examples of items. For a complete list of theme elements, see the *ggplot2* website. The appearance of an element is controlled by the theme function.

To display information on the episodes, the long data format is produced first:

```
D <- Biograph.long (GLHS)
```

Recall that the attributes format.date, format.born and param must have been assigned to the data frame GLHS. To check the presence of the attribute, use str(GLHS). The object D has two components: D$Devent and D$Depisode.

For plotting the duration of each episode, or state occupied, distinguishing between open and closed episodes and between N and J episodes, D$Depisode is used:

```
DE <- D$Depisode
```

An identification number is created for each episode and the duration (time) variable is created:

```
DE$id <- 1:nrow(DE)
DE$Duration <- DE$Tstop-DE$Tstart
DE$StateOccupied <- DE$OR
DE$Status <- factor (DE$status,
            labels=c("Open","Closed"))
```

The choice of the name of the duration variable ('Duration') and the state occupied ('StateOccupied') is in anticipation of the legend in the plot. By default the variable name is used as the title of the legend. The class of the variable status is changed from numeric and continuous to factor because the shape aesthetic is applicable to discrete variables only.

The following code plots the data (982 points), using default shapes and default colours:

```
p.e <- ggplot (DE,
        aes(x=id,y=Duration,shape=Status,
        colour=StateOccupied))
p.e + geom_point()
```

Let us overwrite some defaults. The following code replaces the default shape and default colour:

5.3 Basic Graphics with *ggplot2*

```
p.e2 <- p.e +
geom_point(aes(shape=Status,colour=StateOccupied))
+ scale_shape_manual(values=c(1,19))
+ scale_colour_manual(values=c("N"="red","J"="blue"))
```

The second line specifies the aesthetics to be changed. The third and fourth lines are scale functions that control the shape and colour of the points that represent the ages at labour market entry. The shape is specified by an integer between 0 and 25. Shape 1 is a small open circle and shape 19 is a filled circle (Wickham 2009, p. 196ff). The plot shows the default legend. The title of the legend is the name of the variable, and the categories are the category names in the data. In the data ED, the name of the variable specifying the state occupied during a given episode is OR. The easiest way to change the title of the legend is to change the variable name. Let us change OR to StateOccupied, redefine the aesthetics and get a new plot:

```
p.e <- ggplot (DE,
       aes(x=id,y=Duration,shape=Status,
       colour=StateOccupied))
p.e2 <- p.e + geom_point(
       aes(shape=Status,colour=StateOccupied)) +
       scale_shape_manual(values=c(1,19)) +
scale_colour_manual(
           values=c("N"="red","J"="blue"))
p.e2
```

The result is shown in Fig. 5.4.

The default colour of background of the panel is light grey (theme_grey ()) and the gridlines are white. To get a white background with grey gridlines, use the built-in theme theme_bw ():

```
p.e2 + geom_point() + theme_bw()
```

Adding a theme to a plot overwrites the theme for a single plot.

We may add a title to the plot. For instance, the following code displays the title 'Durations of episodes' in red, with a relatively small font and left adjusted:

```
title <- "Durations of episodes in months"
p.e2 <- p.e +  labs (title=title) +
           theme(plot.title=element_text(colour="red",
           size="12",face="bold",hjust=0))
```

The plot is not shown.

Finally, the colour of the entire plot background may be changed to light blue and the border of the plot to black (not shown).

```
p.e2 + theme (
     plot.background=element_rect
         (fill="lightskyblue1",
             colour="black",size=5)) + geom_point()
```

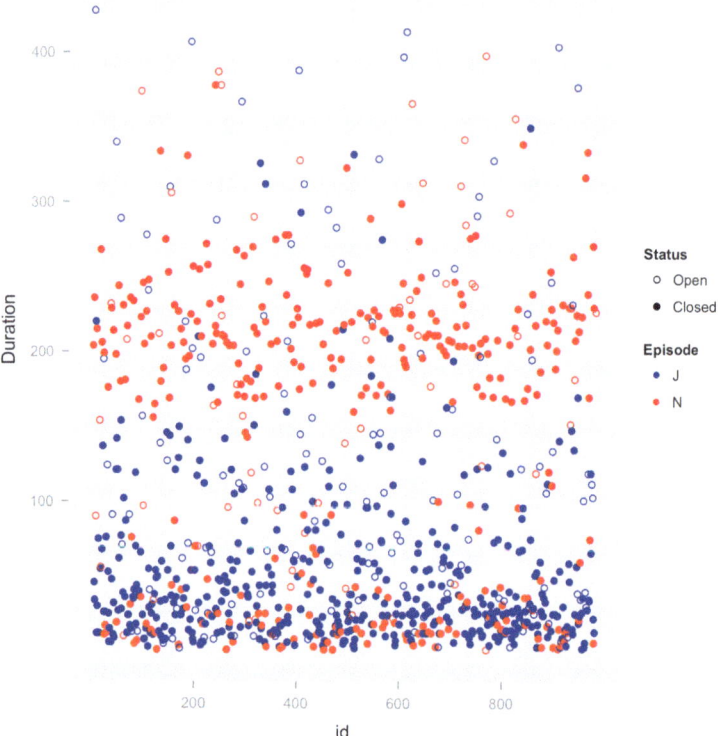

Fig. 5.4 Aesthetic mapping of lengths of episodes in months, by type of episode and state occupied. GLHS

Several of the *ggplot2* functions presented in this subsection are used in *Biograph* to graphically display characteristics of life histories.

5.4 The Lexis Diagram

The Lexis diagram represents transitions and episodes in two time scales: age and calendar time. If age and calendar time are known precisely, the date of birth can be derived. Hence the age-time diagram carries information on birth cohorts. For instance, if we know that a person marries on 20 July 2010 on his 30th birthday, we can derive that the person is born on 20 July 1980. Alternatively, if we know that a person born on 20 July 1980 marries on his 30th birthday, we can derive that the date of marriage is 20 July 2010. Two variables are sufficient to determine the third. The fact is used in drawing Lexis diagrams. It also makes the Lexis diagram an ideal graphical aid for studying how age patterns vary over time and across birth cohorts.

5.4 The Lexis Diagram

In this section Lexis diagrams are produced using functions from two packages in the Comprehensive R Archive Library (CRAN): *Epi*, developed by Carstensen (2007, 2013; see also Carstensen and Plummer 2011; Plummer and Carstensen 2011) for epidemiological and demographic analysis and *ggplot2* developed by Wickham (2009). *Biograph* includes functions to display transitions (points), episodes and state sequences (lines). It also includes functions to display in Lexis diagram event counts and exposure times for individuals, groups of selected individuals and the entire (sample) population. The event count in a given age-time interval and the exposure time during the same interval determine the transition rate during that interval. In this section, the following functions are documented:

- `Lexispoints`: displays ages and dates at transition using functions included in *Epi* package
- `Lexis.points`: displays ages and dates at transition using *ggplot2*
- `Lexislines.episodes`: draws lifelines for selected subjects using functions in *Epi* package
- `Lexis.lines`: draws lifelines for selected subjects using *pplot2*
- `LexisOccExp`: plots Lexis diagram with event counts, exposure times and transition rates by age and calendar year

In the *Epi* package, the main object is the Lexis object. A Lexis object contains the data necessary to display a single episode in a Lexis diagram: the calendar time and age at onset of the episode, the state occupied during the episode and the event marking the end of the episode. The event is a transition to another state or censoring.

Formally, the Lexis object is a data frame with a variable for each time scale and four variables with reserved names starting with lex (see Chap. 3):

(a) `per`: calendar time at start of episode.
(b) `age`: age at start of episode.
(c) `lex.dur`: length of the episode (duration of follow-up).
(d) `lex.Cst`: state occupied during the episode, also referred to as current status and entry status. It is the state in which the follow-up takes place.
(e) `lex.Xst`: exit status (eXit state), i.e. the state taken up after a transition out of lex.Cst. It is also referred to as destination state.
(f) `lex.id`: subject identification number.

Table 5.1 shows the Lexis object of the episode between birth and labour market entry for the first ten respondents in the GLHS subsample. For the computation of the Lexis object, see Chap. 3.

The episode starts at birth. The date of birth is labelled `per`. The age at birth is zero. `per` and `age` represent the entry times on each time scale. The age at labour market entry is the exit time on the age scale. It is the duration of follow-up, denoted by `lex.dur`. At the start of the episode and throughout the episode, the subject is without a job, denoted by 0 (`lex.Cst`). The exit status (`lex.Xst`) is labour market entry, denoted by 1. The last column is the subject identification number.

Table 5.1 Lexis object: data on episodes between birth and labour market entry. GLHS

	per	age	lex.dur	lex.Cst	lex.Xst	lex.id
1	1929.162	0	17.00036	0	1	1
2	1929.666	0	19.66325	0	1	2
3	1939.329	0	17.91823	0	1	3
4	1950.247	0	22.33542	0	1	4
5	1931.329	0	17.16823	0	1	5
6	1940.915	0	16.58070	0	1	6
7	1939.581	0	14.66618	0	1	7
8	1950.666	0	19.08225	0	1	8
9	1931.329	0	17.83323	0	1	9
10	1931.748	0	16.50105	0	1	10

Biograph includes two functions to draw a Lexis diagram: Lexispoints and Lexis.points. First consider Lexispoints. The function uses functions from the *Epi* package. The code

```
data (CLHS)
require (Epi)
z <- Lexispoints (Bdata=GLHS,transition="NJ")
```

creates a Lexis object and draws the Lexis diagram showing ages at labour market entry (transition 'NJ'). The output z contains the Lexis object, augmented by the variables in the GLHS data. The ages may be differentiated by one covariate. In the *Biograph* versions available today, only a single covariate may be used. The values of the covariate are identified by colour. Figure 5.5 shows ages and dates of labour market entry by sex. It is produced by the following code:

```
z <- Lexispoints (Bdata=GLHS,
            transition="NJ",
            title="Calendar time and age at labour
                    market entry",
            cov="sex",
            legend="topleft")
```

The legend is positioned in the top left corner.

To plot the ages and dates at exit from the first job (first JN transition), the code is:

```
z <- Lexispoints (Bdata=GLHS,
        transition="JN",
        title="Calendar time and age at exit from first
                job",
        cov="sex",
        legend="topleft")
```

The figure is not shown. A total of 134 respondents experience the event, and 67 are still in their first job at survey date.

5.4 The Lexis Diagram

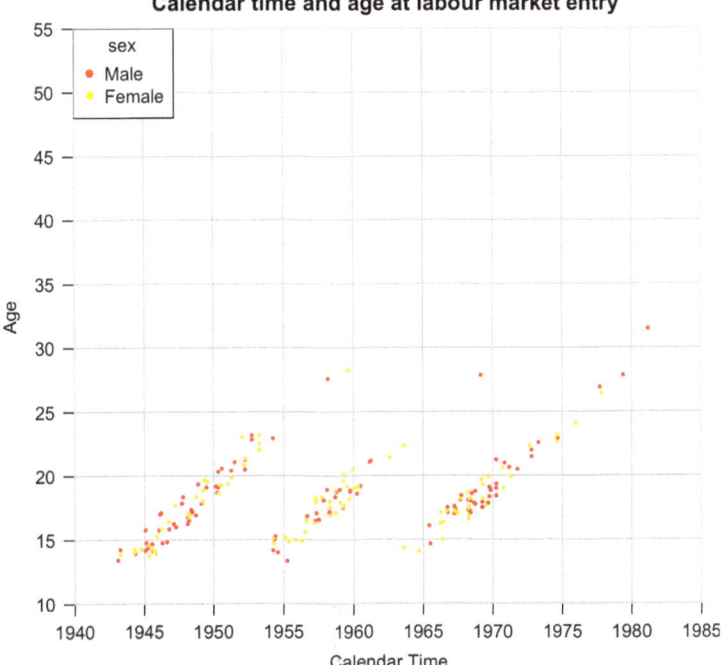

Fig. 5.5 Lexis diagram: scatter plot of calendar years and ages at labour market entry by sex. GLHS

The following call uses the Lexis.points function to display labour market entry by sex and birth cohort. Sex is the covariate and cohort is the group variable. The function uses the *ggplot2* package.

```
library (ggplot2)
z <- Lexis.points (Bdata=GLHS,
    transition="NJ",
    title="Labour market entry by sex and cohort",
    cov="sex",
    group="cohort",
    legend.pos=c(0.9,0.95),
    pdf=FALSE)
```

The legend is positioned in the top right corner. The option to save the plot in a PDF file is not used. The plot is shown in Fig. 5.6.

Now we turn to `Lexislines.episodes` and `Lexis.lines`. Figure 5.7 shows for five subjects the lifelines with the transitions marked. Subject with ID 46 is born in 1951, enters the labour market in 1972 at age 21, leaves the first job in 1975 at age 24 and gets another job in 1979 at age 28. The observation is censored in 1981 (c). The plot is produced by the function `Lexislines.episodes` and the following commands:

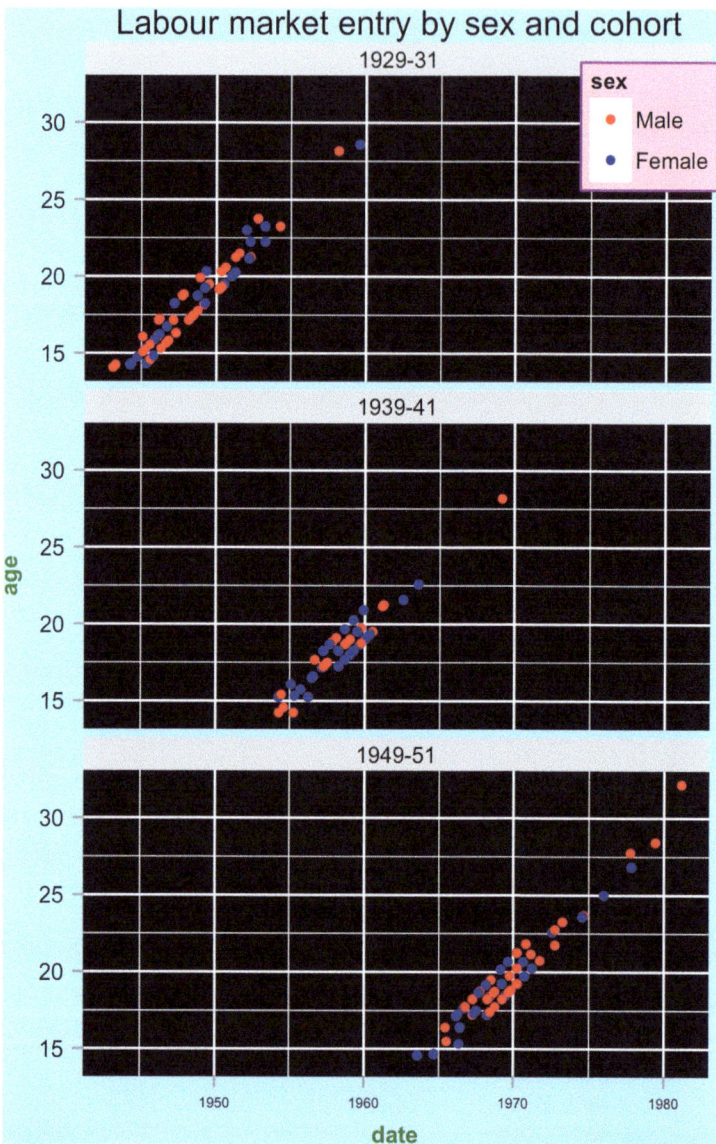

Fig. 5.6 Lexis diagram: scatter plot of calendar years and ages at labour market entry by birth cohort and sex. GLHS

```
subjectsID <- c(1,19,46,208)
title1 <- "Lifelines for selection of respondents. GLHS"
D <- Biograph.long (Bdata=GLHS)
z <- Lexislines.episodes
            (GLHS,D$Depisode,subjectsID,title1)
```

5.4 The Lexis Diagram

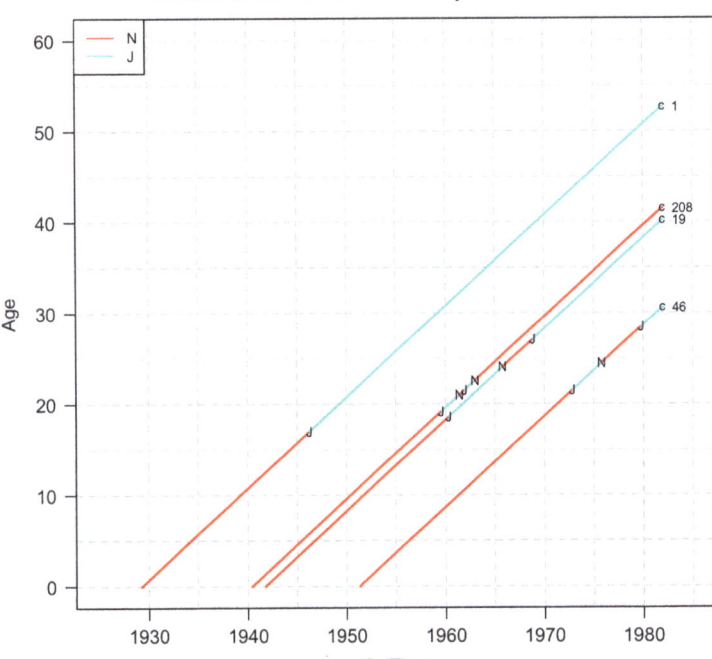

Fig. 5.7 Lexis diagram: employment careers of selected GLHS respondents. Display A, using *Epi* package

The function Lexislines.episodes requires episode data (long format). The function returns the object z$Loc, which is the Lexis object for the subjects selected. The Lexis object is augmented by the raw data (GLHS).

The employment careers for individuals with ID 1, 19, 46 and 208 are displayed. The data for these subjects are obtained by:

```
D$Depisode[D$Depisode$ID %in% c(1,19,46,208),]
```

The Lexis.lines function uses *ggplot2*. It requires data in long format too. In addition, it requires data in decimal calendar years. The following code produces the plot (Fig. 5.8).

```
GLHS.yr <- date_b(Bdata=GLHS,
          selectday=1,format.out="year")
D <- Biograph.long (GLHS.yr)
subjects <- c(1,78,120,208)
z <- Lexis.lines (Bdata=GLHS.yr,
          Dlong=D$Depisode,
          subjectsID = subjects,
          title = " ")
```

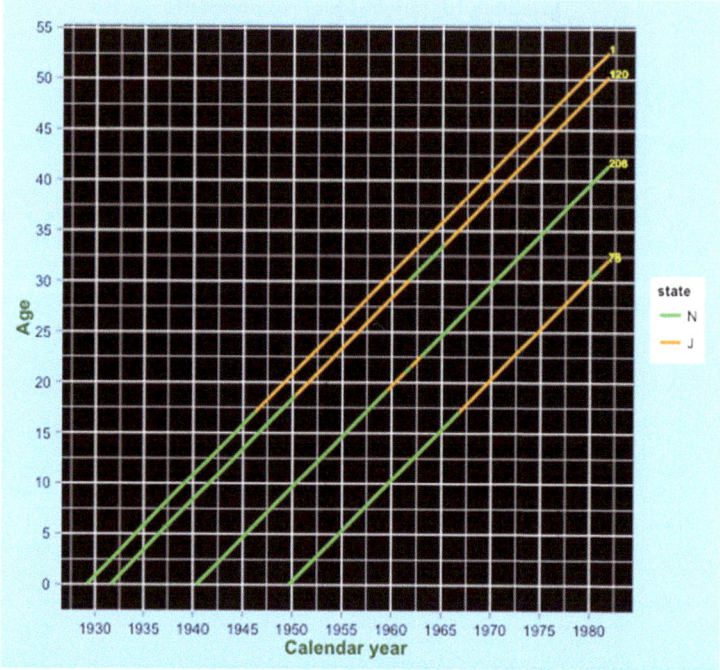

Fig. 5.8 Lexis diagram: employment careers of selected GLHS respondents. Display B, using *ggplot2* package

The function LexisOccExp draws a Lexis diagram with transition counts, exposure times and transition rates for age groups with an interval provided by the user. The interval variable is generally equal to 1 or 5. Consider the transition from Job to NoJob. The transition is denoted by JN. A transition occurs when a respondent leaves his or her job for a period or non-employment. A person is exposed to the risk of the transition when employed. It starts after entry into employment.[2] Some periods of exposure end in the JN transition, while other periods end at survey date. We are interested in plotting in the Lexis diagram transition counts, exposure time and transition rates. The counts, exposures and rates are plotted by 5-year age groups and calendar periods of 5 years. The following command draws the Lexis diagrams:

```
w <- LexisOccExp (Bdata=GLHS,transition= "JN",
                    nyear=5)
```

The function produces three Lexis diagrams, one each for counts, exposures and rates (Fig. 5.9). After each plot, the user needs to press the return key. The function

---

[2] For an exposition of the measurement of risk periods in multistate models, see Beyersmann et al. (2012, p. 175).

5.4 The Lexis Diagram

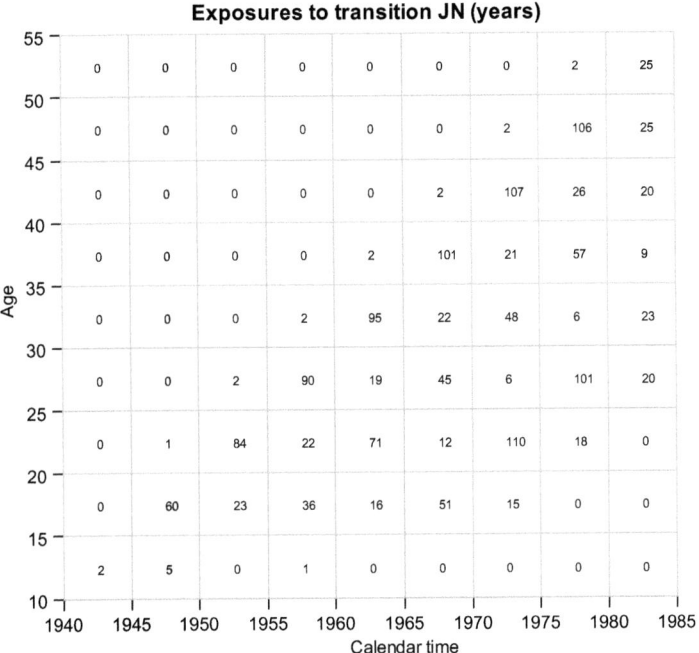

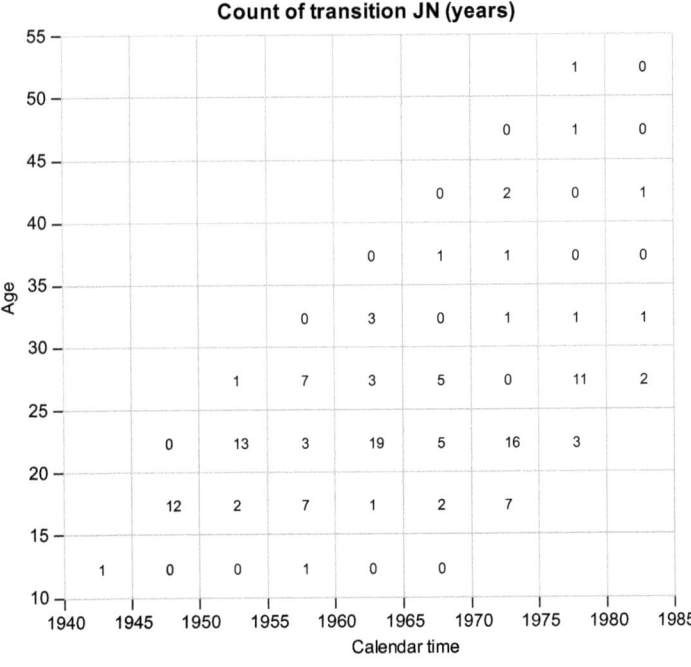

Fig. 9 (continued)

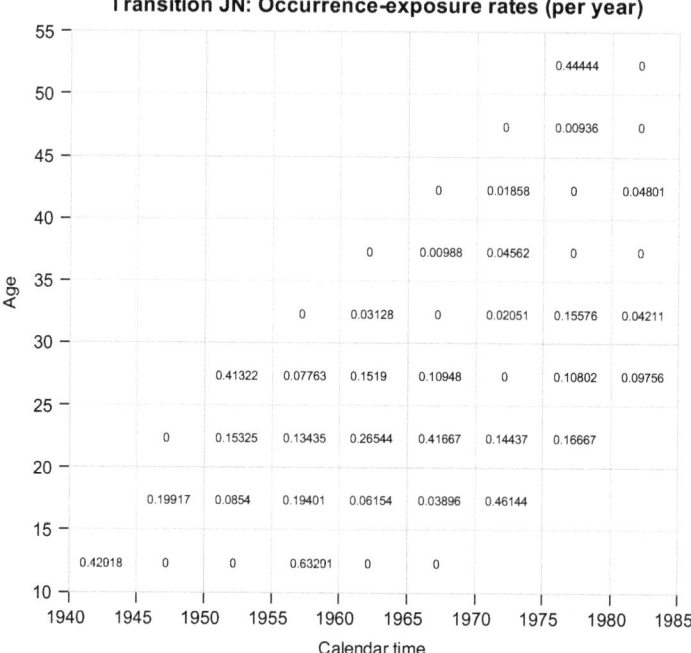

Fig. 5.9 Lexis diagram: job exits and exposure times by calendar period and age: exposure times, transition counts and occurrence-exposure rates. GLHS

uses the par function of R to set the graphical parameter that tells the function to pause until you hit a key:

$$par\ (ask=TRUE)$$

This function requires an input from the user before a new figure is drawn. The LexisOccExp function displays three Lexis diagrams and returns the following objects:

(a) w$surv: the survival object which shows for each respondent and for the first job episode, the starting date of the episode (in this illustration the date of labour market entry), the ending date (the date of the first job exit) and the type of exit (event or censoring).
(b) w$Lcoh: the Lexis object.
(c) w$nevents: the number of transitions by calendar period and age group.
(d) w$ndur: the exposure time by calendar period and age group.
(e) w$rates: the transition rates by calendar period and age group. The transition rates (occurrence-exposure rates) are obtained by dividing transition counts by the durations of exposure.

5.4 The Lexis Diagram

The function `LexisOccExp` uses a particularly useful function of the *Epi* package, the `splitLexis` function. This function divides each interval into disjoint subintervals according to breakpoints supplied by you. As a consequence, each row of the Lexis object is split in several rows, one for each subinterval. Event counts and exposure times may be determined for subintervals. What follows is a technical description that may be skipped. Consider the first job episodes and let `Lcoh` denote the Lexis object. Calendar time varies from 1930 (`PerLow`) to 1985 (`PerHigh`), and age varies from 0 (`AgeLow`) to 60 (`AgeHigh`). The following functions divide the job episodes in intervals of length `nyear`, which in this case is equal to 5. The first function generates intervals along the calendar time axis. The second function adds age intervals.

```
Lcoh <- w$Lcoh
PerLow <- 1930
PerHigh <- 1985
AgeLow <- 0
AgeHigh <- 60
nyear <- 5
Lcoh_tr1_p <- splitLexis(Lcoh,
            breaks=seq(PerLow,PerHigh,nyear),
            time.scale="CalTime" )
Lcoh_tr1_ap <- splitLexis(Lcoh_tr1_p,
            breaks=seq(AgeLow,AgeHigh,nyear),
            time.scale="Age" )
```

where p refers to period and ap to age-period. The breakpoints are 1940, 1945, ..., 1985 and ages 0, 5, ..., 60. The Lexis object `Lcoh` is produced internally in `LexisOccExp`. The ages and the calendar times at the start of the intervals are obtained by the following expressions:

```
Lcoh_tr1_ap$AGE <- timeBand(Lcoh_tr1_ap,"Age","left")
Lcoh_tr1_ap$PER <- timeBand(Lcoh_tr1_ap,"CalTime","left")
```

The number of transitions in each age-period interval from a job to a period without a job is given by

```
nevents <- tapply (status(Lcoh_tr1_ap,"exit")==1,
          list(Lcoh_tr1_ap$AGE,Lcoh_tr1_ap$PER),sum)
```

and the exposure time, i.e. the duration of the job episode, by

```
ndur <- round(tapply (dur(Lcoh_tr1_ap),
          list(Lcoh_tr1_ap$AGE,Lcoh_tr1_ap$PER),sum),2)
```

The sum of the transitions should be equal to 134, the number of persons who experienced the JN transition. The sum is `sum(nevents,na.rm=TRUE)`. The total sojourn time in the first job episode should be 2095.6.

5.5 State Distribution and State Sequences

The subject of this section is to show how to plot state occupancies of the sample population at different ages. A person who is employed (J) at interview started out at age 0 without a job (N) and may have switched between states N and J several times. The state distribution plot displays the collective history of the sample population up to the highest age (54 in this case). Individuals who are not 54 yet at interview occupy the fictitious state 'being censored' between the age at interview and 54. Methods are presented to display state distributions. The first uses the *ggplot2* package, and the second uses the *TraMineR* package. The *TraMineR* package includes a number of useful functions to display life history data.

In Chap. 4 the `plot.occup.S` function was used to display the state occupancies by age. The function makes use of the *ggplot2* package. Figure 4.2 is produced by the code

```
occup <- Occup(GLHS)
z<- plot (x=occup$state occup,
      namstates.desired=c("N","J","Censored"),
      colours=c("red","green","lightgrey"),
      title="States occupancies. GLHS",
      area=TRUE,
      xmin=10,
      xmax=55)
```

The arguments of the function are:

(a) The object `occup$state_occup` contains the state occupancies in the sample population. The object is of class 'occup.S'.
(b) `namstates.desired` is a list of states in a desired sequence. 'Being censored' is treated as a state. A person who is 35 at interview spends 19 years in the state of being censored (between 35 and the highest age 53; note that for plotting 55 is used).
(c) `colours` is the vector of colours representing the states. The last element is the colour of the background of the panel.
(d) `area` is a logical variable. If area is TRUE, then an area plot is displayed (using geom_area of *ggplot2*). If area is FALSE, a bar plot is displayed (using geom_bar of *ggplot2*).
(e) `xmin` and `xmax` are the minimum and maximum ages shown on the x-axis (55 is used instead of 53).

The output of the function is an object with two components. The first contains the state occupancies. The second component is the plot. To display the plot, use z $plot.

The function `seqplot` of the *TraMineR* package displays state occupancies. To use the function, a sequence object needs to be prepared first. The `seqdef` function creates a sequence object in a format accepted by the plotting function of *TraMineR*. *Biograph* produces a sequence object too. The object occup

5.5 State Distribution and State Sequences

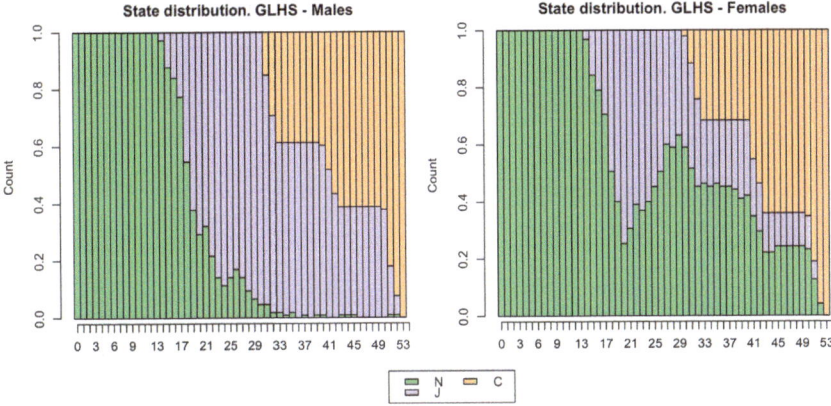

Fig. 5.10 State occupancies by age and sex, using *TraMineR*. GLHS

$st_age_1 shows, for each individual under observation, the state occupied at each birthday during the period of observation. It is a matrix with for each individual (row) the state occupied at exact ages 0–53 (column). *TraMineR* requires that the matrix is converted to a character string, with each state separated by a separator. The *TraMineR* function seqconc may be used for that purpose. The function seqdef creates a state sequence object. The following code produces a state sequence object starting from the raw GLHS data. The time scale is age and the time unit is year.

```
occup <- Occup(GLHS)
require(TraMineR)
DTraMineR <- seqconc (occup$st_age_1,sep="-")
namst <- c(Parameters(GLHS)$namstates,"Censored")
D.seq <- seqdef (DTraMineR,states=namst)
```

with states the short state labels.

The state distribution plot by sex is produced by the code (with group variable sex):

```
seqplot(D.seq, type="d",
title="State distribution. GLHS",
ylab="Count",
xtlab=0:54,
group=GLHS$sex)
```

Figure 5.10 shows the result. The figure clearly illustrates the age pattern of labour force participation of women in the GLHS cohorts. Around age 20, women start leaving jobs. The decline of women without jobs, starting at age 30, is due to the censoring of observations (C).

The function seqiplot plots individual sequences. The following function plots the sequences for subjects with ID 1, 20 and 208 (figure not shown):

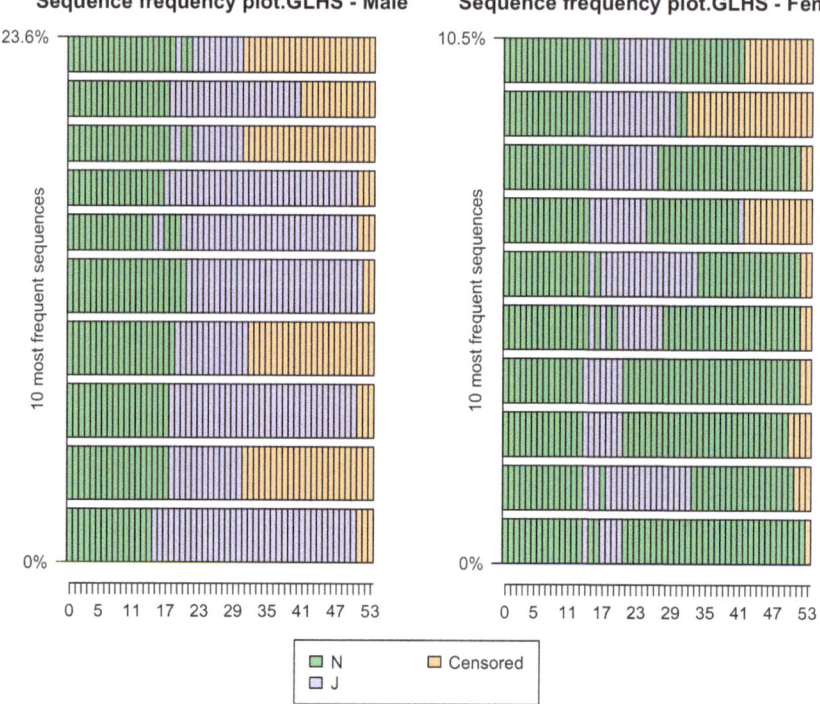

Fig. 5.11 Frequency plot of state sequences, by sex, using *TraMineR*. GLHS

```
seqiplot(D.seq,tlim= GLHS$ID%in%c(1,20,208))
```

The following statement produces a sequence frequency plot, displaying the ten most frequent state sequences for males and females:

```
n <- 10
seqfplot(D.seq,
    group=GLHS$sex,
    tlim=1:n,
    title="Sequence frequency plot.GLHS",
    xtlab=c(0:54),
    ltext=c("N","J","Censored"),
    las=1,
    ylab=paste(n,
        " most frequent sequences (%)",sep="") )
```

The result is shown in Fig. 5.11. Clearly, women have more differentiated employment careers than men. *TraMineR* requires that, if a covariate is a numeric variable, it is converted to a factor variable:

```
GLHS$sex <- factor (GLHS$sex,labels=c("Male","Female"))
```

5.6 Conclusion

One of the strengths of the R computing environment is graphics. R is rich with utilities for creating and developing interesting graphics. Some of the utilities are illustrated in this chapter. It represents first steps towards visualisation of life history data. Effective graphical displays of the complex information in life history data remain a major challenge. Effective visualisation requires adequate conceptualisation of the life course and mapping of life history data to objects displayed in a graphic and their aesthetic attributes. The Lexis diagram (two dimensions) and its extension to the Lexis surface (three dimensions) are a good point of departure. The display of life history data in two time scales, usually age and calendar time or age and birth cohort, may reveal patterns that are difficult to detect otherwise. In the diagram, intercohort variation of life histories become manifest, and effects of age, calendar period and cohort can be revealed relatively easily.

Chapter 6
Statistical Packages for Multistate Life History Analysis

6.1 Introduction

The Comprehensive R Archive Network (CRAN) (http://cran.r-project.org/) has a number of statistical packages for multistate analysis of event histories (multistate survival analysis). These packages focus on statistical inference, i.e. the estimation of transition rates and transition probabilities from empirical data. In this Chapter, the following packages are covered: *survival* by Therneau and Lumley, *eha* by Broström, *mvna* and *etm* by Allignol et al., *mstate* by Putter et al. and *msm* by Jackson. For an up-to-date overview of packages for survival analysis, the reader is referred to the CRAN Task View on Survival Analysis, maintained by Allignol and Latouche. The Task View has a section on multistate models. For a review of methods for estimating multistate models, the reader is referred to Chap. 2 and, for a more extensive treatment, to Aalen et al. (2008, in particular Chap. 3), Beyersmann et al. (2012), and a special issue of the *Journal of Statistical Software* (January 2011), edited by Putter. For recent advances in demography, see Willekens and Putter (2014). Mills (2011) offers a brief introduction to multistate models using R. In essence, the method consists of counting transitions (events) and numbers of persons at risk of a transition just before the transition occurs or in the observation interval. The chapter consists of five sections, in addition to the introduction. Section 6.2 describes the *survival* package, Sect. 6.3 the *eha* package, Sect. 6.4 the *mvna* and *etm* packages, Sect. 6.5 the *mstate* package and Sect. 6.6 the *msm* package.

6.2 The *Survival* Package

The *survival* package was developed in S by Therneau (1999), ported to R by Lumley (2004) and maintained by Therneau (2014). It is a general package for survival analysis with an emphasis on the Cox model. It considers right censoring and left truncation. The core object in the package is the survival object. The object is described in the first subsection. The object is usually used as the response variable in survival models such as the Cox model. By way of illustration, I present the Kaplan-Meier estimation, the exponential transition rate model and the Cox model. These models are covered by Blossfeld and Rohwer (2002) and I compare the output of the *survival* package with the output of the TDA package published by Blossfeld and Rohwer. For an introduction to these models using R, see Mills (2011).

6.2.1 The Survival Object

The survival object documents individual risk periods by starting time, ending time and reason for ending. The object is created by the function Surv. It uses three variables: Tstart, Tstop and status. Tstart is the starting date of an episode, Tstop is the ending date and status is the reason for ending, the occurrence of the transition of interest or censoring. The presence of Tstart indicates that observations on episodes are left truncated. If Tstart is zero for all episodes or the original time scale does not need to be conserved, only two variables are required: time and status. Tstop is replaced by the duration variable time. Consider the first respondent in the GLHS data. The person, a male, enters his first job at CMC 555. He did not leave that job before survey date, which is CMC 983. The function call Surv(555,983,0) produces the survival object: (555,983+], where the first element in the brackets is the starting time of the episode and the second element the ending time. The *survival* package and R assume that intervals are open on the left and closed on the right. A+ refers to an interval that ends because the observation is terminated (censoring). The episode is an open episode. When the + is absent, the interval ends because the event of interest occurs. The episode is a closed episode. The second respondent, a female, enters her first job at CMC 593. At CMC 639 she moves on to another job. The survival object, which is produced by Surv(593,639,1), is (593,639].

The function Biograph.long converts data in *Biograph* format to a counting process data structure that includes the Tstart, Tstop and status variables. The data format is a long format with one record for each risk period or episode. Covariates are copied from the original data set. The function was documented in Chap. 3:

```
D <- Biograph.long (GLHS)
```

The data frame D$Depisode can be used as input for the *survival* package. It has 982 rows (intrastate transitions not removed). Each record pertains to an episode. There are 600 job episodes and 382 episodes without a job. For illustration the 600 job episodes, which are analysed by Blossfeld and Rohwer (2002), are selected. The data are obtained by the following command:

6.2 The *Survival* Package

```
DJ600 <- subset (D$Depisode,D$Depisode$OR=="J")
```

or

```
DJ600 <- D$Depisode[D$Depisode$OR=="J",]
```

The object DJ600 has 600 rows, one for each job episode. There are 348 males and 252 females. These figures can be obtained by table (DJ600$sex) or length(DJ600$ID[DJ600$sex=="Male"]) and length(DJ600$ID [DJ600$sex=="Female"]). There are 458 closed job episodes and 142 open episodes. Job episodes end in (1) another job, (2) NoJob or (3) censoring.

To enable comparison with Blossfeld and Rohwer (2002), the variable time is computed and four attributes of job episodes are added to the data file DJ600. They are: the line number of job episode (NOJ), the prestige of the current job (pres), the prestige of the next job (presn) and the labour market experience (LFX).

```
DJ600$time <- DJ600$Tstop-DJ600$Tstart
data(rrdat) # the data are included in the Biograph
                package
rrdat <- data.frame(rrdat)
DJ600$pres <- rrdat[,10]
DJ600$NOJ <- rrdat[,2]
DJ600$LFX <- DJ600$Tstart-DJ600$LMentry
DJ600$PNOJ <- DJ600$NOJ-1
```

The following code produces the survival object:

```
require (survival)
surv  <- Surv(DJ600$Tstart,DJ600$Tstop,DJ600$status)
surv2 <- with(DJ600, Surv(Tstart,Tstop,status))
```

The survival object is the dependent (response) variable in survival models such as the Kaplan-Meier estimation (function survfit), the transition rate model (function survreg) and the Cox model (function coxph). These models are considered next.

6.2.2 Kaplan-Meier Estimator

The Kaplan-Meier estimation of the survivor function is obtained by the code:

```
KM <- survfit (Surv(time,status)~sex,
        data=DJ600)
```

Fig. 6.1 Kaplan-Meier estimator of job duration, by sex. GLHS

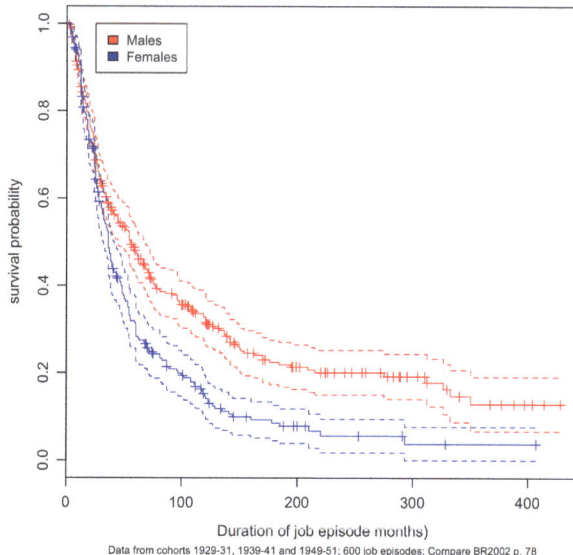

The empirical survival function by sex is given by summary(KM). Figure 6.1 contains the plot of the survivor functions for men and women with 95 % confidence intervals. The plot has been generated with the following code:

```
plot(KM,
     conf.int=TRUE,
     xlab="Duration of job episode months)",
     ylab="survival probability",
     col=c("red","blue"),
     sub="Data from cohorts 1929-31, 1939-41 and 1949-51;
     600 job episodes; Compare BR2002 p. 78",
     cex.sub=0.7)
legend(300/12,1,
     c("Males","Females"),
     col=c("red","blue"),
     fill=c("red","blue"),
     cex=0.9,
     bg="white",
     mark.time=FALSE)
```

The plot is the same as shown by Blossfeld and Rohwer (2002, p. 78).

6.2.3 Exponential Transition Rate Model

The exponential transition rate model predicts the job exit rate. It is one of the parametric transition models reviewed by Blossfeld and Rohwer (2002). It can be estimated in R using the survreg function of the *survival* package:

6.2 The *Survival* Package

```
z <- survreg (formula=Surv(time,status) ~ 1,
              data=DJ600,
              dist="exponential")
```

where time = DJ600$Tstop − DJ600$Tstart. For an introduction to the exponential transition rate model using R, see Mills (2011, pp. 125ff).

The regression coefficient is estimated at 4.488636. The job exit rate is exp $(-4.488636) = 0.0112$ per month. The estimate is the same as the one obtained by Blossfeld and Rohwer, but in Blossfeld and Rohwer (2002, p. 93) the regression coefficient has the opposite sign. When comparing the output of the survival package with the output of TDA and published in Blossfled and Rohwer, note that the regression coefficients in the survival package measure the effects on the duration of the episode (survival time), whereas in TDA the regression coefficients measure the effects on the transition rate. Since the expected duration is one over the transition rate, the regression coefficients are minus the coefficients produced by TDA.

The expected duration of an episode is one over the transition rate. That explains the opposite sign since $\exp(-a)$ is $1/\exp(a)$. The expected (predicted) duration of a job episode is 89 months with a standard deviation of 4.16 years. This result is obtained by the code

```
zp <- predict (z,se.fit=TRUE)
```

Covariates are easily introduced, e.g.

```
zs <- survreg (Surv(time, status) ~ as.factor(sex),
               data=DJ600,
               dist="exponential")
```

with sex as a categorical variable. The first category (male) is the reference category.

The result is obtained with summary(zs) (see Box 6.1). The antilogarithm of the regression coefficient is known as the *alpha effect*.

Box 6.1: Basic Exponential Transition Rate Model with Covariate Sex. GLHS

```
survreg(formula = Surv(time, status) ~ as.factor(sex), data = D,
    dist = "exponential")
                Value Std. Error      z         p
(Intercept)     4.715    0.0639   73.81  0.00e+00
as.factor(sex)2 -0.573   0.0937   -6.11  9.76e-10

Scale fixed at 1

Exponential distribution
Loglik(model)= -2495.6   Loglik(intercept only)= -2513.8
        Chisq= 36.4 on 1 degrees of freedom, p= 1.6e-09
Number of Newton-Raphson Iterations: 5
n= 600
```

The job exit rate for males is exp(−4.715) = 0.00896 and it is exp(−(4.715−0.573)) = 0.01589 for females. Females leave their job at a rate that is 77 % higher than that of males [100*(exp(0.573)−1) = 77.4 %]. When we add the birth cohort as a covariate and control for the cohort effect, females leave their job at a rate that is 65 % higher than that of males [100*(exp(0.507)−1) = 65.0 %]. The difference is due to the distribution of females over cohorts. Females are a little better represented in cohorts that change jobs more often. Cohorts 1939–1941 and 1949–1951 have a rate of leaving a job that is more than twice that of the cohort 1929–1931. The proportion of females in the birth cohort 1929–1931 is 41.6 %; it is 42.2 % in the two mobile cohorts combined. As a result, part of the greater mobility of females relative to males can be attributed to the share of females in the mobile cohorts. The possible effects of cohort differences in the mobility of females relative to males are not considered. That requires interaction effects. The exponential model with two covariates (sex and cohort) is

```
EM <- survreg (Surv(time, status) ~
                    as.factor(sex)+as.factor(cohort),
                    data=DJ600,
                    dist="exponential")
```

The regression coefficients and their standard errors are shown in Box 6.2.

Box 6.2: Basic Exponential Model with Covariates Sex and Birth Cohort. GLHS

```
                         Value Std. Error     z         p
(Intercept)              5.011     0.0843 59.45  0.00e+00
as.factor(sex)2         -0.507     0.0943 -5.37  7.68e-08
as.factor(cohort)1939-41 -0.534    0.1120 -4.76  1.90e-06
as.factor(cohort)1949-51 -0.674    0.1152 -5.85  4.95e-09
```

Consider the full exponential model, discussed by Blossfeld and Rohwer (2002, p. 98). The model is:

```
EM_full <- survreg (Surv(time,status) ~
                    +edu+cohort+LFX+PNOJ+pres,
                    data=DJ600,
                    dist="exponential")
```

The regression coefficients of the full model are listed in Box 6.3.[1] The results are produced by `summary(EM_full)`.

---

[1] The variables NOJ and pres are taken from the original data file `rrdat`. Their values are suppressed in the wide data format.

Box 6.3: Basic Exponential Model with Several Covariates (Full Model). GLHS

```
                          Value Std. Error     z         p
(Intercept)             4.48818   0.279523 16.06  5.14e-58
edu                    -0.07721   0.024708 -3.12  1.78e-03
as.factor(cohort)1939-41 -0.60793 0.113548 -5.35  8.61e-08
as.factor(cohort)1949-51 -0.61222 0.118542 -5.16  2.41e-07
LFX                     0.00317   0.000937  3.38  7.23e-04
PNOJ                   -0.05958   0.044129 -1.35  1.77e-01
pres                    0.02802   0.005530  5.07  4.02e-07
```

The effect of an additional year of schooling on the exit rate is an increase with 8.04 %. The expression is `100*(exp(-EM_full$coefficient[2])-1)`. Three additional years of schooling increases the exit rate by 26.1 %:

```
100*(exp(-3 * EM_full$coefficient[2])-1)
```

The job exit rate for those with the highest education (edu = 19) is:

```
100*(exp(-(max(DJ600$edu)-min(DJ600$edu)) *
       EM_full$coefficient[2])-1)
```

It is 116.4 % higher than that of persons with the lowest education (edu = 9).

The basic exponential model may be used as a predictive model, i.e. to predict the job duration for a person with a given set of characteristics. For instance, the model predicts that an individual born in 1929–1931, with 13 years of education, just entering the labour force (LFX = 0 and PNOJ = 0) into a job with prestige level pres = 60 has an exit rate of r = exp(−4.4894 + 0.07721 * 13−0.02802 * 60) = 0.0057. The mean job duration is 1/0.0057 = 175 months or 15 years. The median job duration is 121 months. The median is the duration at which 50 % has left the job. It is derived from the survival function 0.50 = exp(−0.0057 * t); hence, t = −ln(0.50)/0.0057.

The `survreg` function incorporates several parametric waiting time distributions in addition to the exponential distribution. It does not support time-dependent covariates. It does not support left truncation either. It supports only time = Tstop − Tstart data. The `coxph` function of the *survival* package, however, can handle data that are left truncated and right censored. It can be used to fit any transition of a multistate model.

6.2.4 The Cox Model

The Cox proportional hazard model with job duration as the time variable and a single covariate (sex) is:

```
Cox_s <- coxph(Surv(time,status) ~ sex,
               data=DJ600,
               method="breslow")
```

where `time = Tstop - Tstart`. The result is shown in Box 6.4.

Box 6.4: Cox Proportional Hazard Model. GLHS

```
             coef  exp(coef)  se(coef)     z       p
sexFemales  0.424      1.53    0.0948   4.47  7.6e-06

Likelihood ratio test=19.7  on 1 df, p=8.99e-06   n= 600
```

The variable sex is a categorical variable. By default the first category (males) is the reference category. The dependent variable in the Cox model is the transition rate, in this case the job exit rate. Hence, there is no difference in the sign of the regression coefficients between the *survival* package and TDA. The result indicates that, if the gender effect does not vary with job duration, females leave their job at a rate that is 53 % higher than the job exit rate of males. The `exp(coef)` is the ratio of the job exit rate of females and males (reference category). In other words, it is the job exit rate of females relative to that of males. The ratio of two hazard rates is known as the risk ratio or the hazard ratio. For a thorough discussion of the Cox model, see Therneau and Grambsch (2000). The rate of job exit may vary with job duration, but in the Cox model duration dependence is left unspecified. The proportional hazard model assumes that the effects of the covariates on the transition rate are the same for all durations. How the transition rates vary with duration is beyond the scope of the proportional hazard regression model. The duration dependence is captured in the baseline hazard.

In many applications, such as the prediction of the probability of leaving a job in a given interval or the expected length of a job episode, hazard rates are used. The cumulative baseline hazard rates associated with the Cox model `Cox_s` are produced by the function `basehaz` with argument `Cox_s`. The baseline hazard is determined for a hypothetical individual with covariate values that are the average in the data set, after deletion of any observations with missing values (Therneau and Grambsch 2000, p. 266). Since the average of categorical variables has no meaning, the baseline hazard cannot be interpreted. Therneau and Grambsch make it quite clear: 'users should not expect anything really interpretable from the "mean" curve' (p. 266). The primary reason why the function is included in the survival package is that 'users will look for the phrase "baseline hazard"' (Therneau 2014). The covariate values of the 'mean' subject are given by `Cox_s$mean` (or `Cox_s $means`). The characteristics of the hypothetical individual can be influenced partly. By adding the argument `centered = FALSE`, a baseline hazard is estimated for a hypothetical individual zero values of covariates:

6.2 The *Survival* Package

```
basehaz (Cox_s, centered=FALSE)
```

A much better alternative is to estimate the survival function for individuals with given covariate characteristics (using the `survfit.coxph` function) and to derive the cumulative hazard from the survival function.

The function `survfit.coxph` creates a survival function from a previously fitted Cox model. The survival curve gives the probability that a job episode experienced by an individual with given characteristics exceeds x, where x varies from 0 to the maximum job duration. The survival curve is for a 'mean' individual. However, there are two ways to obtain the survival curve for individuals with given covariates: segmentation and stratification. Segmentation involves the selection of individuals with given characteristics and to estimate the survival curve for each group. For instance, `Dm <- DJ600[DJ600$sex=="Male",]` is the subset consisting of males and `Df <- DJ600[DJ600$sex=="Female",]` is the subset of females.[2] Applying `coxph` to `Dm` and `Df` without covariates fits null models, `Coxm` and `Coxf`, say. The survival function for males and females is created from the results of the null model by the `survfit.coxph` function. These survival curves are the empirical survival curves for males and females. The survival probability is given at every time point at which the survival curve has a step. There are 105 steps in the male data (`Dm`) and 89 in the female data (`Df`). Application of `basehaz` with the argument `Coxm` and `Coxf` gives the cumulative hazard function for males and for females separately.

A second way to obtain the survival curve for individuals with given covariates is stratification. The following code estimates a stratified Cox model with a separate baseline hazard for each stratum (male and female sample population):

```
Cox_s <- coxph(Surv(time,status) ~ +strata(sex),
               data=DJ600,
               method="breslow")
```

The survival curves for males and females separately are produced by:

```
sfits <- survfit(Cox_s)
```

The object `sfits` that is returned by the `survfit` function has several components, the most important being the survival function and the associated upper and

---

[2] Note that the variable sex may be denoted by 1 and 2. To convert the numeric value of the categories to labels, use

```
if (!is.null(survey$sex) & !is.factor(DJ600$sex))
    DJ600$sex <-factor(DJ600$sex,levels=c(1,2),
        labels=c("Males","Females"))
```

lower confidence intervals. To display the components, type str(sfits). The components are explained in the manual of the *survival* package (see survfit. object).

The survival curves are plotted by plot(sfits). Arguments are added to get useful features, such as the 95 % confidence interval:

```
plot (sfits[1],
            conf.int=TRUE,
            lty=c(1,2,2),
            xlab="Job duration (months)",
            ylab="Survival probability",
            col="red",
            mark.time=FALSE)
lines (sfits[2]$time,sfits[2]$surv,
            lty=1,
            col="blue")
lines (sfits[2]$time,sfits[2]$lower,
            lty=2,
            col="blue")
lines (sfits[2]$time,sfits[2]$upper,
            lty=2,
            col="blue")
legend ("topright",
            legend=c("Males","Females"),
            col=c("red","blue"),
            fil=c("red","blue"),
            cex=0.9,bg="white")
```

The resulting plot is shown in Fig. 6.2.

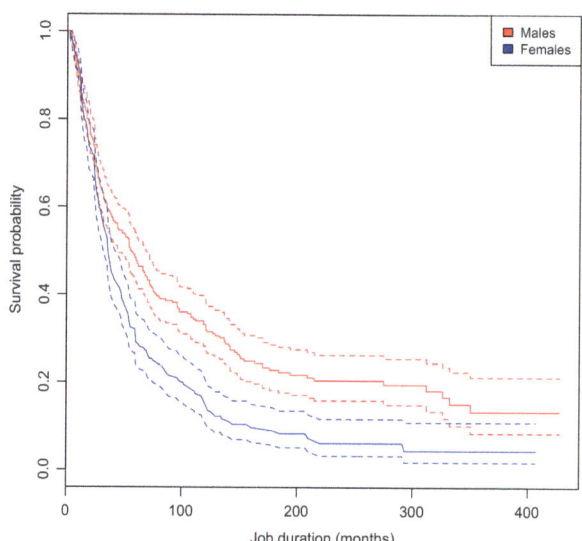

Fig. 6.2 Probabilities that job spells exceed given durations based on the stratified Cox model with single covariate (sex). GLHS

6.2 The *Survival* Package

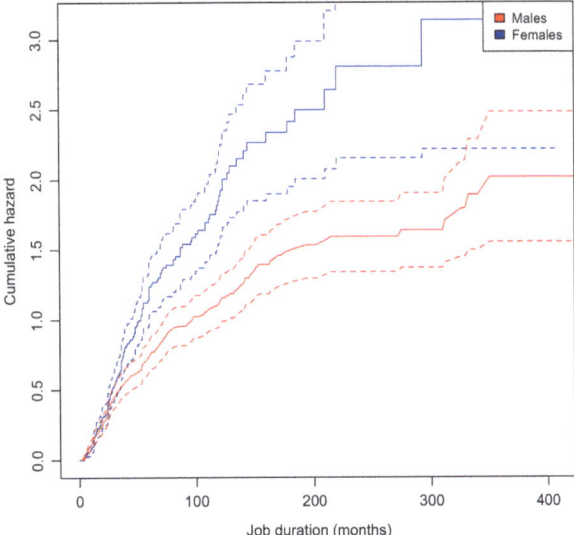

Fig. 6.3 Cumulative hazard based on the stratified Cox model with a single covariate (sex). GLHS

If the survival function has been estimated, then the cumulative hazard is plotted by the following code:

```
plot (sfits[2],
          conf.int=T,
          lty=c(1,2,2),
          fun="cumhaz",
          xlab="Job duration (months)",
          ylab="Cumulative hazard",
          col="blue",
          mark.time=FALSE)
lines (sfits[1]$time,-log(sfits[1]$surv),
          lty=1,
          col="red")
lines (sfits[1]$time,-log(sfits[1]$lower),
          lty=2,
          col="red")
lines (sfits[1]$time,-log(sfits[1]$upper),
          lty=2,
          col="red")
legend ("topright",
          legend=c("Males","Females"),
          col=c("red","blue"),
          fil=c("red","blue"),
          cex=0.9,bg="white")
```

The result is shown in Fig. 6.3.

The Cox proportional hazard model with all covariates is:

```
Cox_full <- coxph(Surv(Tstop-Tstart,status)~
    edu+as.factor(cohort)+LFX+PNOJ+pres,
    data=DJ600,
    method="breslow",
    na.action=na.exclude,
    iter.max=100)
```

Note that `Tstop-Tstart` is the `time` variable. The result is shown in Box 6.5. The regression coefficients are the same as those obtained by Blossfeld and Rohwer (2002, p. 233).

The survival function and other useful measures are produced by `survfit (Cox_full)` and the cumulative baseline hazard is produced by `basehaz (Cox_full)`. Note that the baseline hazard is for a hypothetical subject whose covariate values are the corresponding means from the original data. The duration-specific job exit rates are produced by

```
ms<- coxph.detail(Cox_full)
```

and stored in `ms$hazard`. Details of the Cox model are produced using the `coxph.object(Cox_full)` and `coxph.detail(Cox_full)` functions. For instance, the cumulative baseline hazard is obtained by the expression `basehaz(Cox_full)` and the hazard increments by `coxph.detail (Cox_full)$hazard`.

To test the proportionality assumption of the Cox proportional hazard model, a graphical check using Schoenfeld residuals may be applied. The assumption holds if the effect of a covariate on the transition rate does not vary with the time variable, in this case job duration. The impact of a covariate does not change with duration if the scaled Schoenfeld residuals for that covariate are a horizontal line (Therneau and Grambsch 2000, p. 136; Mills 2011, p. 153). The measure is produced by the `cox.zph` function. Consider the effect of education. The Schoenfeld residual plot is shown in Fig. 6.4 along with the fitted least squares line and the 90 % confidence

---

Box 6.5: Cox Proportional Hazard Model with Several Covariates. GLHS

	coef	se(coef)	Pr(>|z|)	
edu	0.0667012	0.0249169	0.007430	**
as.factor(cohort)1939-41	0.4102979	0.1153436	0.000375	***
as.factor(cohort)1949-51	0.3055312	0.1219753	0.012250	*
LFX	-0.0039771	0.0009315	1.96e-05	***
PNOJ	0.0686945	0.0441625	0.119829	
pres	-0.0261477	0.0055000	1.99e-06	***

6.2 The *Survival* Package

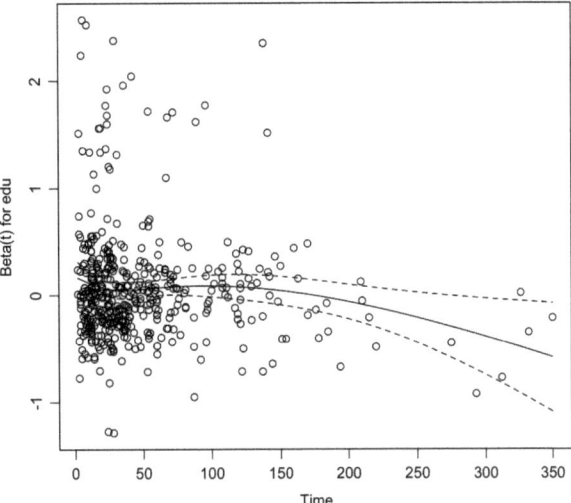

Fig. 6.4 Scaled Schoenfeld residuals for effect of education on job exit rate by job duration. GLHS

intervals. The impact of education does not vary with job duration up to about 150 months. At higher durations, the effect of education diminishes although, because of few observations, the change in the effect of education with job duration is not significant. The Schoenfeld residual plot is produced by the following code:

```
Cox_full.zph <- cox.zph(Cox_full,
            transform="identity",
            global=TRUE)
   plot (Cox_full.zph[1])
```

One function in the *survival* package performs functions similar to the Occup function in *Biograph*: pyears. The function computes the person-years of follow-up contributed by a cohort of subjects, stratified into subgroups. It also computes event counts and numbers of subjects in each cell of the output table. The results of pyears are normally used as input to further calculations. The following code generates the total duration of exposure:

```
pyears(Tstop-Tstart ~ tcut(born,c(0,1000)),
            data=DJ600,scale=1)
```

The scale argument assures that the exposure time is expressed in the same unit as the data. The total duration time is 40,762 months. That figure is the same as the figure produced by *Biograph* and shown in Table 4.2. The function pyears also produces the number of episodes: 600. The function does not give the number of job exits (458).

If the response variable is a Surv object, the pyears function gives for each combination of covariates the exposure time, the number of episodes and the number of events. Consider the Cox model with two covariates: sex and cohort.

The events and durations of exposure by combination of covariates are obtained in two steps. The first step is the estimation of the Cox model:

```
Cox_sc <- coxph(Surv(Tstop-Tstart,status)~
    sex+cohort,data=DJ600,method="breslow",
    na.action=na.exclude,iter.max=100)
```

The second step is the estimation of person-years of exposure:

```
y <- pyears (Cox_sc,DJ600,data.frame=TRUE,scale=1)
```

The results are stored in the object y$data. Events are stored in y$data $event, exposure times in y$data$pyears and numbers of episodes contributed to a given cell of the array in y$data$n. Males born in 1929–1931 contribute 132 job episodes to a total of 600 episodes. Together they experience 92 job exits and their combined exposure time is 15,867 months. Their job exit rate is $92/15{,}867 = 0.0058$. The rates for a given covariate combination are the ratio of events over exposure time. The total number of job exits is sum(y$data $event) = 458, the total exposure time is sum(y$data$pyears) = 40,762 and the overall job exit rate is $458/40{,}762 = 0.0112$.

Once a Cox model has been estimated, the survfit.coxph function predicts the survival probabilities for persons with given characteristics. The covariates are stored in the newdata data frame. Consider the second individual in the data set. The individual was born in 1929–1931 and has 10 years of education. She is a female but that information is not included in the Cox model presented as Cox_full. When the respondent entered the labour force (LFX = 0 and PNOJ = 0), she got a job with prestige level 22 (pres = 22). During the observation period she had three jobs. The second and third jobs had a much higher prestige level, namely, 46. The first job episode lasted 46 months (Tstop-Tstart), the second 34 months and the third 220 months. What are the expected durations predicted by the model? The prediction of the mean survival time is not an option in survfit. coxph and, because of censoring, there is no good estimate of the mean survival time. We estimate the survival function, which is the probability that a job episode lasts at least a given number of months. Consider the first job episode. The survival curve is estimated in two steps (Therneau and Grambsch 2000, p. 264). First, a separate data set is created that contains the covariate values of the individual. In this case, it is individual with ID 2:

```
ID.2.1 <- data.frame(edu=10,
                cohort="1929-31",
                LFX=0,
                PNOJ=0,
                pres=22)
```

Second, the expected individual survival curve is obtained using the covariate values of the individual and the Cox model labelled Cox_full:

6.2 The *Survival* Package

```
sfit.2.1 <- survfit (Cox_full,newdata=ID.2.1)
```

The survival curve and the confidence interval are given by summary (sfit.2.1). The probability that the individual keeps her job for at least 10 years (120 months) is predicted by the Cox_full model at 15.2%. The probability of job exit within 10 years is 84.8 %. The probability of job exit within 4 years (48 months) is 62.8 %. The figures are obtained using the following code:

```
z <- cbind(sfit.2.1$time,sfit.2.1$surv)
100*z[which(z[,1]==120),2]
100*(1-z[which(z[,1]==48),2])
```

The object sfit.2.1$time contains the job durations at which survival probabilities are estimated. Survival probabilities are estimated at time points at which the curve has a step. The object sfit.2.1$surv is the survival probability. The entire survival curve, which gives the probability that a job episode lasts at least x months, for x varying from 0 to the maximum job duration, is graphically displayed by the plot.survfit function. The function draws the survival curve sfit.2.1$surv and the 95 % confidence intervals sfit.2.1$upper and sfit.2.1$lower. The function plot(sfit.2.1) plots the survival curve and the confidence intervals. The following code adds labels, a title and a legend:

```
plot (sfit.2.1,
      las=1,
      xlab="Job duration (month)",
      ylab="Survival probability",
      mark.time=FALSE,
      cex.main=0.9,
      conf.int=T,
      col="black")
zv <- cbind(colnames(ID.2.1),t(ID.2.1))
legend (250,1.0,legend=zv[,1],box.lty=0,cex=0.9)
legend (280,1.0,legend=zv[,2],box.lty=0,cex=0.9)
```

The legend identifies the hypothetical individual in terms of his/her covariates. In the legend, the names of the covariates are displayed at job duration 250 and survival probability one. The values of the covariates are displayed at job duration 280 and survival probability one.

The job exit rate of the hypothetical individual is derived using the predict.coxph function. The function computes fitted values and regression terms for a model fitted by coxph. Two important values that are predicted are the linear predictor ('lp') and the risk score ('risk'). The linear predictor is the value predicted by the Cox model. The risk score is the exponent of the linear predictor, exp(lp).

The code is:

```
lp.2.1 <- predict (Cox_full,
                   newdata=ID.2.1,
                   type="lp",
                   se.fit=TRUE)
```

where `type` is the type of predicted value. The linear predictor is 0.3130 and the standard deviation is 0.1083. The linear predictor is derived from the regression equation $x'_i \hat{\beta}$ where x_i is the covariate vector of individual i and $\hat{\beta}$ is the vector of estimated regression coefficients. The terms of the linear predictor associated with each of the observations (600 job episodes) are generated by the expression

```
uu <- predict (Cox_full,type="terms",se.fit=TRUE)
```

The terms associated with the observation on the first job episode of respondent with ID 2 are uu$fit[2,] and uu$se.fit[2,] (Box 6.6).

A comparison of the predicted job survival curves of individuals with different characteristics is done by plotting different survival curves. The survival curves for four different hypothetical individuals are shown in Fig. 6.5. The four individuals differ in period of birth and years of education. Two have 9 years of education and 2 have 19 years. Two are born in 1929–1931 and two in 1939–1941. The individual characteristics are given in the following data set:

```
indiv <- data.frame(
    edu=c(9,9,19,19),
    cohort=c("1929-31","1939-41","1929-31","1939-41"),
    LFX=0,
    PNOJ=0,
    pres=44)
```

The data frame is:

```
  edu  cohort LFX PNOJ pres
1   9 1929-31   0    0   44
2   9 1939-41   0    0   44
3  19 1929-31   0    0   44
4  19 1939-41   0    0   44
```

It is displayed by `print(indiv)`.
The survival curves are obtained by

Box 6.6: Terms of Cox Model Used to Predict Length of the First Job Episode for Respondent with ID 2. GLHS

```
$fit
          edu      cohort       LFX        PNOJ       pres
1 -0.08471053 -0.2231001 0.2972321 -0.1021258 0.4257716

$se.fit
         edu      cohort       LFX        PNOJ       pres
1 0.03164449 0.06329048 0.06961654 0.06565494 0.0895576
```

6.2 The *Survival* Package

Fig. 6.5 Predicted job survival for individuals with given characteristics based on the Cox model. GLHS (confidence intervals omitted)

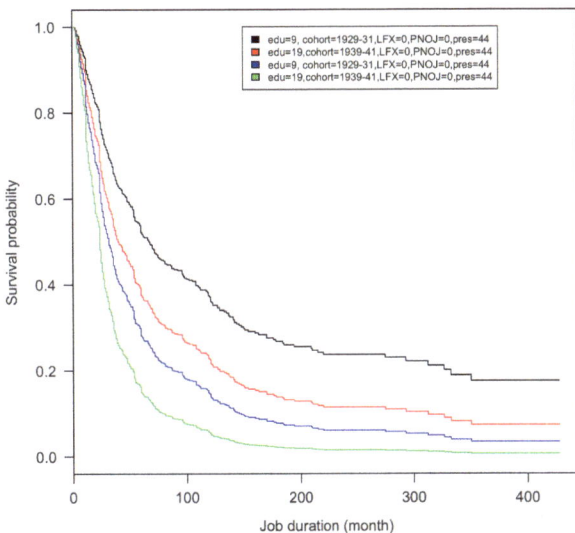

```
sfit <- survfit(Cox_full,newdata=indiv)
```

and the plot by

```
colours <- c("black","red","blue","green")
plot (sfit,
      las=1,
      col=colours,
      xlab="Job duration (month)",ylab="Survival
probability",
      main="Effects of covariates on job duration,Cox model.
GLHS (BR2002)",conf.int=F)
legend (150,1.0,legend=c(
      "edu=9, cohort=1929-31,LFX=0,PNOJ=0,pres=44",
      "edu=19,cohort=1939-41,LFX=0,PNOJ=0,pres=44",
      "edu=9, cohort=1929-31,LFX=0,PNOJ=0,pres=44",
      "edu=19,cohort=1939-41,LFX=0,PNOJ=0,pres=44"),
      cex=0.7,
      col=colours,
      fill=colours)
```

The confidence intervals are not shown. Figure 6.6 shows the confidence interval around the first survival curve. It is produced by:

Fig. 6.6 Predicted job survival for individuals with given characteristics based on the Cox model. GLHS (with confidence intervals)

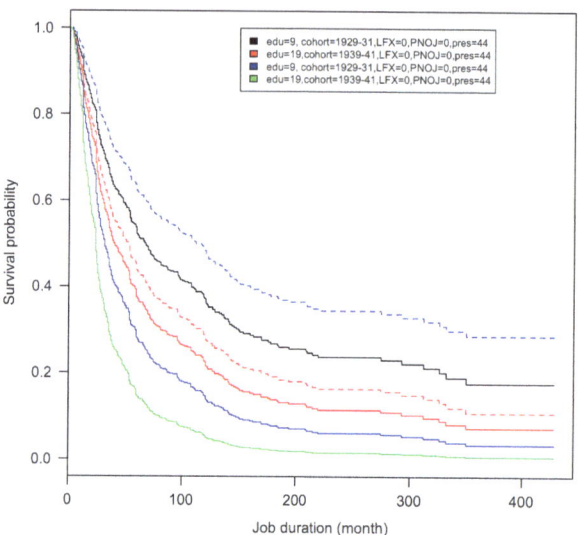

```
plot (sfit[1],las=1,
      conf.int=TRUE,
      col=colours,
      xlab="Job duration (month)",ylab="Survival
probability",
      mark.time=FALSE)
lines(sfit[2],col="red")
lines(sfit[3],col="blue")
lines(sfit[4],col="green")
legend (150,1.0,legend=c(
      "edu=9, cohort=1929-31,LFX=0,PNOJ=0,pres=44",
      "edu=19,cohort=1939-41,LFX=0,PNOJ=0,pres=44",
      "edu=9, cohort=1929-31,LFX=0,PNOJ=0,pres=44",
      "edu=19,cohort=1939-41,LFX=0,PNOJ=0,pres=44"),
      cex=0.7,col=colours,fill=colours)
```

The ratio of the job exit rates of the four hypothetical persons relative to the sample mean job exit rate is derived using the predict.coxph function. The code is:

```
z1 <- predict (Cox_full,
              newdata=indiv,
              type="risk",
              se.fit=TRUE)
```

where type is the type of predicted value. In this case it is the risk score exp (lp) ('risk'), with lp being the linear predictor. The relative risks (ratio of job exit rates) and their confidence intervals are given in Box 6.7.

6.3 The *eha* Package

Box 6.7: Predicted Cumulative Job Exit Rate with Confidence Intervals. Selection of Hypothetical Individuals. GLHS

```
$fit
        [,1]
1 0.7197271
2 1.0848207
3 1.4023212
4 2.1136721

$se.fit
        [,1]
1 0.1089391
2 0.1230591
3 0.2242662
4 0.3027850
```

If no secondary data set (newdata) is provided to the survfit function, then the curve produced is that for the 'mean' subject.

6.2.5 Nelson-Aalen Estimator

The *survival* package does not produce the Nelson-Aalen estimator of the cumulative hazard rate, but the estimator can be obtained indirectly. An easy way is to use the baseline hazard estimator of a Cox model without covariates:

```
NeAa <- basehaz(coxph(Surv(time,status)~1,data=DJ600))
```

An alternative way is to compute the cumulative hazard from the object returned by the survfit function:

```
fit <- survfit (Surv(time,status)~1,data=DJ600)
cumhaz <- cumsum(fit$n.event/fit$n.risk)
```

6.3 The *eha* Package

eha is a package for survival and event history analysis with an emphasis on Cox regression and extensions. It was developed and is being maintained by Broström (2012, 2014) (http://tal.stat.umu.se/~gb/eha/index.html). The package was first uploaded to CRAN in 2003. Its main focus is on proportional hazards modelling in survival analysis, and in that respect, *eha* can be regarded as a complement and an extension of the *survival* package (Broström 2003). In fact *eha* requires *survival*. The package contains several functions for proportional hazards analysis: `coxreg`, `mlreg` and `weibreg`. The function `coxreg` performs Cox regression, almost as `coxph` in the *survival* package. The function `mlreg` is a discrete-time proportional hazards model. The function `weibreg` is a Weibull regression for left-truncated and right-censored data that allows for stratification with different shape and scale parameters in the strata. The function `phreg` estimates a proportional hazard model with parametric baseline hazard. The function `aftreg` estimates parametric models of duration dependence. In addition, *eha* contains a number of functions for data checking and exploratory data analysis. They include the `check.surv` function that checks whether individuals experience *at most* one event, that spells do not overlap and that exit occurs after entry and `join.spells` that cleans up successive spells. Overlapping spells are 'polished' and spells that are cut unnecessarily are glued together. Functions for exploratory analysis include `age.window` and `cal.window` that cut, respectively, age and (calendar) time spells into intervals of given length and `piecewise` that calculates piecewise hazards, number of events and exposure times in each interval. The `perstat` function calculates occurrence-exposure rates for given time periods and ages.

The *eha* package uses the same input data structure as the *survival* package. The package allows for left-truncated and right-censored data.

The package allows the display, for each event time point, of the time point, the event count and the risk set just prior to the event time. The code is

```
ev <- table.events(exit=DJ600$time,event=DJ600$status)
```

The object ev has three components:

(a) ev$times: event (transition) times
(b) ev$events: transition counts
(c) ev$riskset.sizes: risk set

In this section, three functionalities of the *eha* package are discussed: estimation of transition rate models, estimation of Cox models with parametric baseline hazard and the functions to change the observation window.

6.3.1 Transition Rate Models

The *eha* package is particularly useful for parametric models of duration dependence, such as the Gompertz model, the Weibull model, the log-normal model, the log-logistic model and the extreme value distribution. All these models, except the extreme value distribution, are covered by Blossfeld and Rohwer (2002). The models are estimated using the `aftreg` function. The name of the function derives from accelerated failure time regression.

6.3 The *eha* Package

Box 6.8: Weibull Regression Model (*eha*), Without Covariates. GLHS

```
Call:
aftreg(formula = Surv(time, status) ~ 1, data = D, dist = "weibull")

Covariate           W.mean      Coef  Time-Accn   se(Coef)    Wald p
Baseline parameters:
log(scale)                     4.461     86.568      0.054     0.000
log(shape)                    -0.149      0.862      0.036     0.000
Baseline mean:

Events                          458
Total time at risk            40762
Max. log. likelihood         -2504.6
```

The basic exponential model is a Weibull model with the shape parameter fixed at 1. The parameter estimate is 4.489. The average waiting time to a job exit is exp $(4.489) = 89$ months and the monthly job exit rate is $\exp(-4.489) = 0.01124$. The Weibull model without covariates is:

```
z<- aftreg(Surv(time,status)~1,
           dist="weibull",
           data=DJ600,
           shape=0)
```

The argument shape of the function is 0, indicating that the shape parameter needs to be estimated. The results are shown in Box 6.8.

The results of the Weibull regression with one covariate and with several covariates are also shown in Box 6.9. The Weibull model with all covariates considered by Blossfeld and Rohwer (2002) is estimated using the following code:

```
z<- aftreg(Surv(time,status)~
           edu+cohort+LFX+PNOJ+pres,
           dist="weibull",
           data=DJ600)
```

The results are similar to those presented by Blossfeld and Rohwer (2002, p. 195). The coefficients include the two parameters of the Weibull function (the scale parameter and the shape parameter) and the effects of the covariates. The sign of the scale parameters is opposite to that in the model presented by Blossfeld and Rohwer. The reason is that *TDA* considers the job exit rate as the dependent variable in the transition rate model, whereas *eha* considers the failure time, or waiting time, as the dependent variable. The job exit rate is $r(t) = b\, a^b\, t^{b-1}$ where a is the scale parameter and b the shape parameter. The scale parameter depends on the covariates. Consider the individual with ID $=2$ entering the labour market, i.e. the first job episode. The respondent is born in 1929–1931 and has 10 years of education. The first job has a prestige score of 22. The scale parameter is:

Box 6.9: Weibull Regression Model (*eha*), with Covariates. GLHS

```
a. With one covariate (sex)
Covariate          W.mean      Coef  Time-Accn  se(Coef)    Wald p
sex
        Males       0.671      0        1        (reference)
        Females     0.329      0.586    1.797    0.106       0.000

Baseline parameters:
log(scale)                     4.701    110.049  0.072       0.000
log(shape)                    -0.119      0.888  0.036       0.001

c. With several covariates (full model)
Covariate          W.mean      Coef  Time-Accn  se(Coef)    Wald p
edu                11.098      0.078    1.081    0.027       0.004
cohort
        1929-31     0.543      0        1        (reference)
        1939-41     0.256      0.606    1.833    0.124       0.000
        1949-51     0.201      0.578    1.783    0.130       0.000
LFX                74.943     -0.004    0.996    0.001       0.000
PNOJ                1.405      0.064    1.066    0.048       0.184
pres               39.103     -0.029    0.971    0.006       0.000

Baseline parameters:
log(scale)                     4.405    81.858   0.307       0.000
log(shape)                    -0.091     0.913   0.036       0.012
```

$$a = \exp(-4.38702+0.0778*10-0.029169*22) = 0.01425$$

The shape parameter is:

$$b = \exp(-0.091) = 0.913$$

The job exit rate varies with job duration following the Weibull distribution:

$$r(t) = 0.913 * 0.01425^{0.913} \, t^{0.913-1}$$

The function hweibull of *eha* calculates the hazard rate at different durations of the job spell. The code is:

```
w <- hweibull(x=1:428,shape=exp(-0.091),
              scale=1/0.01425)
```

The first argument is a vector or quantiles. The function Hweibull calculates the cumulative hazard rates. Note that in this model specification the scale parameter is 1 over the scale parameter in the Blossfeld and Rohwer specification of the Weibull model. The function plot.aftreg plots the Weibull hazard rate (not shown):

6.3 The *eha* Package

```
plot.aftreg(z,fn="haz",
    ylim=c(0.01,0.018),
    ylab="Job exit rate",
    xlab="Job duration (months)")
```

6.3.2 The Cox Model with Parametric Baseline Hazard

Now I introduce covariates to determine the effect of covariates on the hazard rates. Consider a Cox model with a single covariate (sex). The code is:

```
zs<- coxreg(Surv(time,status)~sex,data=DJ600)
```

The result is shown in Box 6.10. Females leave their job at a rate that is 53 % higher than the job exit rate of males. The same result was obtained with coxph function of the *survival* package. The baseline remains unspecified. The hazard rates are in Cox_s$hazards.

The stratified Cox model, with sex as a covariate, is:

```
Cox_s <- coxreg(Surv(time,status)~strata(sex),
         data=DJ600,
         method="breslow")
```

The number of events in the data is Cox_s$events (458) and the observed total exposure time is Cox_s$ttr (40,762 months). The same figures are produced by the function pyears of the *survival* package. The estimated baseline hazard (not cumulative) is included in the object Cox_s.

The full model, as specified by Blossfeld and Rohwer, is:

```
Cox_full <- coxreg(Surv(time,status)~
           edu+
           as.factor(cohort)+
           LFX+PNOJ+pres,
           data=DJ600,
           method="breslow",
           na.action=na.exclude)
```

The results are shown in Box 6.11. The package has a function for printing the results of the Cox model. It is print.coxreg(Cox_full).

The function phreg estimates a proportional hazard model with parametric baseline hazard. The Weibull distribution is one of the functions describing duration dependence.

Assume that the duration dependence of the job exit rate (i.e. baseline) can be described by a Weibull model. The following command fits a proportional hazard model with a baseline following the shape of a Weibull distribution:

Box 6.10: Impact of Gender on Job Exit Rate: Cox Regression Model. GLHS

```
Covariate           Mean        Coef      Rel.Risk     S.E.      Wald p
sex
         Male       0.673       0         1 (reference)
         Female     0.327       0.428     1.535        0.095     0.000

Events                          458
Total time at risk              -40304
Max. log. likelihood            -2570.6
LR test statistic               20.1
Degrees of freedom              1
Overall p-value                 7.31958e-06
```

Box 6.11: Impact of Several Covariates on Job Exit Rate: Cox Model (*eha*). GLHS

```
Call:
coxreg(formula = Surv(time, status) ~ edu + as.factor(cohort) +
    LFX + PNOJ + pres, data = D, na.action = na.exclude, method =
"breslow")

Covariate           Mean        Coef      Rel.Risk     S.E.      Wald p
edu                 11.098      0.067     1.069        0.025     0.007
as.factor(cohort)
         1929-31    0.543       0         1 (reference)
         1939-41    0.256       0.410     1.507        0.115     0.000
         1949-51    0.201       0.306     1.357        0.122     0.012
LFX                 74.943      -0.004    0.996        0.001     0.000
PNOJ                1.405       0.069     1.071        0.044     0.120
pres                39.103      -0.026    0.974        0.005     0.000

Events                          458
Total time at risk              40762
Max. log. likelihood            -2547
LR test statistic               75.2
Degrees of freedom              6
Overall p-value                 3.4861e-14
```

```
w <- phreg (Surv(time,status) ~ sex,
    data=DJ600,
    dist="weibull",
    shape=0)
```

The argument `shape` of the function is 0, indicating that the shape parameter needs to be estimated. The result, obtained by `print(w)` or `print.phreg(w)`, is shown in Box 6.12. The job exit rates are obtained with `w$hazards`.

6.3 The *eha* Package

Box 6.12: Impact of Several Covariates on Job Exit Rate: Cox Proportional Hazard Model with Weibull Baseline Hazard (*eha*). GLHS

```
a. Single covariate
Call:
phreg(formula = Surv(D$time, D$status) ~ sex, data = D, dist =
"weibull",
    shape = 0)
```

Covariate		W.mean	Coef	Exp(Coef)	se(Coef)	Wald p
sex						
	Males	0.671	0	1	(reference)	
	Females	0.329	0.521	1.683	0.095	0.000
log(scale)			4.701	110.044	0.072	0.000
log(shape)			-0.119	0.888	0.036	0.001

```
Events                       458
Total time at risk         40762
Max. log. likelihood      -2489.8
LR test statistic            29.5
Degrees of freedom            1
Overall p-value           5.65384e-08
```

```
b. Full model
Call:
phreg(formula = Surv(D$time, D$status) ~ edu + as.factor(cohort) +
    LFX + PNOJ + pres, data = D)
```

Covariate	W.mean	Coef	Exp(Coef)	se(Coef)	Wald p
edu	11.098	0.071	1.074	0.025	0.004
as.factor(cohort)					
1929-31	0.543	0	1	(reference)	
1939-41	0.256	0.553	1.739	0.115	0.000
1949-51	0.201	0.528	1.696	0.123	0.000
LFX	74.943	-0.003	0.997	0.001	0.000
PNOJ	1.405	0.058	1.060	0.044	0.187
pres	39.103	-0.027	0.974	0.006	0.000
log(scale)		4.404	81.808	0.306	0.000
log(shape)		-0.091	0.913	0.036	0.012

```
Events                       458
Total time at risk         40762
Max. log. likelihood      -2462.5
LR test statistic            84.1
Degrees of freedom            6
Overall p-value           5.55112e-16
```

The function `check.disk` is used to compare the semi-parametric model (unspecified baseline hazard) with the parametric model (baseline hazard described by a parametric model of duration dependence).

The following command produces the same results as the Weibull regression model without covariates.[3] The results are shown in Box 6.13.

---

[3] The model is also discussed by Blossfeld and Rohwer (2002).

Box 6.13: Weibull Model of Job Exit Rates; Null Model Without Covariates. GLHS

```
Call:
weibreg(formula = Surv(Tstop - Tstart, status) ~
    1, data = DJ600)

Covariate           Mean      Coef  Exp(Coef)  se(Coef)   Wald p
log(scale)                   4.461     86.569     0.054    0.000
log(shape)                  -0.149      0.862     0.036    0.000

Events                        458
Total time at risk          40762
Max. log. likelihood       -2504.6
```

```
w <- weibreg (Surv(Tstop-Tstart,status) ~ 1,
    data=DJ600)
```

Note that the scale parameter is minus the value shown by Blossfeld and Rohwer (2002, p. 193). The reason is that in *eha* (as in *survival*) the dependent variable is the time to job exit rather than the job exit rate. The shape parameter, however, has the same sign.

To get the exponential model, the shape parameter is fixed to unity:

```
weibreg (Surv(Tstop-Tstart,status) ~ 1,
            shape=1,
            data=DJ600)
```

The regression coefficient is 4.489, which is minus the value shown by Blossfeld and Rohwer (2002, p. 93), for the same reason given before.

The following command estimates the transition rate model with Gompertz hazard:

```
g <- aftreg (Surv(Tstart,Tstop,status) ~ sex,
             data=DJ600,
             dist="gompertz")
```

The function `piecewise` produces event counts and exposure times for given time intervals. It also calculates piecewise constant transition rates (occurrence-exposure rates). The command

`piecewise(DJ600$Tstart,DJ600$Tstop,DJ600$status,c(0,10000))`

gives the number of job exits (458) during the entire observation period (from time 0 to a very large number, in this case 10,000), the total exposure time (40,762) and the job exit rate (0.01124). The same results are produced by *Biograph*. To calculate

6.3 The *eha* Package

> **Box 6.14: Numbers of Job Exits, Exposure Times and Job Exit Rates, by Duration Intervals of 1 Year. GLHS**
>
> ```
> $events
>  0 88 94 82 40 41 24 13 10 11 10 11 10  5  2  4  2  1  3  1  0  0  0  1  0  1
>  1  0  2  0  1  0  0  0  0  0  0
>
> $exposure
>  0 6808 5458 4181 3300 2788 2290 1921 1769 1582 1368 1116  965  803  726  664
> 617  546  481  426  388  368  336  319  285  232  206  168  139  112   98
>  91   77   64   44   18    8
>
> $intensity
>  NA 0.012925969 0.017222426 0.019612533 0.012121212 0.014705882 0.010480349
> 0.006767309 0.005652911 0.006953224 0.007309942 0.009856631 0.010362694
> 0.006226650 0.002754821 0.006024096 0.003241491 0.001831502 0.006237006
> 0.002347418 0.000000000 0.000000000 0.000000000 0.003134796 0.000000000
> 0.004310345 0.004854369 0.000000000 0.014388489 0.000000000 0.010204082
> 0.000000000 0.000000000 0.000000000 0.000000000 0.000000000
> ```

job exit rates by duration on the job in single years, the following command may be used:

```
piecewise(enter=0,exit=DJ600$Tstop-DJ600$Tstart,
          event=DJ600$status,
          cutpoints=seq(0,430,by=12))
```

Note that the maximum job episode is 428 months. The results are shown in Box 6.14.

An alternative way to generate the number of events by duration intervals of 1 year is:

```
DJ600$period<-cut((DJ600$Tstop-DJ600$Tstart),
                  breaks=seq(0,440,by=12),
                  include.lowest=T)
table(DJ600$status,DJ600$period)
```

The *eha* package includes a number of utilities for data checking and data exploration. The check.surv function checks whether the ending time of an episode is not before the starting time and that each individual experiences at most one event. The function has been applied to the GLHS with data in *Biograph* format (wide format) and to the data set DJ600, which is the episode file of job episodes used by Blossfeld and Rohwer (2002) (long format). For the first application, a status variable of one has been added to the data file. The first application is evoked by the statement:

```
Z <- GLHS
Z$status <- 1
check.surv(Z$start,Z$end,Z$status,Z$ID)
```

The application responds with TRUE meaning that there are no inconsistencies identified in the data.

6.3.3 Change Observation Window

The functions `age.window` and `cal.window` are particularly useful to change the observation window to an age interval or a time interval. The function `age.window` cuts episodes or spells in age intervals and `cal.window` cuts episodes in time intervals. The function requires a specification of the age and time interval and a list of age and time cutpoints. The function cannot be applied to data in the *Biograph* format (wide format) because it does not adjust the state sequence and the transition dates. It can be applied, however, to data in the long format. Consider the data file `DJ600` (long format). The variable `Tstart` gives the data in CMC at onset of an episode and `Tstop` gives the ending date in CMC. To be able to cut episodes in age intervals and time intervals, we change the date of birth in year and fraction of year and calculate the ages at start and end of episodes. The year of birth is:

```
DJ600$birthY <- cmc_as_year(DJ600$born)
```

The ages at onset and end of the episode are:

```
       DJ600$Tstarta <-
cmc_as_age(DJ600$Tstart,DJ600$born,"cmc")$age
       DJ600$Tstopa  <-
(cmc_as_age(DJ600$Tstop,DJ600$born,"cmc")$age
```

The age `Tstarta` is the age a person reaches during the month in which the transition occurs. The following command creates an observation window that starts at age 20 and ends at age 40:

```
D.agew <- age.window(DJ600,c(20,40),
            surv=c("Tstarta","Tstopa","status"))
```

`surv` is the survival object, which includes the age at onset of the episode, the age at the end of the episode and the status at the end. Records with data on episodes that end before age 20 or start after age 40 are removed from the data file. The data set that results contains observations on exposures and transitions between ages 20 and 40. Note that the variables `Tstart` and `Tstop` are not adjusted. They do not need to be adjusted as long as they are not used in subsequent analysis. The following code may be used to change `Tstart` and `Tstop` to be consistent with the new observation window:

6.3 The *eha* Package

```
    D.agew$Tstartnew <- (D.agew$birthY
        +D.agew$Tstarta-1900)*12
    D.agew$Tstopnew  <- (D.agew$birthY
        +D.agew$Tstopa-1900)*12
```

The same function may be used to select an observation window between given values of `Tstart` and `Tstop`. For instance, the following command selects observations between CMC 500 and 600:

```
    D.cmcw <- age.window(DJ600,c(500,600),
        surv=c("Tstart","Tstop","status"))
```

The following code cuts the time in the interval from 1 January 1950 to 1 January 1970:

```
D.calw <- cal.window(DJ600,c(1950,1970),
        surv=c("Tstarta","Tstopa","status","birthY"))
```

In this case `surv` is a survival object with additional information. It includes the date of birth. In *eha*, it is referred to as the extended survival object.

To adjust the CMC at entry and CMC at exit, the following code may be used:

```
    D.calw$Tstartnew <- (D.calw$birthY
                    +D.calw$Tstarta-1900)*12 + 1
    D.calw$Tstopnew  <- (D.calw$birthY
                    +D.calw$Tstopa-1900)*12
```

Note that January 1950 is CMC 601 (=50*12+1) and December 1970 CMC 840 (=70 * 12). Recall that the first month (CMC = 1) is January 1900. Consider respondent with ID 4. He is born in CMC 604 (April 1950) and enters the labour market in CMC 872 (August 1972), which is after the end of the 1950–1970 observation period. The observation on the first episode of life is censored on 1 January 1970, which is at CMC 840 (=70*12). At that date he is 19.67 years of age. Respondent with ID 4 contributes only one spell to the new data set. Note that the function `cal.window` changes the status variable from 1 to 0 because the first episode no longer ends in an event but in censoring. The destination state (DES) is not changed from J to cens because `cal.window` does not consider the destination state.

The function `perstat` calculates, for a given time period and age interval, the number of events, the duration at risk or exposure time and the occurrence-exposure rate. Suppose we want to estimate the number of job exits, the total exposure time in a job and the job exit rate for individuals aged between 20 and 30 years during the period from 1970 to 1980. The input is an extended survival object (see above). The following code creates the extended survival object `surv.extended`:

Box 6.15: Transitions, Exposure Times and Occurrence-Exposure Rates of Respondents Who Are Aged 20–30 Years During the Period 1970–1980. GLHS

```
$events
                [,1]
(1970 - 1980]    95

$exposure
                [,1]
(1970 - 1980]  479.1667

$intensity
                [,1]
(1970 - 1980]  0.1982609
```

```
surv.extended <- cbind(enter=DJ600$Tstarta,
            exit=DJ600$Tstopa,
            event=DJ600$status,
            birthdate=DJ600$birthyear)
```

By way of control, let us compute the total number of job exits, the total duration of employment and the job exit rate during the entire period for all ages. It is:

```
z <- perstat (surv.extended,
            period=c(1920,2000),
            age=c(0,100))
```

The total number of job exits is 458, the total exposure time is 3,397 years and the job exit rate is 0.1348 per year. The sojourn time is expressed in the time unit used in the extended survival objects, which is years. Hence, although the month is the time unit in the original data, the intensity is the number of transitions per person-years. The same results may be obtained by *Biograph*. Table 4.2 shows an exposure time of 40,762 months, which is 3,397 years.

The job exit rate (occurrence-exposure rate) for individuals aged 20–30 years during the period 1970–1980 is computed by the code:

```
z <- perstat (surv.extended,
            period=c(1970,1980),
            age=c(20,30))
```

The result is shown in Box 6.15. The observation window is an age-period observation window. During the period 1970–1980, persons aged 20–30 spent a total of 479 years employed; 95 left their job, resulting in a job exit rate of 0.20. The job exit rate between 1950 and 1970 was lower, 0.17.

The function may be used to compute age-specific transition rates from transitions and durations of exposure. If age intervals are 1 year, the measures produced by the perstat function are the same as those produced by *Biograph* and shown in Table 4.8. Consider persons aged between 40 and 41. The function perstat computes an exposure time of 83.17 months and three job exits, the same figures obtained by *Biograph* (see Table 4.8).

6.4 The *mvna* and *etm* Packages

The *mvna* and *etm* packages were developed by Allignol (2013, 2014). The mvna package generates Nelson-Aalen estimates of the cumulative hazard in multistate models from data that may be right censored and left truncated (see also Allignol et al. 2008). The *etm* package generates Aalen-Johansen estimates of transition probabilities (Allignol et al. 2011). The two packages are documented in Beyersmann et al. (2012). The Aalen-Johansen estimator is also called the empirical transition matrix. The transition probabilities are derived from the Nelson-Aalen estimates. For that reason they are combined in this section. I present the Nelson-Aalen estimator first, followed by the Aalen-Johansen estimator.

6.4.1 mvna: Nelson-Aalen Estimator in Multistate Models

The Nelson-Aalen estimator is a non-parametric estimator (see Chap. 2). It is an increasing right-continuous step function with increments d_j/r_j at observation time j, with d_j the number of transitions at j and r_j the number of individuals at risk just prior to j. For a discussion of the estimator in the context of multistate models, see Andersen and Keiding (2002), Andersen et al. (1993), Aalen et al. (2008) and Beyersmann et al. (2012). For a comparison with related estimators (Kaplan-Meier and Aalen-Johansen), see Borgan (1998). The *mvna* package allows time-dependent covariates.

The Biograph.mvna function prepares the input data for the *mvna* package (see Chap. 3):

```
Dmvna <- Biograph.mvna(GLHS)
```

The object returned by the function is Dmvna and the data are in the component Dmvna$D. Transitions from one job to another job (intrastate transitions) are removed, as required by the *mvna* and *etm* packages.

The *mvna* package is called by the following expression:

```
na <- mvna(data=Dmvna$D,
           state.names=c("N","J"),
           tra=attr(Dmvna$D,"param")$trans_possible,
           cens.name=Dmvna$cens)
```

The output of mvna includes the number of individuals at risk in each state just prior to a given transition (n.risk), the number of transitions at each event time (n.event) and the number of censored cases at each censoring time (n.cens). That information may be used to construct a table similar to the ratetable $Stable table produced by the Ratetable function of *Biograph*. The table includes event counts and exposure times. To produce the table from *mvna* output, a few steps need to be taken. In the first step, create a data frame with the variables that are required. Note that in this application, age is the time variable. The variables are: age (time) at transition, risk set in each state at that point in time, number of transitions and number of censored cases at each age. The code is:

```
# risk set at event time
am <-cbind(round(na$time,4),na$n.risk)
#transitions at event time
ab <- aperm(na$n.event,c(3,1,2))
hh <- data.frame(row.names=c(1:nrow(am)),
           cbind(Time=am[,1],
                 AtRisk_N=am[,2],
                 AtRisk_J=am[,3],
                 NJ=ab[,1,2],
                 JN=ab[,2,1],
                 NC=na$n.cens[,1],
                 JC=na$n.cens[,2]))
```

In the second step, numbers of events by single years of age are computed. Records with event times in the same age are combined. The code is:

```
hh$Time2 <- cut(hh$Time,
            breaks=c(0,seq(10,55,by=1)),
            include.lowest=TRUE,
            right=FALSE)
hh$Time3 <- match (hh$Time2,unique(hh$Time2))
tt<- aggregate(hh[,4:7],list(Count=hh$Time2),sum)
```

An individual of exact age x is included in the age interval [x,x + 1). In demographic analysis and most other studies, the lowest value is included in the interval and the highest value is excluded. The interval is said to be closed on the right and open on the left. That requirement is operationalised with the arguments include.lowest=TRUE and right=FALSE. The variable Time3 is an indicator variable. It is one if the record in the data object is the first of an age interval (of one year) and it is zero otherwise. It is produced to select the first record

6.4 The *mvna* and *etm* Packages

Table 6.1 Sample population at risk, by age, and transitions, by age, produced by *mvna*. GLHS

	Age	AtRiskN	AtRiskJ	NJ	NC	JN	JC
1	0	201	0	0	0	0	0
2	13	201	0	6	0	0	0
3	14	195	6	24	0	2	0
4	15	173	28	12	0	3	0
5	16	164	37	21	0	6	0
6	17	149	52	44	0	1	0
7	18	106	95	37	0	9	0
8	19	78	123	34	0	11	0
9	20	55	146	16	0	24	0
10	21	63	138	20	0	17	0
11	22	60	141	19	0	9	0
12	23	50	151	10	0	10	0
13	24	50	151	7	0	15	0
14	25	58	143	3	0	11	0
15	26	66	135	8	0	14	0

of each age interval. The function `aggregate` determines the number of events in an age interval.

The third step is to determine the population at risk at the beginning of each age interval. The code is:

```
hh$test <- rep(1,length(hh$Time3))
hh$test[2:length(hh$Time3)] <- ifelse
    (diff(hh$Time3[1:length(hh$Time3)],lag=1)==0,
    0,1)
hh2 <- subset(hh,hh$test==1)
```

In the fourth step, the relevant data are combined into a data frame:

```
Stable <- cbind(Age=trunc(hh2$Time),
        AtRiskN=hh2$AtRisk_N,
        AtRiskJ=hh2$AtRisk_J,
        tt[,2:5])
```

The results are shown in Table 6.1 (selected ages). Note that *mvna* excludes transitions to the same state.

Table 6.2 shows `ratetable$Stable` (produced by *Biograph*) for selected ages.

The Nelson-Aalen estimator of the cumulative hazard is shown in Fig. 6.7. The plot is produced by the `xyplot.mvna` function. This function also plots several types of pointwise confidence intervals (Andersen et al. 1993, p. 208). For details, see the description of the *mvna* package. The `xyplot` function is from the *lattice* package.

Table 6.2 Sample population at risk, by age, and transitions, by age, produced by *Biograph*. GLHS

```
, , State = N

            Case
Age         Occup        PY  Leaving       N       J  Censored
  0          201     201.00        0       0    0.00      0.00
 13          201     199.17        6       0    6.00      0.00
 14          195     181.42       24       0   24.00      0.00
 15          173     167.50       12       0   12.00      0.00
 16          164     157.83       21       0   21.00      0.00
 17          149     122.75       44       0   44.00      0.00
 18          106      89.75       37       0   37.00      0.00
 19           78      63.08       34       0   34.00      0.00
 20           55      62.75       16       0   16.00      0.00
 21           63      56.92       20       0   20.00      0.00
 22           60      50.83       19       0   19.00      0.00
 23           50      50.50       10       0   10.00      0.00
 24           50      55.17        7       0    7.00      0.00
 25           58      62.00        3       0    3.00      0.00
 26           66      66.08        8       0    8.00      0.00

, , State = J

            Case
Age         Occup        PY  Leaving       N       J  Censored
  0            0       0.00        0    0.00    0.00      0.00
 13            0       1.83        1    0.00    1.00      0.00
 14            6      19.58        4    2.00    2.00      0.00
 15           28      33.50        7    3.00    4.00      0.00
 16           37      43.17        8    6.00    2.00      0.00
 17           52      78.25        9    1.00    8.00      0.00
 18           95     111.25       22    9.00   13.00      0.00
 19          123     137.92       36   11.00   25.00      0.00
 20          146     138.25       41   24.00   17.00      0.00
 21          138     144.08       34   17.00   17.00      0.00
 22          141     150.17       32    9.00   23.00      0.00
 23          151     150.50       22   10.00   12.00      0.00
 24          151     145.83       28   15.00   13.00      0.00
 25          143     139.00       21   11.00   10.00      0.00
 26          135     134.92       25   14.00   11.00      0.00
```

6.4 The *mvna* and *etm* Packages

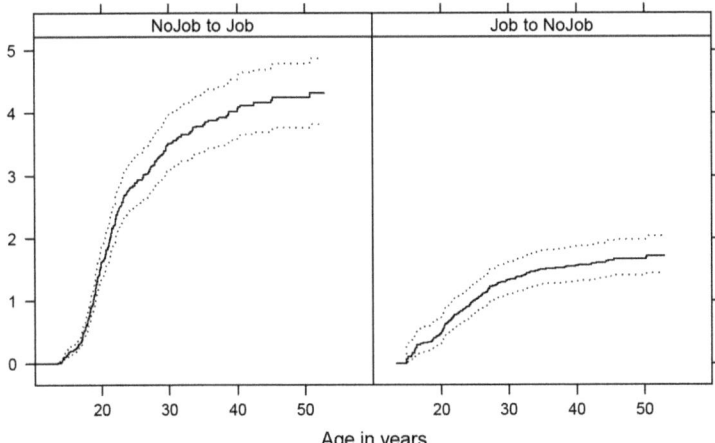

Fig. 6.7 Trellis plot of cumulative hazard rates, produced by *mvna*. GLHS

```
library (lattice)
xyplot(na,tr.choice=c("N J","J N"),
            aspect=1,
            strip=strip.custom(bg="white",
            factor.levels=c("NoJob to Job",
                            "Job to NoJob"),
            par.strip.text=list(cex=0.9)),
            scales=list(alternating=1),
            xlab="Age in years",
            xlim=c(10,60),
            ylab="Nelson-Aalen esimates")
```

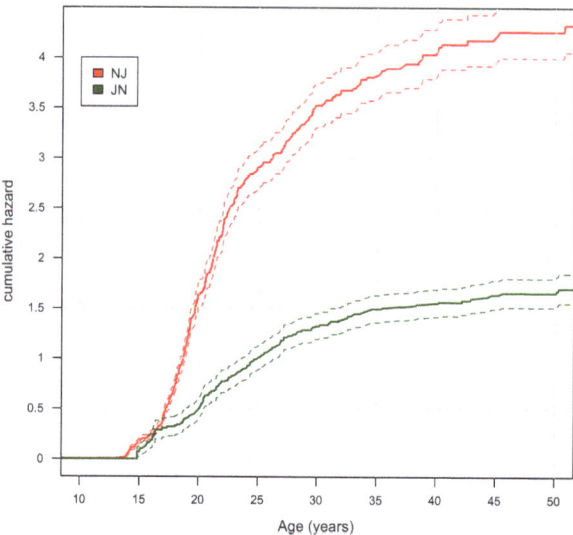

Fig. 6.8 Cumulative hazard rates. GLHS

The function plot.mvna plots the cumulative transition rates in one panel: plot(na). It does not show confidence intervals.

The following code produces a similar plot (Fig. 6.8) but does not require the *lattice* package:

6.4 The *mvna* and *etm* Packages

```
plot(c(0, na$'N J'$time),c(0,na$'N J'$na),
     type="l",
     xlab="Age (years)",
     ylab="cumulative hazard",
     xlim=c(10,50),
     main="GLHS Labour market transitions",
     col="red",
     axes=F,
     lwd=2)
 lines (c(0, na$'N J'$time),
        c(0,na$'N J'$na-sqrt(na$'N J'$var.aalen)),
        col="red",lty=2,lwd=1)
 lines (c(0, na$'N J'$time),
        c(0,na$'N J'$na+sqrt(na$'N J'$var.aalen)),
        col="red",lty=2,lwd=1)
  axis (side=1,at=seq(10,50,by=5),
        labels=seq(10,50,by=5),
        cex.axis=0.8)
  axis (side=2,las=1,at=seq(0,max(na$'N J'$na),by=0.5),
        labels=seq(0,max(na$'N J'$na),by=0.5),
        cex.axis=0.8)
box()
  abline (h=seq(0,max(na$'N J'$na),by=0.5),lty=2,col="lightgrey")
  abline (v=seq(10,50,by=5),lty=2,col="lightgrey")  # line at median
age
 lines (c(0,na$'J N'$time),c(0,na$'J N'$na),
        col="darkgreen",
        lty=1,
        lwd=2)
 lines (c(0,na$'J N'$time),c(0,na$'J N'$na-sqrt(na$'J N'$var.aalen)),
        col="darkgreen",
        lty=2)
 lines (c(0,na$'J N'$time),c(0,na$'J N'$na+sqrt(na$'J N'$var.aalen)),
        col="darkgreen",
        lty=2)
 legend(10,4,c("NJ","JN"),
        col=c("red","darkgreen"),
        fill=c("red","darkgreen"),
        cex=0.9,
        bg="white")
```

The cumulative hazard rates at given ages may be derived using the `predict` function of the *mvna* package. The cumulative hazard rate at consecutive birthdays from 0 to 53 is obtained by:

```
cumh.1 <- predict (na,times=seq(0,53,by=1))
```

The cumulative rates of transition from NoJob to Job are `cumh.1$'N J'$na`; the rates for the Job to NoJob transition are `cumh.1$'J N'$na`. Note that, while close in value to each other, the cumulative transition rate at a given age differs from the cumulative occurrence-exposure rate. The latter is the sum of transition rates that are averages in age intervals. From the cumulative transition rates, age-specific transition rates may be derived for further analysis, e.g. for the construction of multistate life tables.

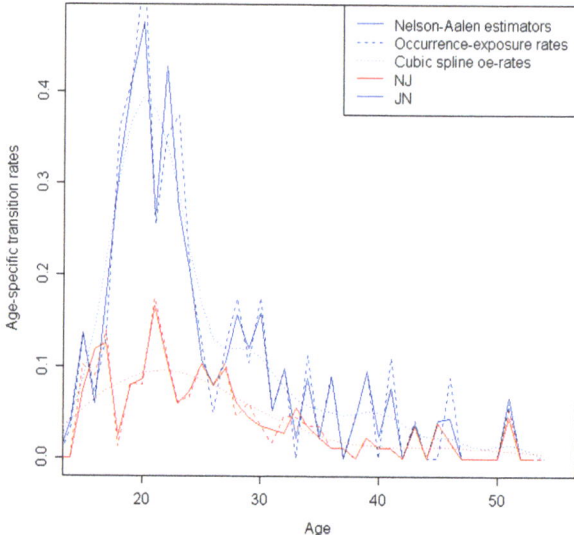

Fig. 6.9 Age-specific transition rates from NoJob to Job (NJ) and from Job to NoJob (JN): Nelson-Aalen estimates and occurrence-exposure rates. GLHS

Figure 6.9 shows the Nelson-Aalen estimators of the age-specific transition rates, produced by the *mvna* package, and the occurrence-exposure rates by single years of age, produced by *Biograph*. The two sets of rates are very similar as expected (Borgan and Hoem 1988, p. 888). The figure also shows the values of the occurrence-exposure rates smoothed by a cubic spline.

The cumulative transition rates are the basis for the multistate survival function and the sojourn time function. These functions and the multistate life table (MSLT), of which they are part, are discussed in Chaps. 2 and 7.

6.4.2 etm: Aalen-Johansen Estimator in Multistate Models

The transition rates are input to transition probabilities. The empirical transition probabilities or Aalen-Johansen estimators are obtained by product integration (Allignol et al. 2011; Beyersmann et al. 2012, p. 32ff), implemented in the *etm* package. The packages *etm* and *mvna* use the same input data. The following code produces the probability that an individual has a job at age 26.

```
etm <- etm::etm(data=Dmvna$D,
                state.names=c("N","J"),
                tra=attr(Dmvna$D,"param")$trans_possible,
                cens.name=Dmvna$cens,
                s=0,t=26)
```

The probability of being employed at 26 is 67.66 %. The probability may also be computed using the multistate life table. The multistate life table is also based on transition rates. The multistate life table based on Nelson-Aalen estimates of the cumulative hazard gives 70.41 % and the multistate life table based on occurrence-exposure rates gives 67.62 %. The latter is very close to the Aalen-Johansen estimate at age 26. The Aalen-Johansen estimator of being employed at age 50 is 69.41 %; the multistate life table gives 69.22 % if based on the Nelson-Aalen estimator and 69.74 % if based on the occurrence-exposure rates.

6.5 The *mstate* Package

The *mstate* package was developed by Putter and colleagues (Putter 2014; Putter et al. 2007, 2011; de Wreede et al. 2011). It estimates multistate models by using a Cox proportional hazard model for the transition rates. The method is described by Therneau and Grambsch (2000) and implemented in the `coxph` function of the *survival* package (see Sect. 6.2). In the proportional hazard model, the transition rate for an individual with given covariates is proportional to the transition rate of a reference individual, i.e. an individual with all covariate values equal to reference categories (see Putter et al. 2007, p. 2418). To accommodate different baseline hazards for different transitions, the data are stratified by transition.

Putter et al. discuss a particularly interesting application of multistate models, namely, the estimation of transition rates in the presence of a time-dependent covariate. The *mstate* package includes a function to predict the outcome of a process for persons with particular characteristics and histories. The process Putter et al. consider is a disease process. The prediction is in terms of conditional probabilities of some future events, given an event history and possibly a set of values for prognostic variables of the subject being considered. The prediction probabilities are special cases of the Aalen-Johansen estimator.

The *mstate* package requires data in the 'msdata' format (see Chap. 3). An object of class 'msdata' is a data frame with one row for each *possible* transition, i.e. for each transition *for which the subject is at risk*. In other words, there is one record of data for each competing risk. In addition, the data frame has the transition matrix as a '`trans`' attribute. Note that the data frame in the *Biograph* format has the same attribute, inspired by Putter et al. The need for one record for each transition for which the subject is at risk implies that several records refer to transitions that do not occur (indicator variable 0). That data requirement serves the flexibility in model specification. In *mstate* it is particularly easy to specify different transition models and to estimate the parameters of the models. That flexibility is a major strength of *mstate*.

The `Biograph.mstate` function produces a data frame in the 'msdata' format:

```
Dmstate <- Biograph.mstate (GLHS)
```

The function removes intrastate transitions, calls the `Parameters` function to determine the transition matrix, calls the `Biograph.long` function to produce a data frame in the long format and adds the attributes 'param', 'trans', 'format.date', and 'format.born' to create a data frame of class 'msdata':

```
attr(Dmstate, "param") <- Parameters(GLHS)
attr(Dmstate, "trans") <- Parameters(GLHS)$tmat
attr(Dmstate, "format.date") <- attr(GLHS,"format.date")
attr(Dmstate, "format.born") <- attr(GLHS,"format.born")
class(Dmstate) <- c("msdata", "data.frame")
```

The third command defines the class of the object. These three expressions are part of `Biograph.mstate`. The data frame `Dmstate` is of class 'mstate' (to check, use `str(Dmstate)`). The long format differs from that required by the *survival* package and *mvna* package. The *mstate* package requires one line for each *possible* transition. It implies that for every censored observation, one record is included for every possible destination. For instance, if a job episode is censored, one record is included for the transition from Job to NoJob (Job to Job is not possible). In that record the status variable is 0 indicating that the observation is censored. The transition matrix shows the transition numbers and is returned by the `Parameters` function as the 'tmat' component. In *mstate*, the intrastate transitions should be omitted. In the transition matrix, only NAs are allowed on the diagonal.

The `msprep` function of *mstate* creates an object of class 'msdata' from a data frame in a wide format, provided the Markov chain is irreversible acyclic (Putter et al. 2011, p. 18). States cannot be visited more than once. The illness-death model is an illustration of an irreversible Markov chain. The wide format has one record per subject. A record includes a subject identification number and the following information for each of the possible transitions: (a) time at transition or censoring and (b) indicator variable (status variable), which is 1 if the transition occurs and 0 otherwise. The wide format also contains covariates. In the long format (episode file), a record includes a subject identification number, the starting time and stopping time of the episode, a status variable to denote whether the episode ends in a transition (1) or not (0), the origin state and the destination state. A selection of covariates is copied to the long format. The selection is determined by the `keep` argument of the `msprep` function. If a (from-to)transition occurs, the destination state (receiving state) is visited. The transition time is equivalent to the time at which a state is visited.

Consider two illustrations. The first is an irreversible Markov chain. The illness-death model, extensively studied by Putter and colleagues, belongs to this category. The second is a reversible Markov chain, where subjects may leave a state and enter the state again at a later date. Most attention is paid to the first illustration.

6.5.1 Illness-Death Model

Suppose we want to study the employment path that starts at labour market entry (first job), includes second and higher-order jobs, and ends with entry in the NoJob state. Some persons exit their first job (J1) for the NoJob (N) state, while others have a second or third job (J2) before they enter the NoJob state. The second and higher-order jobs are denoted by second+ job. Some persons never enter the NoJob state. They are with a job at time of survey and they never experience a jobless period. The NoJob state is an absorbing state, which, once entered, cannot be left. We do not distinguish between second and higher-order jobs. This case is analogous to a model widely studied in epidemiology and known as the illness-death model, which has three states: healthy, diseased and death. It is shown in Fig. 6.10.

The transition matrix of the above diagram is shown below:

```
              to
from        Job1(J1)  Job2(J2)  NoJob(N)
   Job1(J1)    NA        1         2
   Job2(J2)    NA        NA        3
   NoJob(N)    NA        NA        NA
```

Transition 1 is the transition from the first job to a second job. It is also denoted as J1J. Transition 2, also denoted as J1N, is the transition from the first job to an episode without a job. Transition 3, also denoted as J2N, is the transition from the second or higher-order job to an episode without a job. We first discuss the data preparation. Data analysis is illustrated next. The transition matrix is produced by the function GLHS.trans():

```
trans <- GLHS.trans()
```

The function returns the transition matrix, which is stored in the object `trans`.

The function GLHS.IllnessDeath derives from the GLHS data the input data for the illness-death model with the three states Job1, Job2 and NoJob. The duration variable measures time since labour market entry. The function is included in *Biograph*. The following code produces a data frame in wide format to be used as input in the illness-death model:

```
tg <- GLHS.IllnessDeath (GLHS)
```

The data for the first 10 respondents in the wide format are shown in Table 6.3. ID is the identification number, and J1Jt is the time at transition from the first job to the second job or censoring. J1Js is the status variable indicating whether the respondent had a second job. JNt is the time at transition from Job (first or second+) to NoJob or from Job to censoring, and JNs is the status variable that indicates whether the NoJob state was ever entered. Several covariates are included in the data. The CMC at labour market entry is now treated as a covariate. From that

Fig. 6.10 Illness-death model of job change. GLHS

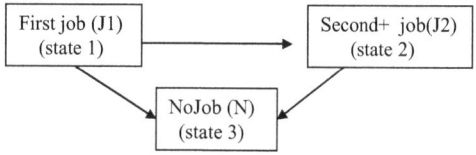

Table 6.3 GLHS data in wide format to be used as input in *mstate*

	ID	J1Jt	J1Js	JNt	JNs	sex	cohort	born	age_entry	edu
1	1	428	0	428	0	Male	1929-31	351	17.00	17
2	2	46	1	300	1	Female	1929-31	357	19.67	10
3	3	12	1	141	1	Female	1939-41	473	17.92	11
4	4	55	0	55	1	Female	1949-51	604	22.33	13
5	5	68	1	400	0	Male	1929-31	377	17.17	11
6	6	26	0	26	1	Male	1939-41	492	16.58	11
7	7	53	1	99	1	Female	1939-41	476	14.67	9
8	8	6	1	145	0	Male	1949-51	609	19.08	11
9	9	11	1	392	0	Male	1929-31	377	17.83	12
10	10	121	1	263	1	Male	1929-31	382	16.50	11

covariate, the age at labour market entry is calculated because later we want to assess whether persons who enter the labour market early have different transition rates than persons who enter at higher ages. A total of 30 persons enter the labour market before age 15 and 102 before age 18. The first respondent enters the labour market at age 17 with a professional college qualification, equivalent to 17 years of education. There is clearly a problem with the data. Although the variable edu is defined as the highest educational attainment before entry into the labour market (Blossfeld and Rohwer 2002, p. 44), it is likely that the variable was measured differently. The age at labour market entry is denoted by age_entry.

The following code produces the data in long msdata format:

```
library(mstate)
tmat <- attr(tg,"param")$tmat
tglong <- msprep(
          time=c(NA,"J1Jt","JNt"),
          status=c(NA,"J1Js","JNs"),
          data=tg,
          keep=c("sex","cohort","born",
          "age_entry","edu"),
          trans=tmat)
```

where tg is the object with the data in the wide format. The argument time is a character vector containing the column names indicating the transition times. Some elements of time may be missing (NA). Status is a character vector containing the column names with the status variables. The wide data structure has 201 records, the long structure 498. The keep argument lists the covariates to be kept in the long format. Data in the long format (tglong) are shown in Table 6.4 (the first 4 respondents).

6.5 The *mstate* Package

Table 6.4 GLHS data in long format to be used as input in *mstate*

	id	from	to	trans	Tstart	Tstop	time	status	sex	cohort	born	age_entry	edu
1	1	1	2	1	0	428	428	0	Male	1929-31	351	17.00	17
2	1	1	3	2	0	428	428	0	Male	1929-31	351	17.00	17
3	2	1	2	1	0	46	46	1	Female	1929-31	357	19.67	10
4	2	1	3	2	0	46	46	0	Female	1929-31	357	19.67	10
5	2	2	3	3	46	300	254	1	Female	1929-31	357	19.67	10
6	3	1	2	1	0	12	12	1	Female	1939-41	473	17.92	11
7	3	1	3	2	0	12	12	0	Female	1939-41	473	17.92	11
8	3	2	3	3	12	141	129	1	Female	1939-41	473	17.92	11
9	4	1	2	1	0	55	55	0	Female	1949-51	604	22.33	13
10	4	1	3	2	0	55	55	1	Female	1949-51	604	22.33	13

The first respondent (male) is in his first job when the observation is censored, 428 months after labour market entry. He did not move to a second job or the NoJob status. The second respondent (female) entered the labour market at CMC 593, changed jobs 46 months after labour market entry (at CMC 639). The competing risk (transition from J1 to N) did not materialise at that time. She left a job episode for an episode without a job in CMC 893, which is 300 months after she entered the labour market and 254 months since she started her second job.

The data in msdata format are used for analysis. For illustrative purposes, a few functions of the *mstate* package are considered. The number of transitions by origin and destination is produced by the following code:

```
z <- events(tglong)
```

Among the sample population, 96 left the first job for a second job, 89 left the first job for an episode without a job and 16 were censored while in their first job. Of those 96 with a second+ job, 45 moved to a period without a job before the survey and 51 had a job continuously between the start of the first job and the survey. The different trajectories that are possible in the multistate model, provided one cannot enter a state more than once, are given by paths(trans) of the *mstate* package. They are:

```
       [,1] [,2] [,3]
[1,]    1   NA   NA
[2,]    1    2   NA
[3,]    1    2    3
[4,]    1    3   NA
```

A major strength of the *mstate* package is the flexible approach to estimating transition models. The flexibility is largely the result of being able to associate covariates with each transition. Covariates may affect transitions differently.

The expand.covs function expands the data set (long format) by adding transition-specific covariates (also called type-specific covariates, Putter et al. 2007, p. 2403). The covariate cov associated with transition s is called cov.s, where s = 1, 2, ..., n with n the number of transitions. The extension s refers to a specific transition. The transition number is given in the transition matrix

Table 6.5 GLHS data in expanded format of *mstate*

	id	from	to	trans	Tstart	Tstop	time	status	sex	cohort	born	age_entry	edu
1	1	1	2	1	0	428	428	0	Male	1929-31	351	17.00	17
2	1	1	3	2	0	428	428	0	Male	1929-31	351	17.00	17
3	2	1	2	1	0	46	46	1	Female	1929-31	357	19.67	10
4	2	1	3	2	0	46	46	0	Female	1929-31	357	19.67	10
5	2	2	3	3	46	300	254	1	Female	1929-31	357	19.67	10
6	3	1	2	1	0	12	12	1	Female	1939-41	473	17.92	11
7	3	1	3	2	0	12	12	0	Female	1939-41	473	17.92	11
8	3	2	3	3	12	141	129	1	Female	1939-41	473	17.92	11
9	4	1	2	1	0	55	55	0	Female	1949-51	604	22.33	13
10	4	1	3	2	0	55	55	1	Female	1949-51	604	22.33	13

(continued)

	sexFemale.1	sexFemale.2	sexFemale.3
1	0	0	0
2	0	0	0
3	1	0	0
4	0	1	0
5	0	0	1
6	1	0	0
7	0	1	0
8	0	0	1
9	1	0	0
10	0	1	0

trans. For example, for the covariate sex, sex.1 is the covariate associated with the first transition (J1J), sex.2 the covariate associated with the second transition (J1N), etc. The expanded long format is produced by the following code:

```
tglonge <- expand.covs(tglong,
          c("sex","cohort","age_entry","edu"))
```

where the covariates are specified in the argument list. The expanded covariates data set can be used in regression models. The object may become quite large. A version with a single covariate is illustrated in Table 6.5. The covariate sexFemale.1 (s.1) impacts on transition 1, covariate sexFemale.2 (s.2) on transition 2 and sexFemale.3 (s.3) on transition 3. The value of sexFemale is 0 if the respondent is male and 1 if the respondent is female. The regression coefficient associated with the covariate gives the effect on the transition rate of being a female relative to the effect of being a male (reference category).

Suppose we want to know whether the effect of gender on the rate of transition varies between transitions. Assume that the three transitions have different baseline hazards, which is implemented by stratifying the data by transition. The line number of a transition is the stratification variable: strata (trans). For a given transition, the rates for males and females are proportional, however. The model is:

```
cx.s <- coxph(Surv(Tstart,Tstop,status) ~
        sexFemale.1+sexFemale.2+sexFemale.3
        +strata(trans),
        data=tglonge,method="breslow")
```

6.5 The *mstate* Package

> **Box 6.16: The Effect of Gender on Transition Rates. Cox Model. GLHS**
>
> ```
> a. Output cx.s
> Call:
> coxph(formula = Surv(Tstart, Tstop, status) ~ sexFemale.1 +
>   sexFemale.2 + sexFemale.3 + strata(trans), data = tglonge,
>   method = "breslow")
>
>               coef exp(coef) se(coef)      z       p
> sexFemale.1 -0.0105    0.99    0.212 -0.0494 0.96000
> sexFemale.2  0.5995    1.82    0.219  2.7330 0.00630
> sexFemale.3  1.0610    2.89    0.314  3.3781 0.00073
>
> Likelihood ratio test=19.5  on 3 df, p=0.000211  n= 498,
> number of events= 230
>
> b. Output cx.s2
>                                               coef  se(coef)       p
> as.factor(sex)Female                       -0.0105    0.212    0.96
> as.factor(trans)2                               NA       NA      NA
> as.factor(trans)3                               NA       NA      NA
> as.factor(sex)Female:as.factor(trans)2   0.6099    0.305   0.0450
> as.factor(sex)Female:as.factor(trans)3   1.0715    0.379   0.0047
> ```

Putter et al. (2007) refer to the model as the Markov stratified hazards model. The results are shown in Box 6.16. The exponentiated coefficients exp(coef) are *hazard ratios*, i.e. ratios of hazard rates of females over hazard rates of males (reference category). Hazard ratios are interpretable as multiplicative effects on the hazard. The example shows that gender has no significant effect on the rate of job change (J1J), but a significant effect on the rate of leaving employment, particularly after the second or higher-order jobs (J2N). The J1N transition rate for women is 82 % higher than the rate for men. For the J2N transition, the rate is 189 % higher. Hence, the effect of gender on the transitions is quite different. The results in the box are produced by summary(cx.s). The cumulative baseline hazards are produced by the basehaz(cx.s) function, which is part of the *survival* package.

The results shown in Box 6.16a may also be obtained by applying the Cox model to subsets of data and by applying an interaction term. First, consider subsets of data and consider the second transition, which is J1N. The following code produces the same effect of gender on the J1N transition rate as the expanded model (regression coefficient 0.599):

```
tg2 <- subset(tglong,tglong$trans==2)
cx.2 <- coxph(Surv(Tstart,Tstop,status)~sex,
         data=tg2,
         method="breslow")
```

The model with an interaction term between gender and the transition is:

```
cx.s2 <- coxph(Surv(Tstart,Tstop,status)~
    as.factor(sex)+strata(trans)
    +as.factor(sex)*as.factor(trans),
    data=tglong,method="breslow")
```

The result is shown in Box 6.16b. The coefficient -0.0105 is the effect of gender on the transition rate J1J (transition 1). Transition is a categorical variable and transition J1J is the reference category. Females are a little less mobile than males ($100*(\exp(-0.0105)-1) = 1\%$). The effect on transition 2 is the effect on the first transition plus the effect of the interaction between gender and transition, $-0.0105 + 0.6099 = 0.5995$, which is the coefficient obtained in the model with expanded covariates. The interaction term is significant, indicating that gender influences transitions 1 (J1J) and 2 (J1N) differently. The NAs in the second and third rows are due to the fact that the main effects of the transition type cannot be estimated since, for each transition, the baseline hazard is freely estimated. By stratifying the data by transition, the transition-specific baseline hazards are not restricted in any way.

For each of the three transitions J1J, J1N and J2N, the cumulative hazard rates are obtained by the basehaz function from the *survival* package.

```
z<- basehaz(cx.s,centered=FALSE)
```

The object z contains the cumulative hazard rates for males (reference category) for durations at which transitions occur (z$time) and for each stratum (z$strata). The cumulative hazards for females are obtained by multiplying the male hazards by the exponent of the appropriate coefficient of the Cox model. For instance, the cumulative J1N transition rates for females are z$hazard[z$strata=="trans = 2"]*exp(0.5995).

The predicted survival functions for the Cox model (the probability that a job duration exceeds a given value) and for each transition are produced by the survfit function, which is part of the *survival* package:

```
y <- survfit (cx.s)
```

The numeric values of the survival function and the confidence intervals are given by summary(y). By default, Survfit estimates the survival function for the average value of the covariates. Average values are not meaningful for categorical variables. Therefore, the survival function needs to be estimated for specific values of the covariates, specified in the newdata argument of the survfit function. The following code estimates survival functions for males (ym) and females (yf):

6.5 The *mstate* Package

```
ym <- survfit (cx.s,
       newdata=data.frame(sexFemale.1=0,sexFemale.2=0,
       sexFemale.3=0),individual=FALSE)
yf <- survfit (cx.s,
       newdata=data.frame(sexFemale.1=1,sexFemale.2=1,
       sexFemale.3=1),individual=FALSE)
```

The `plot` function is the `plot.msfit` function, which plots an object of class 'msfit'.

```
plot(ym$time[1:ym$strata[1]],
     ym$surv[1:ym$strata[1]],
     type="s",col="red",
     xlab="Months since labour market entry",
     ylab="Survival probability",
     ylim=c(0,1),las=1)        # J1J males
lines (ym$time[(ym$strata[1]+1):(ym$strata[1]+ym$strata[2])],
       ym$surv[(ym$strata[1]+1):(ym$strata[1]+ym$strata[2])],
       type="s",col="blue")              # J1N males
lines (ym$time[(ym$strata[1]+ym$strata[2]+1):
       (ym$strata[1]+ym$strata[2]+ym$strata[3])],
       ym$surv[(ym$strata[1]+ym$strata[2]+1):
       (ym$strata[1]+ym$strata[2]+ym$strata[3])],
       type="s",col="green")             # J2N males
lines (yf$time[1:yf$strata[1]],yf$surv[1:yf$strata[1]],
       type="s",col="red",lty=2)         # J1J females
lines (yf$time[(yf$strata[1]+1):(yf$strata[1]+yf$strata[2])],
       yf$surv[(yf$strata[1]+1):(yf$strata[1]+yf$strata[2])],
       type="s",col="blue",lty=2)        # J1N females
lines (yf$time[(yf$strata[1]+yf$strata[2]+1):
       (yf$strata[1]+yf$strata[2]+yf$strata[3])],
       yf$surv[(yf$strata[1]+yf$strata[2]+1):
       (yf$strata[1]+yf$strata[2]+yf$strata[3])],
       type="s",col="green",lty=2)       # J2N females
legend ("topright",
        legend=c("J1J","J1N","J2N"),
        col=c("red","blue","green"),
        fil=c("red","blue","green"),
        cex=0.9,bg="white")
legend (180,1,
        legend=c("Males","Females"),
        lty=1:2,bg="white")
```

The resulting survival functions are shown in Fig. 6.11.

An alternative to `survfit` is the `msfit` function in the *mstate* package. The msfit function estimates individual cumulative hazards. An individual is characterised by covariate values. Consider a single covariate: sex. The following code produces the estimated cumulative hazard for each transition together with the estimated variances and covariances. The measures are evaluated at the durations at which transitions occur in any of the strata. The code is:

Fig. 6.11 Survival functions for J1J, J1N and J2N transitions, by sex. GLHS

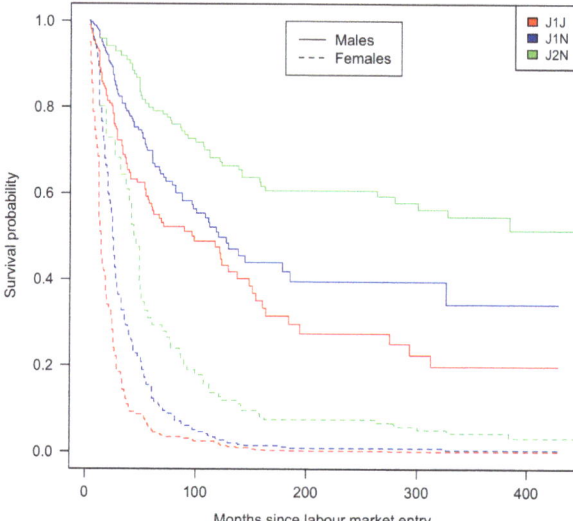

```
newdm <- data.frame(trans=1:3,
      sexFemale.1=c(0,0,0),sexFemale.2=c(0,0,0),
      sexFemale.3=c(0,0,0),strata=1:3)
msfm <-msfit(cx.s,newdata=newdm,
      trans= attr(tglonge,"trans"))
newdf <- data.frame(trans=1:3,
      sexFemale.1=c(1,0,0),sexFemale.2=c(0,1,0),
      sexFemale.3=c(0,0,1),strata=1:3)
msff <-msfit(cx.s,newdata=newdf,
      trans= attr(tglonge,"trans"))
```

The individual characteristics are specified in the newdata frame. The data frame newdm has the information for males and newdf has the information for females. The first column shows the line number of the transitions. The second, third and fourth columns show the covariate values of males (newdm) and females (newdf). Since 'males' is the reference category, the values are 0. The last column of the newdata frame specifies to which stratum in the coxph object a transition belongs. This is needed in msfit but not in survfit.

In the previous application (model cx.s), I assumed that each transition corresponds to a separate stratum (stratification variable trans). Suppose now that two transitions have a common baseline hazard. The research question is: What are the rates of leaving a second or higher-order job for a jobless period by job duration if the rates are proportional to the rates of leaving for persons in their first job (first-job holders)? The assumption of proportionality is introduced by grouping the J1N and J2N transitions in the same stratum. The transitions J1N and J2N have a common destination state (N). Therefore, the stratum variable is the destination state (to). The interpretation of common baseline hazard is: Persons in their second or higher-order job have a rate of leaving that job for a jobless period that is

6.5 The *mstate* Package

proportional to the rate of leaving for first-job holders. The proportionality holds irrespective of job duration. Persons in their second or higher-order job have z times the rate of first-job holders. Persons are at risk of the J2N transition only after entering a second or higher-order job. J1J is an intermediate event that impacts on the rate of transition to N. The occurrence of the intermediate event (J1J) is a time-dependent covariate (Putter et al. 2007, p. 2418; Putter 2014, p. 7). The time-dependent covariate (newjob) equals 0 before the transition from the first to the second job (J1J) and 1 after the job change. It means that the time-dependent covariate equals 0 when the subject is at risk for the J1J and J1N transitions, and it is 1 if the subject is at risk of the J2N transition. Hence,

```
tglonge$newjob <- ifelse(tglonge$trans==3,1,0)
```

I first consider the model without covariates. The model is:

```
vv <- coxph(Surv(Tstart,Tstop,status)~
    newjob+ strata(to),
    data=tglonge,method="breslow")
```

The model predicts three transition rates (J1J, J1N and J2N) for various job durations when the rates of transitions J1N and J2N are forced to be proportional. The coefficient of newjob is the effect of being in a second or higher-order job on the rate of leaving a job for a jobless period. It is -0.278. The baseline hazards are given by the basehaz(vv) function. The baseline hazard in the (to=2) stratum gives the cumulative rates of J1J transition by job duration. The baseline hazard in the (to=3) stratum gives the cumulative rates of transition J1N, which is the reference category (newjob $= 0$). The cumulative rates of transition J2N are the cumulative rates of transition J1J multiplied by $\exp(-0.278)$. The cumulative transition rates are shown in Fig. 6.12.

Now I distinguish males and females. The research question is: Do males and females have different rates of transition if the rate of moving to a jobless period from a second or higher-order job is proportional to the rate of moving to a jobless period from the first job? The combination of the two transitions results in the following model:

```
cx.s.p <- coxph(Surv(Tstart,Tstop,status)~
    sexFemale.1+sexFemale.2+sexFemale.3
    + newjob + strata(to),
    data=tglonge,method="breslow")
```

The model predicts the effect of sex on the three transition rates (J1J, J1N and J2N), when the J1N and J2N transitions are forced to share a common baseline hazard. It means that the rates of the transitions J1N and J2N are proportional. The output is shown in Box 6.17. The effect of sex on the J1J transition is the same as in the Cox model with the data stratified by transition (Box 6.16). The baseline hazard

Fig. 6.12 Cumulative hazards of J1J, J1N and J2N transitions. GLHS

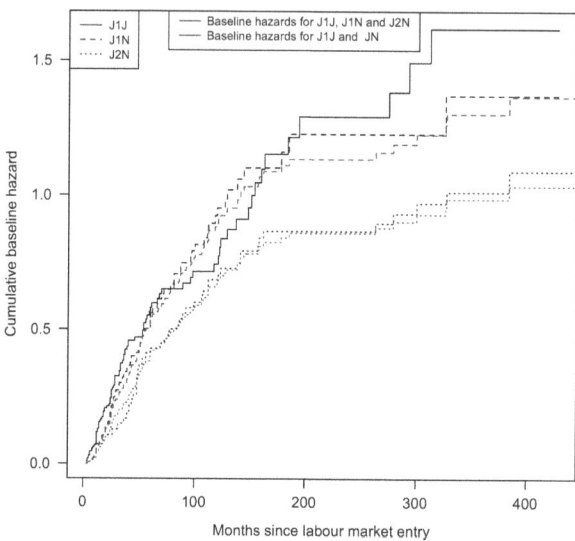

Box 6.17: Effect of Gender on J1J, J1N and J2N Transition Rates. Cox Model with Stratification by Destination State. GLHS

```
Call:
coxph(formula = Surv(Tstart, Tstop, status) ~ sexFemale.1 +
sexFemale.2 + sexFemale.3 + newjob + strata(to),
data = tglonge, method = "breslow")

              coef exp(coef) se(coef)       z      p
sexFemale.1 -0.0105    0.990    0.212 -0.0494 0.9600
sexFemale.2  0.6074    1.836    0.217  2.7944 0.0052
sexFemale.3  1.0547    2.871    0.311  3.3883 0.0007
newjob      -0.5411    0.582    0.303 -1.7842 0.0740

Likelihood ratio test=21.6  on 4 df, p=0.000238  n= 498,
number of events= 230
```

of the J1N and J2N transitions does not affect the J1J transition. The regression coefficients associated with the J1N and J2N transitions are comparable to the those of the Cox model with data stratified by transition, as expected (Putter et al. 2007, p. 2420). The hazard ratio of newjob (0.582) indicates that respondents (male or female) are less likely to leave a job for a jobless period if they are in the second or a higher-order job. The effect of job change on the rate of leaving a job for a jobless period is however not statistically significant.

The validity of the proportionality assumption can be inspected graphically or tested more formally using the cox.zph function from the *survival* package (result not shown):

6.5 The *mstate* Package

```
cox.zph(cx.s.p)
```

Although a transition from a first to a second job does not affect the rate of transition to a jobless period significantly, the time of job change may. Time is measured as the duration since entry in the first job (labour market entry). Persons who leave their first job at short durations may have a higher risk of becoming jobless than persons who stay relatively long with their first job. The start of a second job is the onset (Tstart) of the risk period for the J2N transition. Hence,

```
tglonge$tnewjob.3 <- ifelse (tglong$trans==3,
             tglonge$Tstart[tglonge$trans==3],0)
```

The model is:

```
cx.s.p2 <- coxph(Surv(Tstart,Tstop,status)~
    sexFemale.1+sexFemale.2+sexFemale.3
    + newjob + tnewjob.3
    + strata(to),
    data=tglonge,
    method="breslow")
```

The result is not shown. The coefficients for sex and the move to a second or higher-order job are about the same as in the previous model. The timing of job change has no effect.

Stratification results in separate and unrelated baseline hazards. If we assume that the baseline hazards are proportional, then the transitions are not used as strata but as covariates for which relative risks are estimated. The model is:

```
cx.s3 <- coxph(Surv(Tstart,Tstop,status)~
        as.factor(sex)+
        as.factor(trans),
        data=tglong,method="breslow")
```

The regression coefficients are not shown. For a discussion of these and other models, see Putter et al. (2007).

Males and females may have different transition rates because of other covariates, such as birth cohort, level of education, age at entry in the labour market and marital status. Marital status is a time-varying covariate. Consider the additional effects of birth cohort and education. The following code estimates a separate Cox model for each transition (transition 1 is J1J, 2 is J1N and 3 is J2N):

```
cx.sce <- coxph(Surv(Tstart,Tstop,status)~
    sexFemale.1+cohort1939.41.1+cohort1949.51.1 + edu.1
    +sexFemale.2+cohort1939.41.2+cohort1949.51.2 + edu.2
    +sexFemale.3+cohort1939.41.3+cohort1949.51.3 + edu.3
    +strata(trans),
    data=tglonge,method="breslow")
```

The result of this model estimation is shown in Box 6.18. The introduction of period of birth and level of education does change the effect of sex, but not much. If one controls for birth period and level of education, then the rate at which females leave a first job for a jobless period relative to males increases slightly (91 % compared to 82 %; compare Boxes 6.18 and 6.16). The effect of education on leaving the first job for a jobless period is statistically significant with each year of education raising the rate of leaving by 10 %. Education has no effect on the rate of changing jobs, however.

The model may be used to predict the cumulative transition rates for two groups of males, born in 1939–1941. The first group has 17 years of education (professional college). The second group has 11 years of education (lower secondary school with vocational training). The characteristics of the subpopulation selected are provided in the `newdat` object:

Box 6.18: Effect of Gender, Birth Cohort and Level of Education on Timing of Job Change. Cox Model. GLHS

```
Call:
coxph(formula = Surv(Tstart, Tstop, status) ~ sexFemale.1 +
cohort1939.41.1 + cohort1949.51.1 + edu.1 +
sexFemale.2 + cohort1939.41.2 + cohort1949.51.2 + edu.2 +
sexFemale.3 + cohort1939.41.3 + cohort1949.51.3 + edu.3 +
strata(trans), data = tglonge, method = "breslow")

                  coef exp(coef) se(coef)      z       p
sexFemale.1    -0.0323    0.968   0.2181  -0.148 0.88000
cohort1939.41.1 0.3838    1.468   0.2607   1.472 0.14000
cohort1949.51.1 0.2910    1.338   0.2524   1.153 0.25000
edu.1           0.0230    1.023   0.0453   0.508 0.61000
sexFemale.2     0.6457    1.907   0.2284   2.826 0.00470
cohort1939.41.2 0.5295    1.698   0.2768   1.913 0.05600
cohort1949.51.2 0.3727    1.452   0.2582   1.443 0.15000
edu.2           0.1003    1.106   0.0430   2.333 0.02000
sexFemale.3     1.0799    2.944   0.3154   3.424 0.00062
cohort1939.41.3 0.2745    1.316   0.3800   0.722 0.47000
cohort1949.51.3 0.1849    1.203   0.3972   0.465 0.64000
edu.3          -0.0546    0.947   0.0797  -0.685 0.49000

Likelihood ratio test=31.6  on 12 df, p=0.00159   n= 498, number of
events= 230
```

6.5 The *mstate* Package

```
# Male born in 1939-41, with professional college
# qualification
    newdat17 <- data.frame(trans=1:3,
        sexFemale.1=c(0,0,0),
        cohort1939.41.1=c(0,1,0),
        cohort1949.51.1=c(0,0,0),
        edu.1=17,
        sexFemale.2=c(0,0,0),
        cohort1939.41.2=c(0,1,0),
        cohort1949.51.2=c(0,0,0),
        edu.2=17,
        sexFemale.3=c(0,0,0),
        cohort1939.41.3=c(0,0,1),
        cohort1949.51.3=c(0,0,0),
        edu.3=17,
        strata=1:3)

# Male, born in 1939-41 with secondary school
# qualifications with vocational training
    newdat11 <- data.frame(trans=1:3,
        sexFemale.1=c(0,0,0),
        cohort1939.41.1=c(1,0,0),
        cohort1949.51.1=c(0,0,0),
        edu.1=11,
        sexFemale.2=c(0,0,0),
        cohort1939.41.2=c(0,1,0),
        cohort1949.51.2=c(0,0,0),
        edu.2=11,
        sexFemale.3=c(0,0,0),
        cohort1939.41.3=c(0,0,1),
        cohort1949.51.3=c(0,0,0),
        edu.3=11,
        strata=1:3)
```

The following code produces the cumulative transition rates and the variances:

```
msf.sce17 <-msfit(cx.sce,newdata=newdat17,
        trans= attr(tglonge,"trans"))
msf.sce11 <-msfit(cx.sce,newdata=newdat11,
        trans= attr(tglonge,"trans"))
```

The cumulative transition rates are not shown.

The *mstate* package includes a function that predicts state and transition probabilities for subjects with a given set of covariates (including prognostic factors and life history or medical history) (Putter et al. 2007, p. 2421ff). For example, consider a male born in 1939–1941 with a professional college qualification and another person with the same characteristics except for the level of education. The following code predicts the state probabilities. The prediction starts at labour market entry ($predt = 0$) and yields state probabilities for successive points in time (direction forward).

Fig. 6.13 Multistate survival curve for male, born in 1939–1941 and with lower secondary school with vocational training. GLHS

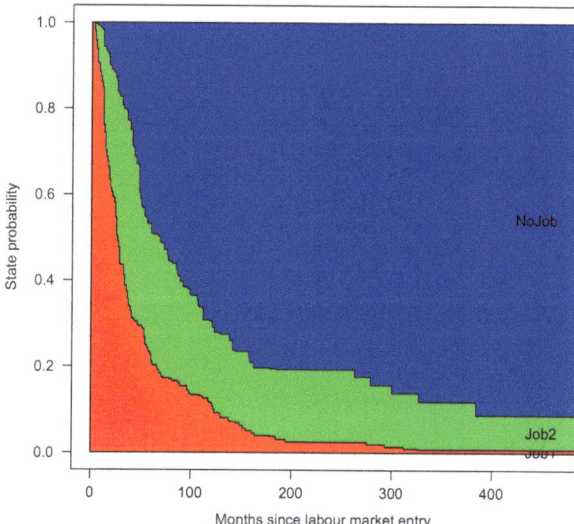

```
pt17 <- probtrans(msf.sce17,direction="forward",predt=0)
pt11 <- probtrans(msf.sce11,direction="forward",predt=0)
```

The `probtrans` function produces a list object with probabilities of transition from the state [[s]] at time `predt` to the states listed in the columns at durations listed in the rows. The object `pt17[[1]]` shows the state probabilities (state occupation probabilities) and their standard errors for males born in 1939–1941 and with professional college qualification. After 12 months of entry into the first job, the probability that a member of that group is still in the first job is 0.70 or 70% with a very large standard error (0.7). The probability that he is without a job is 11 % and the probability that he is in a second or higher-order job is 19 %. The standard errors are exceptionally high, however, due to the small sample size (201 respondents) and the small number of transitions. After 10 years (120 months), the probability of having entered the absorbing jobless state is 87 %. Note that a return from a jobless state to a job is not accounted for in this 'illness-death' model. A male born in the same period but with lower secondary school vocational training has a probability of 76 % to be in the first job 12 months after entry, 18 % to be in a second or higher-order job and 6 % to be without a job. The multistate survival function for a male, born in 1939–1941 and with lower secondary school with vocational training, is displayed in Fig. 6.13. The plot is produced by the function `plot.probtrans`, which plots an object of class '`probtrans`':

```
plot (pt11,type="filled",ord=c(1,2,3),las=1,
      xlab="Months since labour market entry",
      ylab="State probability",
      cex.main=0.9)
```

6.5.2 Reversible Markov Chain

The second application is a reversible Markov chain in which a state may be left and entered again at a later date. It is sometimes viewed as an illness-death model with recovery. It was considered by de Wreede et al. (2010). Reversible Markov chains have been studied extensively in mobility (e.g. migration) modelling. The state space is shown in Fig. 6.14. There are 323 NJ transitions and 181 JN transitions. Intrastate transitions are removed.

Biograph.mstate produces a data structure in 'msdata' format, excluding transitions to the same state. The param, trans and format.date attributes of the *Biograph* object are transferred to the object of class 'msdata':

```
Dmstate <- Biograph.mstate (GLHS)
```

The transition matrix of the reversible Markov chain can be retrieved from the Dmstate object as follows:

```
trans <- attr(Dmstate,"trans")
```

The transition matrix is:

```
          To
From   N   J
   N  NA   1
   J   2  NA
```

The first transition is the NJ transition; the second is JN. The transition count is produced by the events function of *mstate*, i.e. events (Dmstate) (Box 6.19).

Note that for 142 Job episodes and 59 NoJob episodes, observation ends at survey date. The function paths does not produce the sample paths in the multistate model, but gives an error message (*infinite recursion*). The reason is the infinite number of possible paths in a reversible Markov chain.

To study the impact of covariates on each of the NJ and JN transitions separately, the data set must be expanded by specifying transition-specific covariates. The expanded data set is created by the expand.covs function of the *mstate* package. Four covariates are considered for illustration: sex, birth cohort, level of education and age at marriage.

To facilitate the interpretation of the regression coefficients, Dmstate includes age. The ages at start and end of episodes with and without a job are:

```
Dmstate$Tstarta <-
round(cmc_as_age(Dmstate$Tstart,Dmstate$born,"cmc")$age,2)
Dmstate$Tstopa <-
round(cmc_as_age(Dmstate$Tstop,Dmstate$born,"cmc")$age,2)
```

Fig. 6.14 The reversible Markov chain model

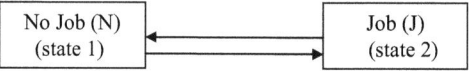

No Job (N) (state 1) ← → Job (J) (state 2)

Box 6.19: Transitions in the Reversible Markov Chain Model. GLHS

```
$Frequencies
       to
from    N    J  no event  total entering
  N     0  323        59              382
  J   181    0       142              323

$Proportions
       to
from          N          J   no event
  N  0.0000000  0.8455497  0.1544503
  J  0.5603715  0.0000000  0.4396285
```

Age at marriage is specified as:

```
Dmstate$agem <- round ((Dmstate$marriage-
                        Dmstate$born)/12,2)
```

Redundant variables are removed:

```
Dmstate$Tstart <- Dmstate$Tstop <-
      Dmstate$pres <- Dmstate$NOJ <-
      Dmstate$TE <- Dmstate$marriage <- NULL
```

The code that produces the expanded data set is:

```
Dcov <- expand.covs(Dmstate,
        c("sex","cohort","edu","agem"))
```

A selection of the expanded data set is shown in Table 6.6.

First, we estimate the NJ and JN transition rates separately by specifying a Cox model with stratum variable and without covariates. The msfit function is used to create data frames containing cumulative hazards:

6.5 The *mstate* Package

Table 6.6 Expanded data set for reversible Markov chain model, with selection of covariates. GLHS

	ID	OR	DES	status	trans	edu	LMentry	cohort	OD	Episode	Tstarta	Tstopa	from	to	agem	sexFemale.1	sexFemale.2
1.2	1	N	J	1	1	17	555	1929-31	NJ	1	0.00000	17.00000	1	2	27.33	0	0
1.15	1	J	N	0	2	17	555	1929-31	cens	2	17.00000	52.66667	2	1	27.33	0	0
2.2	2	N	J	1	1	10	593	1929-31	NJ	1	0.00000	19.66667	1	2	33.75	1	0
2.3	2	J	N	1	2	10	593	1929-31	JN	2	19.66667	44.66667	2	1	33.75	0	1
2.15	2	N	J	0	1	10	593	1929-31	cens	3	44.66667	52.16667	1	2	33.75	1	0
3.2	3	N	J	1	1	11	688	1939-41	NJ	1	0.00000	17.91667	1	2	33.08	0	1
3.3	3	J	N	1	2	11	688	1939-41	JN	2	17.91667	29.66667	2	1	33.08	1	0
3.15	3	N	J	0	1	11	688	1939-41	cens	3	29.66667	42.50000	1	2	33.08	1	0
4.2	4	N	J	1	1	13	872	1949-51	NJ	1	0.00000	22.33333	1	2	22.33	1	0
4.3	4	J	N	1	2	13	872	1949-51	JN	2	22.33333	26.91667	2	1	22.33	0	1

```
c1 <- coxph(Surv(Tstarta,Tstopa,status) ~
            strata(trans),
            data=Dmstate,
            method="breslow")
fit1 <- msfit (c1,trans= attr(Dmstate,"trans"),
            vartype="aalen")
```

Now we consider covariates by using the following code:

```
cs <- coxph(Surv(Tstarta,Tstopa,status) ~
            sexFemale.1+sexFemale.2
            +cohort1939.41.1+cohort1939.41.2
            +cohort1949.51.1+cohort1949.51.2
            +edu.1+edu.2
            +strata(trans),
            data=Dcov,
            method="breslow")
```

The results are shown in Box 6.20. To interpret the figures, note that all respondents entered the labour market, i.e. they have at least one job episode.

Box 6.20: Cox Proportional Hazard Model for the NJ and JN Transitions. GLHS

```
Call:
coxph(formula = Surv(Tstarta, Tstopa, status) ~ sexFemale.1 +
    sexFemale.2 + cohort1939.41.1 + cohort1939.41.2 + cohort1949.51.1 +
    cohort1949.51.2 + edu.1 + edu.2 + strata(trans), data = Dcov,
    method = "breslow")

                   coef exp(coef) se(coef)      z       p
sexFemale.1     -0.7940     0.452   0.1345 -5.904 3.5e-09
sexFemale.2      0.9872     2.684   0.1571  6.285 3.3e-10
cohort1939.41.1  0.1328     1.142   0.1386  0.958 3.4e-01
cohort1939.41.2  0.4613     1.586   0.1866  2.472 1.3e-02
cohort1949.51.1  0.0868     1.091   0.1408  0.616 5.4e-01
cohort1949.51.2  0.2576     1.294   0.1977  1.303 1.9e-01
edu.1           -0.1441     0.866   0.0280 -5.139 2.8e-07
edu.2            0.0883     1.092   0.0344  2.564 1.0e-02

Likelihood ratio test=110  on 8 df, p=0  n= 705, number of events= 504
```

Persons who never got a job are excluded from the data. The data show that for females the rate of job entry from a position without a job is 54 % less than the rate for males. Since all females in the data had at least one job, it means that, once they leave a job for a jobless period, they are considerably less likely than males to enter a new job. Their rate of leaving a job for an episode without a job is 168 % larger than for males. The cohort effect is not statistically significant but the effect of education is. Education seems to reduce job entry (NJ) and increase job exit (JN), which is not expected. The effect of education is even stronger and in the same direction if the interaction between gender and education level is introduced in the model. Since all persons in the sample experienced at least one job episode, it means that persons with more education are a little less likely to leave a job, and they are less likely to get a new job once they left a job for a jobless period.

One may expect that, in the cohorts studied, females are likely to leave employment after marriage and never return to a job. Marital status is a time-varying covariate. The following code generates the variable mar for marital status and the variables mar.1 and mar.2 to assess the effect of marital status change on the NJ and JN transitions:

```
Dcov$mar <- ifelse(Dcov$Tstarta >= Dcov$agem,1,0)
Dcov$mar.1 <- ifelse (Dcov$trans==1,Dcov$mar,0)
Dcov$mar.2 <- ifelse (Dcov$trans==2,Dcov$mar,0)
```

The following model estimates the effect of gender, marital status and their interaction on the NJ and JN transition rates:

```
cs.sm <- coxph(Surv(Tstarta,Tstopa,status) ~
        sexFemale.1+sexFemale.2+
        +mar.1+mar.2
        +sexFemale.1*mar.1 +sexFemale.2*mar.2
        + strata(trans),
        data=Dcov,
        method="breslow")
```

Box 6.21 shows the result.

The analysis reveals that the reason for a lower NJ transition rate for females is marital status. Females have a lower NJ rate than males, but the gender effect is not statistically significant. Note that all persons in the subsample have at least one job. Married persons have an NJ rate that is almost twice that of not married persons. It means that married persons are very likely to get another job once they have left a job. This observation applies much less to females than to males, however. Married females have an NJ transition rate that is only 13 % of that of married males. The cumulative hazard rates for females show an interesting pattern. Non-married females have a relatively low rate of job exit and a high rate of job re-entry. The cumulative rate of job entry increases in an approximately linear fashion, meaning that the rate of leaving a jobless period does not decline with age. Married females

6.5 The *mstate* Package

Box 6.21: Effect of Gender and Marital Status on NJ and JN Transition Rates. GLHS

```
                   coef exp(coef) se(coef)        z       p
sexFemale.1     -0.0708     0.932    0.129  -0.550 5.8e-01
sexFemale.2      0.8764     2.402    0.169   5.177 2.2e-07
mar.1            0.5914     1.807    0.234   2.527 1.1e-02
mar.2           -0.4107     0.663    0.466  -0.882 3.8e-01
sexFemale.1:mar.1 -2.0216   0.132    0.285  -7.084 1.4e-12
sexFemale.2:mar.2  0.7027   2.019    0.522   1.346 1.8e-01

Likelihood ratio test=128  on 6 df, p=0  n= 705, number of events= 504
```

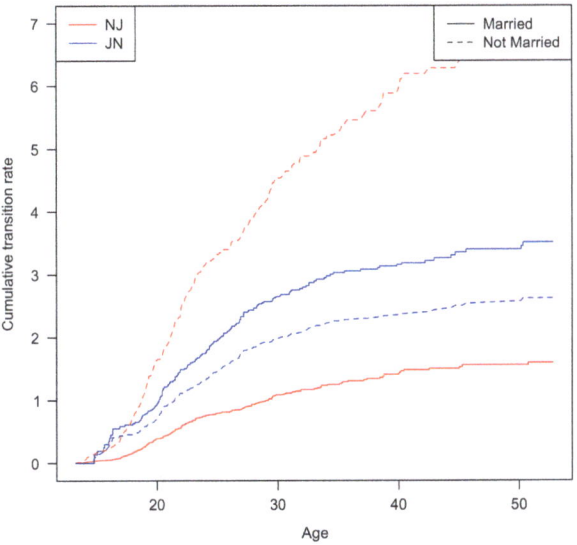

Fig. 6.15 Cumulative job entry and job exit rates of females, predicted by Cox model with predictors gender and marital status, using the msfit function of the *mstate* package. GLHS

have a high rate of job exit and a rather low rate of job entry (exit from jobless episode) (see Fig. 6.15). Note that the data used for the illustration were collected in the early 1980s in Germany and covered cohorts born before 1952. At that time and for that cohort, female labour force participation was less than today and many women left the labour force at time of marriage or childbirth.

The figure is produced by the following code:

```
# married persons
newdat <- data.frame(trans=1:2,
                     sexFemale.1=c(1,0),
                     mar.1=c(1,0),
                     sexFemale.2=c(0,1),
                     mar.2=c(0,1),
                     strata=1:2)
fit.sm1 <- msfit (cs.sm,trans= attr(Dmstate,"trans"),
         vartype="aalen",newdata=newdat)
plot(fit.sm1,las=1,xlab="Age",
         ylab="Cumulative transition rate",
         legend=c("NJ","JN"),legend.pos="topleft",
         col=c("red","blue"),
         cex.main=0.9,ylim=c(0,7))
# no-married persons
newdat <- data.frame(trans=1:2,
                     sexFemale.1=c(1,0),
                     mar.1=c(0,0),
                     sexFemale.2=c(0,1),
                     mar.2=c(0,0),
                     strata=1:2)
fit.sm2 <- msfit (cs.sm,trans= attr(Dmstate,"trans"),
         vartype="aalen",newdata=newdat)
lines (fit.sm2$Haz$time[fit.sm2$Haz$trans==1],
      fit.sm2$Haz$Haz[fit.sm2$Haz$trans==1],
      lty=2,col="red")
lines (fit.sm2$Haz$time[fit.sm2$Haz$trans==2],
      fit.sm2$Haz$Haz[fit.sm2$Haz$trans==2],
      lty=2,col="blue")
legend ("topright",
      legend=c("Married","Not Married"),
      lty=1:2,bg="white")
```

In this section I illustrated the *mstate* package using an illness-death model with three states and unidirectional moves (no re-entry) and a model with two states and re-entry. A major strength of the *mstate* package is the flexible approach to estimating transition models. The long format, in combination with type-specific covariates (expanded data set) and stratified Cox regression, offers great flexibility in modelling the effect of covariates on the different transition rates, while using standard statistical software (the *survival* package). Covariates may affect transitions differently.

6.6 The *msm* Package

The *msm* package was developed by Jackson (2011, 2014a, 2014b). It fits multistate Markov and hidden Markov models in continuous time by maximum likelihood. A variety of observation schemes are supported. Processes may be observed at arbitrary times (panel data) or continuously. In the latter case, the exact times at transition are known. It follows the counting process approach. When data consist of observations at arbitrary times, the likelihood is calculated in terms of transition probabilities, and transition intensities are determined using the method proposed by Kalbfleisch and Lawless (1985). The *msm* package includes a microsimulation utility that simulates Markov processes with piecewise constant intensities that depend on time-varying covariates. A time-varying covariate is described by a step function that remains constant in between observation times. Expected sojourn times in transient states are estimated by using a simple algorithm: the inverse of the rate of exit from the state. The method used in *msm* is described in detail in Jackson (2011, 2014b).

The function Biograph.msm produces a data file for the *msm* package:

```
Dmsm <- Biograph.msm(GLHS)
```

The Dmsm object has three attributes. The first, 'reshapeLong', is given by the reshape function to simplify the reshaping of the long format back to the original wide format (see documentation of reshape function). The other attributes are 'param' and 'format.date', taken from GLHS. The format of the dates of birth is included in the param attribute. The GLHS data in *msm* format are shown in Chap. 2.

In this section some functions of the *msm* package are used. The function statetable.msm creates a table of transitions:

```
transitions <- statetable.msm(state,
                              ID,
                              data=Dmsm)
```

The transition table is shown in Table 6.7. The transitions are shown in the off-diagonal elements. During the period of observation, the 201 subjects in the sample experience a total of 323 transitions from NoJob to Job and 181 transitions from Job to NoJob. The diagonal elements show the sum of intrastate transitions and censored cases. A total of 59 subjects are out of a job at the time of censoring and 419 leave a job for another job (277) or are interviewed while having a job (censoring) (142). The same transition counts are produced by a *Biograph* function: OverviewTransitions (GLHS).

Table 6.7 Number of transitions between states, reported by *msm* package. GLHS

	To	
from	1	2
1	59	323
2	181	419

6.6.1 Multistate Transition Rate Models

The msm function estimates the transition rates of the multistate model. The transition rates are the basis for transition probabilities, expected state probabilities (or state occupation probabilities) and expected state occupation times. These measures are discussed in this section using two illustrations that differ in the time scale used. The first uses calendar time. The second uses age as the time scale. The same data set is used in both cases. The object Dmsm has calendar time, denoted by date (and expressed in Century Month Code), and age, denoted by age. The function needs starting values for the maximum likelihood estimation of transition rates. They are given in the intensity matrix twoway2.q:

```
twoway2.q <- rbind(c(-0.0055,0.0055),c(0.008,-0.008)).
```

For transitions that are not possible, the entry in the initial intensity matrix is zero.

Since the exact transition times are known, the following code estimates the labour market transition rates from the GLHS data (exact time = TRUE and method is BFGS):

```
out.msm <- msm( state ~ date,
       subject=ID,
       data = Dmsm,
       qmatrix = twoway2.q,
       method="BFGS",
       use.deriv=TRUE,
       exacttimes=TRUE,
       control = list (trace = 2, REPORT = 1 ) )
```

The object out.msm has a large number of components. To see the list, use str(out.smsm) and use ?msm for the description of each component. The transition rates and the 95 % confidence intervals are shown in Table 6.8.

The rate of transition from NoJob to Job (NJ) is 0.005455 per month and the rate of transition from Job to NoJob (JN) is 0.004441 per month. The confidence intervals are shown in brackets. The table is produced by the qmatrix.msm (out.msm) function of the *msm* package. The figures are also contained in the objects out.msm$Qmatrices. Note the difference between the JN transition

6.6 The *msm* Package

Table 6.8 NJ and JN transition rates, estimated by *msm*. No covariates and time unit is month. GLHS

From\To	State 1	State 2
State 1	-0.005455 (-0.006084,-0.004892)	0.005455 (0.004892,0.006084)
State 2	0.004441 (0.003839,0.005137)	-0.004441 (-0.005137,-0.003839)

-2 * log-likelihood: 6335.366

rate and the job exit rate shown in Blossfeld and Rohwer (2002). The job exit rate, which is 0.01123 per month, is the rate of leaving a job irrespective of the destination (another job or a period without a job). The JN transition rate is the rate of leaving a job for a period without a job. These rates may be compared with the rates produced by *Biograph*. *Biograph* obtains the transition rates by dividing the number of transitions by the person-years (see the Stable object produced by the RateTable function in *Biograph*). *Biograph* gives an NJ rate of $323/4{,}934 = 0.06546$ per year (since the sojourn time is given in years) and a JN rate of $181/3{,}397 = 0.05328$ per year. These values, divided by 12, are the same as the estimates obtained by the *msm* package. It demonstrates that *Biograph* and *msm* (method BFGS with exact transition times known) yield the same point estimates of the transition rates. *Biograph* does not provide confidence intervals, however. Note that the transition rate matrix produced by *msm* differs from the transition rate matrix in *Biograph* in two ways: (1) the diagonal elements are negative (in *Biograph* they are positive and the off-diagonal elements are negative) and (2) the row variable is the state of origin and the column variable is the state of destination (*Biograph* uses the transpose, i.e. origin in column and destination in row).

The transition rates are the basis for transition probabilities and state probabilities. The probability that an individual in a given state is in another given state t months later is produced by the pmatrix.msm function. The following statement produces probabilities of discrete-time transition during a period of 12 months:

```
p.12 <- pmatrix.msm(out.msm,t=12)
```

The resulting transition rates are shown in Table 6.9.

The probability that a person without a job has a job after a period of 12 months is 6.2 %. The probability that a person with a job is without a job 12 months later is 5.0 %. Transition probabilities are determined by the exponential model assuming that the transition rates are constant during the period (0,t): $\mathbf{P} = \exp[\mathbf{M} * t]$, with $\mathbf{M}$ being the transition rate matrix produced by the *msm* package and t being the length of the period. The same method is used in the multistate life table (see next chapter).

Discrete-time transitions should be distinguished from direct transitions and the probabilities have a different interpretation. The probability of a discrete-time

Table 6.9 NJ and JN transition probabilities for periods of 12 months, estimated by *msm*. GLHS

From\To	State 1	State 2
State 1	0.93827344	0.06172656
State 2	0.05024472	0.94975528

transition is the probability that a person who is in a state (i) at time t_0 is in another state (j) at time $t_0 + t$ where t is the length of the interval. The probability of a direct transition is the probability that the individual transfers from i to j at least once during the interval.

The expected state probabilities (state occupation probabilities) at a given point in time are obtained by multiplying the transition probability matrix and the vector of state probabilities at the beginning of the interval. Suppose that everyone is in the state N (NoJob), which is the first state, at the start of the interval. The state probabilities after a period of 48 months are:

```
t(pmatrix.msm(out.msm,t=48)) %*% c(1,0)
```

The transpose of the transition probability matrix is used because the matrix is postmultiplied by the state vector at the beginning of the interval. The probability of being in N after 48 months is 79 % and the probability of being in J is 21 %.

The expected state probabilities are also produced by the `prevalence.msm` function. The function gives the state probabilities during the entire period of observation. In the GLHS data it is more than 50 years. State probabilities are produced by the following code:

```
z <- prevalence.msm (out.msm)
```

The state probabilities at intervals of 12 months, starting at CMC 349, are estimated by the function:

```
z <- prevalence.msm(out.msm,
        timezero=349,
        initstates=c(1,0),
        times=seq(349+0,349+600,by=12))
```

The object z has four components: the observed state occupancies, i.e. the observed number of respondents in a state at different points in time, the expected state occupancies, the observed percentages in each state and the expected state probabilities.

msm uses the sample population at the initial time to generate state probabilities. The initial distribution is multiplied by the transition probability matrix. The initial time is the first time when the subjects are recorded. In the GLHS data set, it is CMC

6.6 The *msm* Package 199

Table 6.10 NJ and JN transition rates. No covariates and time unit is year. GLHS

```
From\To State 1                       State 2
State 1 -0.06546 (-0.07301,-0.0587)  0.06546 (0.0587,0.07301)
State 2  0.05328 (0.04606,0.06164)  -0.05328 (-0.06164,-0.04606)
```

349. In that month, the two oldest persons in the sample are born (=min(survey $born)) and are in state N (no job). The IDs of these two persons are 119 and 161.

The state probabilities in CMC 361, i.e. after 12 months, are estimated by prevalence.msm, but they may also be obtained by the equation:

```
t(pmatrix.msm(out.msm,t=12)) %*% c(100,0)
```

The state probabilities in CMC 601 are 49.4 % in state N and 50.6 % in state J:

```
t(pmatrix.msm(out.msm,t=(601-349))) %*% c(100,0)
```

The time scale used has been calendar time, expressed in CMC. Switching to age as the time scale is easy since age is included in the data set. The time variable is set to age:

```
out_a.msm <- msm( state ~ age,
      subject=ID,
      data = Dmsm,
      qmatrix = twoway2.q,
      method="BFGS",
      use.deriv=TRUE,
      exacttimes=TRUE,
      control = list (trace = 2, REPORT = 1 ) )
```

The estimates are shown in Table 6.10. The estimates do not differ from previous estimates with month as the time unit. The values are those shown in Table 6.8 multiplied by 12.

The state probabilities by single years of age from 0 to 53 are produced by the following code:

```
z <- prevalence.msm(out_a.msm,
            timezero=0,
            initstates=c(1,0),
            times=c(0:53))
```

The plot.prevalence.msm function plots the state probabilities by age:

```
plot.prevalence.msm(out_a.msm,legend.pos=c(10,100))
```

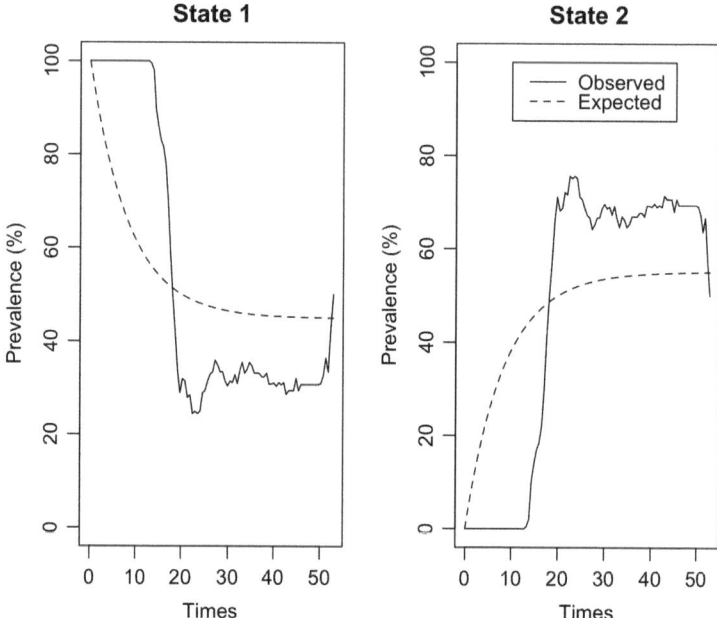

Fig. 6.16 Observed and predicted state occupation probabilities by age. GLHS

The results are shown in Fig. 6.16. State N is state 1 and J is state 2.

Labour market attachment differs between males and females and between birth cohorts. The following code estimates transition rates by sex and birth cohort:

```
out_s.msm <- msm( state ~ age,
    subject=ID,
    data = Dmsm,
    qmatrix = twoway2.q,
    method="BFGS",
    use.deriv=TRUE,
    exacttimes=TRUE,
    covariates  = ~ sex+cohort,
    control = list (trace = 2, REPORT = 1 ) )
```

The extractor functions qmatrix.msm, pmatrix.msm and sojourn.msm display transition rates, expected transition probabilities and expected sojourn times, respectively. By default qmatrix.msm (out_s.msm) shows the transition rates at the mean values of the covariates, which is meaningless if the covariates are categorical variables. To get meaningful transition rates, a covariate list should be added. The transition rates of males born in 1949–1951 are

```
qmatrix.msm (out_s.msm,
    covariates=list(sex="Male", cohort="1949-51"))
```

6.6 The *msm* Package

Table 6.11 NJ and JN transition rates of birth cohort 1949–1951, by sex, predicted by exponential transition rate model (*msm*). GLHS

```
a. Males
              State 1                          State 2
State 1 -0.08413 (-0.1044,-0.06781)   0.08413 (0.06873,0.103)
State 2  0.04597 (0.03313,0.0638)    -0.04597 (-0.06198,-
0.0341)
b. Females
              State 1                          State 2
State 1 -0.05402 (-0.0686,-0.04254)   0.05402 (0.04254,0.0686)
State 2  0.1409  (0.1063,0.1868)     -0.1409  (-0.1868,-0.1063)
```

Time unit is year

and of females

```
qmatrix.msm (out_s.msm,
        covariates=list(sex="Female",cohort="1949-51"))
```

The transition rates are shown in Table 6.11. Females have a much higher rate of job exit for jobless periods than males (0.14 vs. 0.05).

The transition rates of the reference category (males) are produced by the code:

```
qmatrix.msm (out_s.msm,covariates=0)
```

It gives the same results as:

```
qmatrix.msm (out_s.msm,
        covariates=list(sex="Male",cohort="1929-31"))
```

The job exit rates may also be derived using the regression coefficients. The expected JN transition rate of females is:

```
JN-rate for males * exp(1.12) = 0.0212*exp(1.2) = 0.065
```

Women have a rate of leaving a job for a spell without a job that is more than three times that of males.

A very useful indicator is the expected sojourn time in a state. The time a male born in 1949–1951 may expect to spend in the transient states is produced by the following code:

```
sojourn.msm(out_s.msm,
        covariates=list(sex="Male",cohort="1949-51"))
```

Males may expect to spend $1/\text{rate}(NJ) = 1/0.08413 = 11.9$ years in state N and $1/\text{rate}(JN) = 1/0.04597 = 21.8$ years in state J as shown in Table 6.12.

Table 6.12 Expected state occupation times, by sex, predicted by exponential transition rate model (*msm*). GLHS

```
a. Males
         estimates         SE        L         U
State 1  11.88682  1.514860   9.581233  14.74720
State 2  21.75150  7.176548  16.135475  29.32221
b. Females
         estimates         SE        L         U
State 1  18.512009  2.256791  14.577531  23.508404
State 2   7.097741  1.021640   5.353025   9.411114
```

In the above table, SE is the standard error and L and U are lower and upper confidence limits (95 % confidence interval). The expected sojourn times are obtained by $1/m_{i+}$, where m_{i+} is the rate of leaving state i. It is the sum of destination-specific transition rates from i.

6.6.2 Synthetic Individual Life Histories

A particularly interesting function in *msm* is sim.msm. It simulates individual trajectories or life paths. The trajectory is determined by the estimated transition rates and random values drawn from an exponential distribution. The following code simulates an employment career between ages 0 and 53 from time-invariant transition rates estimated from the GLHS data:

```
sim <- sim.msm(qmatrix.msm(out.msm)$estimates,
        mintime=0,
        maxtime=53,
        start=1)
```

The object has three components: the state sequence (sim$states), the sequence of transition times (sim$times) and the transition rate matrix (sim $qmatrix). At age 0, a person occupies state 1 (N). The sim.msm function may include a matrix of time-dependent covariates. Table 6.13 shows a trajectory for an average individual.

The virtual individual enters the first job at age 31 and leaves employment at age 47. The output also shows the transition rate matrix (qmatrix) from which the trajectory is produced.

The *msm* package was designed for panel data but accommodates empirical studies with known exact dates of transitions. In this chapter, two illustrations of the package were presented. They differ in time unit used. Transition rates, estimated

6.6 The *msm* Package

Table 6.13 Simulated individual employment career, generated by *msm* based on aggregate GLHS transition rates

```
$states
[1] 1 2 1 1

$times
[1]  0.00000 31.35283 47.83234 53.00000

$qmatrix
                State 1       State 2
State 1 -0.005455344  0.005455344
State 2  0.004440588 -0.004440588
```

from the data, are used to determine transition probabilities, expected state probabilities and expected sojourn time in each of the states.

Chapter 7
The Multistate Life Table

7.1 Introduction

The multistate life table is a method developed in demography to describe the mortality and mobility experience of a cohort, a group of people born in a same period. The multistate life table is an extension of the life table, which describes the mortality experience. The life table was first developed in the seventeenth century by John Graunt. Graunt was interested in estimating probabilities of survival from observations on deaths. The life table is an established method in demography (see, e.g. Preston et al. 2001). In the 1970s Andrei Rogers extended the life table to include migrations between regions in addition to mortality (Rogers 1975). It soon became clear that regions may be replaced by states and interregional migrations by transitions between states. That resulted in the *multistate* life table and the wider field of multistate demography (Land and Rogers 1982). Today the multistate life table is used to describe life histories from birth to death. In this chapter I present functions for estimating multistate life table indicators. Age is the duration variable used throughout the chapter. The age intervals considered are of 1-year length.

In this chapter the life table method is used to generate cohort employment careers. Cohort careers show the distribution of cohort members by state and age. They also indicate the expected time spent in a state. Microsimulation is used to generate individual employment careers. Aggregation of individual careers of cohort members leads to cohort careers. The aggregate may differ slightly from the expected cohort career produced by the multistate life table because of sample variation.

The data are from the GLHS. The oldest respondent was 52 at survey date. The employment careers are from birth to age 53. The employment career is inferred from transition rates estimated from the GLHS subsample of 201 respondents. Each respondent in the sample contributes data on part of the employment career from age 0 to age 53. By combining data from several respondents, transition rates can be estimated for the entire age range. Since the employment career is estimated using data from different respondents, the cohort experiencing the employment career is a *synthetic* cohort and the individual is a *synthetic* individual. The multistate life table (MSLT) describes the employment experience of that synthetic cohort and the microsimulation describes the employment experience of a synthetic individual. Three classes of indicators are distinguished: counts (cohort members), probabilities and durations (sojourn times). Two types of probabilities are distinguished: state probabilities and transition probabilities. Probabilities and sojourn times may be conditioned on the state occupied at a reference age.

The chapter consists of six sections. The estimation of transition rates is covered in Sect. 7.2. Two estimation methods are implemented. The first is the non-parametric method that yields Nelson-Aalen estimators. The second is the partly parametric method that produces occurrence-exposure rates. The multistate survival function is presented in Sect. 7.3. The multistate survival function gives state occupation probabilities at consecutive ages. Expected state occupation times are derived in Sect. 7.4. The sum of state occupation times beyond a given age for individuals of that age is the life expectancy at that age. Section 7.5 covers the microsimulation and presents distributions of individual employment careers in the synthetic cohort. The last section is a summary with some conclusions.

7.2 Transition Rates

In Chap. 2, two methods were discussed for estimating transition rates: a non-parametric method yielding Nelson-Aalen estimates of cumulative transition rates and a partly parametric method yielding occurrence-exposure rates. The software for estimating transition rates is presented in Chap. 4 (the `RateTable` function to estimate occurrence-exposure rates) and in Chap. 6 (Nelson-Aalen estimator). The two methods are combined in the `Cumrates` function of *Biograph*. That function is a shortcut to the multistate life table.

`Cumrates` uses the *mvna* package to obtain the Nelson-Aalen estimator. The mvna function of the *mvna* package estimates cumulative transition rates for any age where a transition occurs. The multistate life table does not need cumulative transition rates at ages where transitions occur. It needs cumulative transition rates at the beginning of age intervals because age-specific transition rates can be derived from these cumulative transition rates. The *mvna* function `predict` is used to generate cumulative transition rates at the start of age intervals.

The function `Rates.ac` of *Biograph* estimates occurrence-exposure rates. The function can be used separately or as part of `Cumrates`. The `Rates.ac` function produces age-specific occurrence-exposure rates by origin and destination from the information in the `Stable` object produced by the `RateTable` function (see Chap. 3). The function produces transition rates of the age-cohort type. Age-cohort rates are for life tables. They differ from period-cohort rates that are used in population projections (for an introduction, see, e.g. Preston et al. 2001). The following code produces estimates of age-cohort occurrence-exposure rates:

7.2 Transition Rates

```
occup <- Occup(GLHS)
seq.ind <- Sequences.ind
        (GLHS$path,attr(GLHS,"param")$namstates)
trans <- Trans (GLHS)
ratetable <- RateTable(GLHS,occup=occup,trans=trans)
rates <- Rates.ac (Stable=ratetable$Stable)
```

The object `ratetable` is produced by the `RateTable` function. The object `rates` contains the transition rates by age (row variable), state of destination (column variable) and state of origin (layer variable).

The following code generates Nelson-Aalen estimators of the cumulative transition rates for the NJ and JN transitions:

```
GLHSd <- Remove.intrastate(GLHS)
cr <- Cumrates (irate=1,Bdata=GLHSd)
```

The parameter `irate` selects the method. If `irate` is one, the Nelson-Aalen estimator is produced using the *mvna* package. The output includes the expected value of the cumulative hazard and the upper and lower 95 % confidence intervals.

If `irate` = 2, the occurrence-exposure rate is generated. A value of 3 instructs the function to produce both the Nelson-Aalen estimator and the occurrence-exposure rate. The object `cr` is an object of class `cumrates`. It has seven components:

(a) `cr$D`: the *Biograph* object (the data).
(b) `cr$irate`: the method used.
(c) `cr$NeAa`: the Nelson-Aalen estimator, i.e. estimates of cumulative transition rates.
(d) `cr$predicted`: Nelson-Aalen estimates predicted at consecutive birthdays. They are produced by the function `predict.mvna` of the *mvna* package.
(e) `cr$astr`: age-specific transition rates derived from the Nelson-Aalen estimates of cumulative transition rates predicted at consecutive birthdays. Age intervals are 1 year.
(f) `cr$oeCum`: cumulative occurrence-exposure rates.
(g) `cr$oe`: occurrence-exposure rates.

The object `cr$NeAa` is a four-dimensional array with age as the row variable and destination as the column variable. Origin is the third dimension and the variant of the cumulative transition rate is the fourth dimension. The three variants are: expected value, upper 95 % confidence interval and lower 95 % confidence interval. The command `cr$NeAa[,2,1,1]` displays the expected values of the cumulative transition rates by age from origin state N (state 1) to destination state J (state 2). The object `cr$predicted` is a list of two-dimensional arrays, one for each transition. For instance, `cr$predict$"N J"[21:31,]` shows the Nelson-Aalen estimator of transition rates at exact ages from 20 to 30, the variance, the

Fig. 7.1 Cumulative NJ and JN transition rates by age: Nelson-Aalen estimator and cumulative occurrence-exposure rates. GLHS

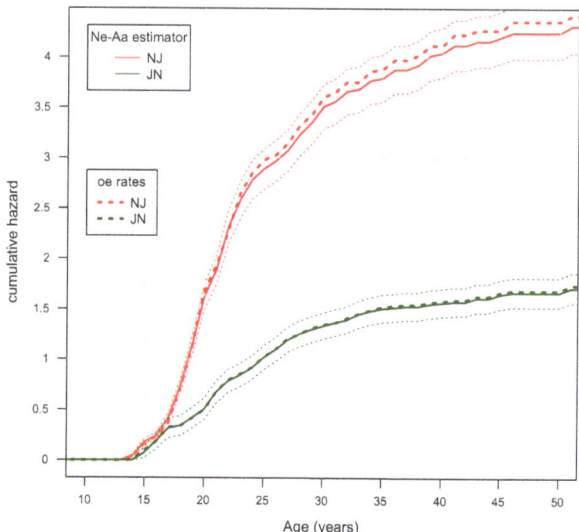

upper and lower 95 % confidence intervals, the number of respondents at risk at that age (risk set) and the number of transitions during the age interval. The objects cr $oeCum and cr$oe are three-dimensional arrays with age as the row variable, destination as the column variable and origin as the layer variable.

The function plot.cumrates plots the cumulative transition rates. The following code computes and plots age-specific cumulative transition rates (Nelson-Aalen estimators and occurrence-exposure rates):

```
cumrates <- Cumrates (irate = 3, Bdata=GLHS)
z<- plot (x=cumrates,ptrans=c("NJ","JN"),title=NULL)
```

The plot is shown in Fig. 7.1. The occurrence-exposure rates do not differ from the age-specific rates predicted by the Nelson-Aalen estimator. The confidence intervals of the Nelson-Aalen estimates are also shown.

7.3 The Multistate Survival Function

The multistate survival function is derived from transition rates. The function MSLT.S produces the multistate survival function:

```
S.na <- MSLT.S(cumrates$astr[,,1])
```

where cr$astr[,,1] is the set of age-specific transition rates computed from the expected cumulative transition rates at consecutive birthdays derived from

7.3 The Multistate Survival Function

Nelson-Aalen estimators. The multistate survival function may also be computed from occurrence-exposure rates:

```
S.oe <- MSLT.S(cumrates$oe)
```

The object S.*, with * denoting na or oe, has two components. The first, S.*$S, is the multistate survival function. The second, S.*$P, is the set of age-specific transition probabilities.

The multistate survival function is a table of state occupation probabilities by age and origin state. The table has three dimensions: age, origin state and current state. In the GLHS, the origin state is the state at birth. At birth, all respondents are outside of employment at birth. The multistate survival function is derived from age-specific transition probabilities using the recursive formula:

$$l(x+1) = \widehat{\mathbf{P}}(x, x+1) \, l(x)$$

where $l(x)$ is the vector of state occupation probabilities at exact age x and $\widehat{\mathbf{P}}(x, y)$ is the estimate of transition probabilities at age x (see Chap. 2). The (i,j)-element $\hat{p}_{ij}$ $(x, x+1)$ of $\widehat{\mathbf{P}}(x, x+1)$ is the probability that an individual in state i at exact age x will be in state j 1 year later, at exact age $x+1$. At the lowest age, state occupation probabilities are fixed exogenously. Since in the GLHS all respondents are outside of employment at birth, the state occupation probability at age 0 is one for N (first state) and 0 for J (second state). It is often convenient to consider a birth cohort and multiply the state occupation probabilities at birth by the cohort size. The measure that results is known as *radix*. The measure is commonly used in demography.

Transition probabilities are estimated from transition rates:

$$\widehat{\mathbf{P}}(x, x+1) = \exp[-\widehat{\mathbf{m}}(x, x+1)]$$

(see Chap. 2). The age-specific transition rates are either derived from cumulative transition rates at consecutive birthdays (Nelson-Aalen estimators) (cr$astr) or they are occurrence-exposure rates (cr$oe).

Since in this application all subjects originate in a single state (state N), only the state probabilities S.*$S[,,1] have meaning. Consider reference age 0 and the state probability at age 30. The object S.*$S[30,2,1] is the probability that a subject who starts in state 1 is in state 2 at age 30. The probability that at age 30 the subject is in state 1 is S.*$S[30,1,1].

7.4 Expected State Occupation Times

The function `MSLT.e` produces expected state occupation times by state and age. They are estimated from the multistate survival function. Because transition rates are assumed to be piecewise constant, the survival function is piecewise exponential. For computation purposes, a piecewise linear survival function is assumed. Since the length of an age interval is 1 year, the approximation is generally adequate. The multistate survival function can be `S.na$S` or `S.oe$S`. The function is invoked by the command

```
e <- MSLT.e (S.*$S,radix)
```

where `radix` is the number of subjects by state at the start of the process (age 0). In this application,

```
radix <- c(10000,0)
```

The object `e` has four components:

(a) `e$L`: the time a cohort member may expect to spend in each state between two consecutive ages that is during an age interval. The element `L[30,2,1]` gives the number of years a subject who is in state 1 (N) at birth may expect to spend in state 2 (J) between exact ages 30 and 31.
(b) `e$e0`: expected number of years a newborn may expect to spend in each state. It is the life expectancy at birth by state.
(c) `e$e.p`: expected number of years an individual aged x may expect to spend in each state beyond age x. It is the population-based life expectancy, which depends on reaching age x and does not depend on the state occupied at age x.
(d) `e$e.s`: expected number of years an individual aged x and occupying a given state may expect to spend in each state beyond age x. It is the status-based life expectancy, which depends on survival to age x and on the state occupied at age x.

For the distinction between population-based and status-based life table measures, see Willekens (1987) and Chap. 2.

Consider an application to the GLHS data. In these data mortality is absent and transition rates are given for all ages up to 52. The highest age is 53, i.e. at 53 observation is censored. If occurrence-exposure rates are used to determine expected state occupation times, then the number of years a newborn may expect to spend outside of employment (state N) is 27.93 years and the number of years with

7.4 Expected State Occupation Times

employment (state J) 25.07 years. A member of a synthetic cohort, whose labour market mobility is governed by the age-specific occurrence-exposure rates estimated from the GLHS subsample, may expect to spend 27.93 years without employment and 25.07 years being employed before reaching age 53 (e.oe$e0 or e.oe$e.p[1,,1]). If age-specific rates are derived from predicted Nelson-Aalen estimates at birthdays, then the expected state occupation times are 27.97 and 25.03, respectively. The difference is negligible.

An individual of age 30 spends 23 years before reaching age 53, 16.6 years with a job and 6.4 years without employment (e$e.p). If the 30-year-old is not employed, the expected years in employment are lower (14.7 years) and the years without employment much higher (8.27 years). If the individual of age 30 is employed, the expected number of years beyond age 30 with a job is 19.7 years and without a job 3.31 years. A 30-year-old person without a job is likely to spend less time employed than a person of the same age who has a job, even if the transition rates at ages above 30 do not depend on the employment status at age 30. The figures for a 30-year-old who is employed are produced by the code:

If, on the other hand, the individual of age 30 has no job, he or she may expect to spend 15.0 years without employment and 8.0 years with employment. The code is:

```
e.oe$e.s[which(dimnames(e.oe$e.s)[[1]]=="30"), ,1]
```

Those without employment at age 30 are more likely to be women who left the labour force than unemployed men. In the subsample, 61 persons are without a job at age 30 and 138 with a job (Occup(GLHSd)$state_occup[31,]). Of the 61 persons without a job, 56 are women and 5 are men. The following code computes the figures:

```
z.f <- state_age (Bdata=GLHSd,age=29.999,
                  ID=GLHSd$ID[GLHSd$sex=="Female"])
z.m <- state_age (Bdata=GLHSd,age=29.999,
                  ID=GLHSd$ID[GLHSd$sex=="Male"])
z.f$state.n
z.m$state.n
```

Note that 3 persons are exactly 30 years old at time of survey (the survey month was the month of their 30th birthday): 1 woman and 2 men. The state_age function allocates the individuals to the state 'censored' because censoring is assumed to occur at the beginning of the month, not different from the age measurement of other transitions.

The expected state occupation times beyond age 30 by state occupied at that reference age are estimated assuming that the transition rates beyond age 30 do not depend on the state occupied at age 30. The transition rates only depend on state occupied just before the transition. This is the Markov assumption. If the transition

Fig. 7.2 The multistate survival function: state occupation probabilities in N and J, predicted by the multistate life table from empirical transition rates. GLHS

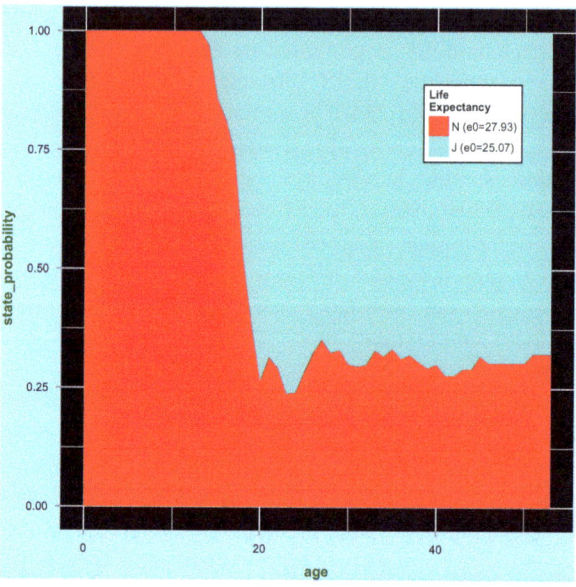

rate at an age beyond 30 depends on the state occupied just before the transition and on the state occupied at age 30, then the result will differ.

The function plot.MSLT.S plots the cumulative hazard:

```
z<- plot (x=S.oe$S,e.oe$e0,
         title = NULL,
         area=TRUE,
         order=c("N","J"))
```

where S.oe$S is an object of class MSLT.S created by MLT.S and e.oe$e0 is a numeric object created by MSLT.e. The package *ggplot2* is used for plotting. State occupation probabilities and life expectancies by state are shown in Fig. 7.2. Since the plot also shows the expected sojourn times in each state, MSLT.e should be called before plotting.

7.5 Synthetic Individual Life Histories

Individual life histories (employment careers) are realisations from continuous-time Markov processes. The parameters are age-specific (i.e. piecewise constant) transition rates, in this chapter occurrence-exposure rates. Microsimulation is used

7.5 Synthetic Individual Life Histories

Table 7.1 Data for generation of employment careers of synthetic individuals

	ID	birth	interview	Start	Stop	st_entry	Sex
1	1	01/03/1929	01/11/1981	0	53	N	Male
2	2	01/09/1929	01/11/1981	0	53	N	Female
3	3	01/05/1939	01/11/1981	0	43	N	Female
4	4	01/04/1950	01/11/1981	0	32	N	Female
5	5	01/05/1931	01/11/1981	0	51	N	Male
6	6	01/12/1940	01/11/1981	0	41	N	Male
7	7	01/08/1939	01/11/1981	0	43	N	Female
8	8	01/09/1950	01/11/1981	0	32	N	Male
9	9	01/05/1931	01/11/1981	0	51	N	Male
10	10	01/10/1931	01/11/1981	0	51	N	Male

to generate the individual life histories. Since transition rates are available for ages 0–53, we could generate employment careers between ages 0 and 54. To compare the aggregation of individual careers over cohort members and the expected cohort employment career produced by the MSLT, 201 individual life histories are produced and individual age ranges are taken from the GLHS subsample. Table 7.1 shows the birth dates and interview dates used in the microsimulation, the age range, the state occupied at the start of the microsimulation (st_entry) and the sex of the individual. The sex is not used. These data are taken from the GLHS subsample. Intrastate transitions, i.e. job changes, are removed.

The function sim.bio is used to generate individual biographies. The function produces a life history for a single individual between two given ages and in a given state at the lowest age. The sequences of states and transitions are based on age-specific transition rates (single years of age). The transition rates may depend on covariates. The two given ages can be any two ages in the age range for which transition rates are available (0 and 53 in the case of the GLHS data). The sim.bio function is based on the sim.msm function of the *msm* package. The function sim.pop coordinates the microsimulation. It calls sim.bio for each individual in the virtual population and saves the individual life histories in a *Biograph* object. The *Biograph* package may then be used to analyse the simulated life histories. The functions sim.bio and sim.pop are not included in *Biograph* (version 2). They may be included in a later version. They are available from the author. The following code produces simulated life histories:

214   7 The Multistate Life Table

```
born.date <- date_convert (d=GLHSd$born,
      format.in="CMC",
      selectday=1,
      format.out="%d/%m/%Y")
born.yr <- date_convert (GLHS$born,
      format.in="CMC",
      selectday=1,
      format.out="year")
interview.date <- date_convert (d=GLHSd$end,
      format.in="CMC",
      selectday=1,
      format.out="%d/%m/%Y")
Age.interview <- trunc(date_convert (d=GLHSd$end,
      format.in="CMC",
      selectday=1,
      format.out="age",
      born=GLHSd$born,
      format.born="CMC"))+1
Age.start <- rep(0,nrow(GLHSd))
state_at_entry <- substr (GLHSd$path,1,1)
V <- data.frame (ID=1:nrow(GLHS),
      birth=born.date,
      born=born.yr,
      interview=interview.date,
      Start=Age.start,
      Stop=Age.interview,
      st_entry=state_at_entry,
      Sex=GLHSd$sex,
      stringsAsFactors=FALSE)
GLHSd.sim <- sim.pop (
      V=V,
      ratesM=rates$M,
      covs=c("Sex","st_entry"))
```

GLHSd is GLHS with the intrastate transitions removed. The first four statements convert dates in a desired format. The dates of birth, the interview dates and the age at interview are determined using functions included in *Biograph*. The decimal year of birth born.yr is not needed in the simulation, but will be included in the *Biograph* object. The data frame V combines the relevant data and is an input to the microsimulation, together with the age-specific transition rates, the states at entry and the covariates. The object rates$M is a component of the object produced by the Rates.ac function of *Biograph*. The object GLHS.sim is a *Biograph* object.

State occupancies of the simulated population are similar to those of the observed population. Of the 201 individuals of age 20, 142 are employed in the simulated population and 146 in the observed sample. Among the individuals aged 30, 139 are employed in the simulated population and 138 in the observed sample. Let us compare the distribution of state sequences in the observed and the simulated populations.

```
seq.sim <- Sequences (GLHSd.sim,mean_median="median")
seq.obs <- Sequences(GLHSd)
```

7.6 Summary

Table 7.2 State sequences: observed and simulated. GLHS

	ncase	%	cum%	age_en	age_ex	ns	case	tr1	tr2	tr3
a.	\multicolumn{10}{l	}{Most frequent sequences in GLHS sample population (no intrastate transition)}
1	67	33.33	33.33	0	41.75	2	NJ	18.08>J		
2	54	26.87	60.20	0	40.96	4	NJNJ	17.88>J	21.71>N	26.17>J
3	44	21.89	82.09	0	42.08	3	NJN	18.17>J	24.88>N	
4	16	7.96	90.05	0	40.42	6	NJNJNJ	17.83>J	20.83>N	23.96>J
5	10	4.98	95.02	0	41.71	5	NJNJN	17.29>J	20.12>N	21.21>J
b.	\multicolumn{10}{l	}{Most frequent sequences in simulated population (no intrastate transition)}
1	61	30.35	30.35	0	43.0	4	NJNJ	17.59>J	21.88>N	25.08>J
2	59	29.35	59.70	0	41.0	2	NJ	18.42>J		
3	35	17.41	77.11	0	42.0	3	NJN	18.51>J	26.05>N	
4	22	10.95	88.06	0	42.0	5	NJNJN	17.21>J	21.51>N	23.91>J
5	12	5.97	94.03	0	41.5	6	NJNJNJ	16.38>J	20.1>N	21.76>J

Table 7.2 shows the most frequent state sequences in the GLHS subsample and the simulated population. The difference is considerable because of small sample size.

The transition rates may be used to generate individual employment histories from birth to a highest age (53 in this case). The results of the microsimulation may be compared to the MSLT. The MSLT indicates that 73 % of the synthetic cohort is employed at age 20 and 70 % at age 30. In the microsimulation of 201 individual life histories, it is 74 % at age 20 and 67 % at age 30.

7.6 Summary

The multistate life table summarises the mobility experience of a synthetic cohort. The life table method is sometimes referred to as a non-parametric method for estimating transition rates for age intervals of fixed length. The life table method is not really non-parametric because it implies an assumption on the distribution of events during unit age intervals. In this chapter, it has been assumed that the transition rate is constant during an interval, which implies a piecewise exponential distribution of events between birth and death or the highest age. Another common assumption in demography, epidemiology and actuarial science is that events are uniformly distributed during a unit interval, which implies a piecewise linear survival function from birth to death or the highest age. In both cases, transition rates are referred to as occurrence-exposure rates because they relate an event count to an exposure time. The truly non-parametric method estimates transition rates each time an event occurs without making any assumption about the variation of the likelihood of event occurrence with age. The non-parametric estimator of transition rates is known as the Nelson-Aalen estimator. The occurrence-exposure rate and the Nelson-Aalen estimator are considered in this chapter.

Age-specific transition rates are used to produce estimates of state occupation probabilities by age and state occupation times by age. *Biograph* incorporates an option to estimate state probabilities and occupation times from occurrence-exposure rates or from Nelson-Aalen estimates. The results differ only slightly.

The multistate life table translates transition rates into probability and duration measures that can be interpreted more easily. Other life history indicators may be derived from these measures. The multistate life table indicators are for a synthetic cohort. They are expected values derived from the continuous-time Markov process model. Distributions of individual values around the expected values are obtained by microsimulation. In this chapter, microsimulation was used to generate individual employment histories. In general, the simulated individual employment histories are similar to observed employment histories, and aggregation of individual employment histories is comparable to the expected employment history of the synthetic cohort. The increased availability of longitudinal data triggered a growing interest in synthetic life histories and the microsimulation technique. A discussion of these developments is beyond the scope of this book. CRAN now includes packages designed to predict individual life trajectories using microsimulation. They include the general-purpose *MicSim* package developed by Zinn (2014) and the *MILC* (Microsimulation Lung Cancer Model) package developed by Chrysanthopoulou (2014) for lung cancer trajectories. *MicSim* is a multistate model and *MILC* is a staging model developed in a competing risk framework.

Chapter 8
Application to the Netherlands Family and Fertility Survey

8.1 Introduction

The aim of this chapter is to illustrate *Biograph* with data from the Netherlands Family and Fertility Survey of 1998 (Onderzoek Gezinsvorming 1998 or NLOG98). Statistics Netherlands organised the survey for information on partnerships, marriage and family. In this chapter *Biograph* is used to study pathways to first birth. What life paths do women in the Netherlands follow between leaving parental home and motherhood? Some leave the parental home for marriage and have a child soon after marriage. Most women have a different pathway, however. The trajectory women follow determines to a large extent the age at which they become a mother. Differences in pathways can be associated with background characteristics. Three covariates are considered: religious denomination (kerk), level of education (educ) and birth cohort (cohort). The pathway to the first child was studied by Matsuo (2003).

The chapter consists of six sections. In Sect. 8.2 I briefly describe the data and review the five steps required to create a *Biograph* object. In Sect. 8.3, summary measures that characterise the data are presented. The summary measures include indicators on episodes, transitions and state sequences. The estimation of occurrence-exposure rates is also discussed. Section 8.4 covers transition rate models. It illustrates the packages *survival*, *mvna* and *mstate*. Multistate life table analysis is discussed in Sect. 8.5. Section 8.6 concludes the chapter.

8.2 Data and Preparation of *Biograph* Object

Between February and May 1998, Statistics Netherlands (CBS) conducted the Netherlands Family and Fertility Survey. Data were collected on 5,450 women and 4,717 men in the Netherlands, born in the period 1945–1979. They were

18–52 years at time of survey. The sample frame consisted of the Municipal Population Administration (Gemeentelijke Bevolkingsadministratie or GBA). The GBA is the main source of statistical information on the population in the Netherlands. The random sample survey was done in two steps. In the first step 262 municipalities were selected from 572 municipalities. GBA data of the selected municipalities were then used to randomly select 14,000 addresses and subsequently men and women born in the period of 1945–1979. (For details on the sampling, see de Graaf and Steenhof 1999, p. 36.) Eventually, 5,450 women and 4,717 men were interviewed using structured questionnaires. About two thirds of women in the sample became a mother before survey date.

DANS (Data Archiving and Networked Services) distributes the survey data for public use (https://easy.dans.knaw.nl/; search for *gezinsvorming*). The data are distributed in two SPSS files. The file BOAV98.SAV contains the data for females, and the file BOAM98.SAV contains the data for males. In this chapter, data on females are used.

The Netherlands Family and Fertility Survey provides extensive information on marital status, living arrangements, partnership and fertility. The information is collected retrospectively and covers the period from birth to survey date. For each respondent, the OG98 reports up to three marriages and up to six cohabitations. Each marriage may be followed by a divorce or widowhood.

The raw data need considerable processing to be useful for *Biograph*. First, the public use file does not include the survey month. Although we know that the survey took place in the period from February to May 1998, the month of interview is not included in the data and is not available to researchers. The age of the respondent at the time of survey is available, however. The survey month is estimated from the age at survey, the month of birth of the respondent and the months in which transitions occur. No transition may occur after the survey date. The estimation procedure includes a random number generation to allocate the survey date to one of several plausible months, taking into account that transitions reported by the respondent could not have taken place after the survey date.

Second, the public use data file is not well suited for life history data analysis. The focus of the questionnaire is on partnership and not on timing of transitions. Life history data analysis requires that the transitions are ordered and defined in terms of origin state, destination state and date of occurrence. The conversion of raw data into an event history data structure is a tedious process that was completed by Matsuo and Willekens (2003). The dates of transitions are recoded in Century Month Codes (CMC). In some cases imputation was necessary. The emphasis on the sequence and timing of transitions did reveal several inconsistencies in the data. Some sequences of transitions are not possible (e.g. the second child is born before the first child) or are not plausible (e.g. remarriage before a divorce). Transitions may be missing (e.g. second marriage is reported, while information on dissolution of first marriage is missing). The inconsistencies were investigated in detail and corrected if it was clear that the inconsistent sequence or timing of transitions was due to errors in recording or coding. The report by Matsuo and Willekens (2003) is limited to the data for females. Starting from the public use file BOAV98.SAV,

8.2 Data and Preparation of *Biograph* Object

inconsistencies are removed and an event history data file prepared in 10 steps. Each step is documented in an SPSS syntax file. The report by Matsuo and Willekens and the SPSS syntax files are available on request. The name of the SPSS file with the event histories is NLOG98_F_CMC.sav. The syntax file also creates a text file in *Biograph* format to be used as input in *Biograph*. The name of that data file is NLOG98cov.DAT. For the illustrations in this chapter, a subsample of 500 women was selected from the 5,450 women in the NLOG98 sample. That R data file is included in the *Biograph* package under the name NLOG98.Rdata. The command data(NLOG98) loads the data set. For convenience, the data object is renamed to OG.

A *Biograph* object is created in five steps. The steps are implemented in the programme create.NLOG98.r, which is distributed with the *Biograph* package (see Documentation folder of the package source Biograph_2.0.2.tar.gz or later version). The first step is the specification of the state space and the possible transitions. The second step is the selection of covariates. The third step is the specification of the observation window for each subject. In the fourth step, the state sequence is determined and the dates at transition are determined. In the fifth and final step, all data are stored in a data frame and three data attributes are attached to the data frame. The state space describes the pathways to the first child, i.e. the set of states a woman may occupy before the first child is born. Figure 8.1 presents the state space and the associated transitions. The path starts with the state of living at the parental home. We assume that the parental home may be left only once, although in reality persons may leave the parental home and return later at least for some time. A respondent may leave home for one of three reasons. The first is independence, which is manifested by leaving home to live alone. The second reason is marriage and the third is cohabitation. Childbearing may occur in any of these states. The state space is determined by a composite variable that combines three domains of life. The first domain of life is the living arrangement with three possibilities: living at the parental home, living alone and living with someone. The second domain of life is the marital status: not married or married. The third domain is motherhood (fertility). The three domains of life are combined into a single state space. Some combinations of states are excluded (e.g. cohabitating at the parental home, married while living at the parental home). The primary states of interest are:

1. Living at parental home (H)
2. Living alone (independently) (A)
3. Married (M)
4. Cohabiting (C)
5. First child (K)

The specification of the state space determines the sequence of states and transitions that can be studied. In this example, a married woman may start cohabitation upon marriage dissolution. She may start living alone instead, but she may not move back to the parental home. Some living arrangements, such as Living Apart Together (LAT) (commuting marriage), are not considered in the state

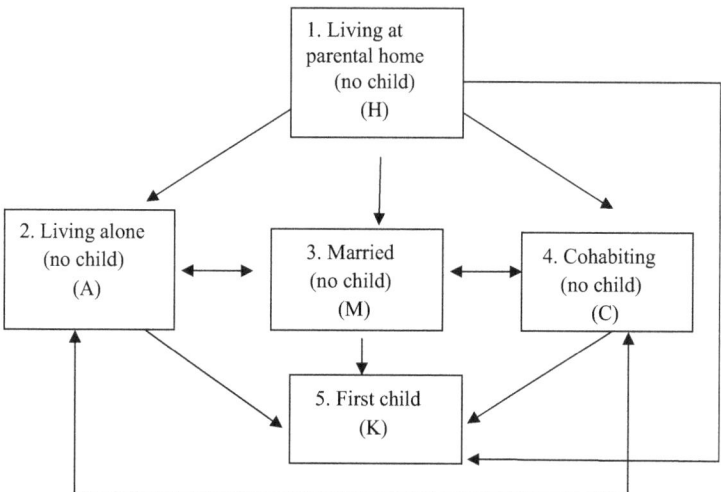

Fig. 8.1 Schematic representation of pathways to the first child

space and can therefore not be studied. To include that arrangement a distinction must be made between partnership status (union status) and residence status, and the timing of the transitions between the states should be known. The focus on pathways to first birth implies that the transitions that occur after the birth of a child are not considered in the analysis. The birth of a child implies entry into an absorbing state.

The NLOG98 reveals some uncommon living arrangements. For instance, some married women do not live with their husband; some live alone and some live with another partner. These living arrangements are not considered in this chapter since we lack information and the state space is too restrictive. To capture these living arrangements, the state space would need to be extended.

The state space has five states with the names 'H' (living at the parental home), 'A' (living alone), 'C' (cohabiting), 'M' (married) and 'K' (with at least one child). The number of possible transitions is 16: HA, HM, HC, HK, AM, AC, AK, CA, CM, CK, MA, MC, MK, AA, CC and MM. Cohabiting or married respondents may change partner without a period of independent living, resulting in transitions CC and MM. That transition is maintained in the data set, but it is disregarded because it is a transition to the same state. In the subsample, 2 women reported a CC transition. The feasible transitions are identified in the transition matrix:

8.2 Data and Preparation of *Biograph* Object

```
          Destination
Origin   H      A      C      M      K
   H  FALSE  TRUE   TRUE   TRUE   TRUE
   A  FALSE  FALSE  TRUE   TRUE   TRUE
   C  FALSE  TRUE   TRUE   TRUE   TRUE
   M  FALSE  TRUE   TRUE   FALSE  TRUE
   K  FALSE  FALSE  FALSE  FALSE  FALSE
```

Most packages for multistate analysis with R use a transition matrix. In *Biograph*, the transition matrix is contained in the object attr (OG, "param") $trans_possible (see below). The calendar dates of transitions are expressed in Century Month Code (CMC).

To determine the dates at transition, the following date variables are extracted from the data file. NLO98_F_CMC

Variable name	Meaning
CMCINT	CMC at interview
CMCB_OP	CMC at birth
CMCLEAVE	CMC at leaving parental home
CMCCO1	CMC at first cohabitation
CMCE1CO	CMC at end first cohabitation
CMCCO2	CMC at second cohabitation
CMCE2CO	CMC at end second cohabitation
CMCCO3	CMC at third cohabitation
CMCE3CO	CMC at end third cohabitation
CMCCO4	CMC at fourth cohabitation
CMCCO5	CMC at fifth cohabitation
CMCMA1	CMC at first marriage
CMCE1MA	CMC at end of first marriage
CMCMA2	CMC at second marriage
CMCE2MA	CMC at end of second marriage
CMCMA3	CMC at third marriage
CMCE3MA	CMC at end of third marriage
CMC_K1	CMC at birth of first child

The second step is the selection of covariates. Two covariates are selected and included in the *Biograph* object: religious denomination (kerk) and level of education (educ). The first covariate is religion (labelled **KERKGEZ** in the original data distributed by Statistics Netherlands). The following categories are distinguished, with the original code in brackets and the number of respondents n in the original sample of 5,450 respondents:

1. No religion [1] (n = 2,395)
2. Roman Catholic [2] (n = 1,677)
3. Protestant [3, 4, 5 and 6] (n = 1,014)
4. Other religion [7, 8, 9 and 10] (n = 357)
NA. Missing data [98, 99] (n = 7)

The second covariate is the highest completed education. In the original data set, the covariate is called OPL_HB. The following categories are distinguished, with the original codes in brackets and the number of respondents n:

1. Primary [2] (n = 363)
2. Secondary lower [3] (n = 1,250)
3. Secondary higher [4] (n = 2,489)
4. First step high [5] (n = 869)
5. Second step high [6] (n = 238)
6. Third step high [7] (n = 20)
NA. Missing data [9] (n = 221)

In addition, two birth cohorts are derived from the dates of birth. The first cohort is born before 1960, and the second cohort is born in 1960 or later.

The third step is the specification of the observation window for each subject. The life history is recorded retrospectively starting at birth and ending at interview date. The interview date is given in CMC, and the assumption is made that interview is at the end of the month, estimated using the procedure described above. Since *Biograph* assumes that transitions, including censoring, occur at the beginning of a month, a one is added to the interview month.

In the fourth step, the state sequence is determined and the dates at transition are recorded. The *Biograph* function Sequences.ind.0 is used. The function orders dates chronologically and determines the state sequence. The output is an object with three components. The first component is the state space. The second is a character string denoting the state sequence (Sequences.ind.0$path). The third is the sequence of the CMCs at transition (Sequences.ind.0$d).

In the fifth and final step, all data are stored in a data frame and three data attributes are attached to the data frame: the format of the dates at transition ('format.date'), the format of the date of birth ('format.born') and the output produced by the Parameters function of *Biograph* ('param').

A selection of the subsample of 500 respondents is shown in Table 8.1. The variables ID, born, start, end and Tr* are numeric. The variable path is a character variable and the covariates are factors.

Table 8.1 *Biograph* object: selection of NLOG98 data

	ID	born	start	end	kerk	educ	cohort	path	Tr1	Tr2	Tr3	Tr4	Tr5
2	2	630	630	1184	no religion	5	<1960	HAC	966	1002	NA	NA	NA
8	8	707	707	1180	Roman Catholic	NA	<1960	HCMK	894	906	910	NA	NA
24	24	813	813	1179	Roman Catholic	4	1960+	HCK	1004	1040	NA	NA	NA
28	28	673	673	1180	no religion	2	<1960	HMCK	939	990	1066	NA	NA
34	34	789	789	1179	no religion	6	1960+	HACA	1016	1105	1150	NA	NA
43	43	609	609	1179	Protestant	NA	<1960	HK	840	NA	NA	NA	NA
52	52	895	895	1182	no religion	5	1960+	HA	1118	NA	NA	NA	NA
82	82	689	689	1181	no religion	6	<1960	HACM	973	1003	1013	NA	NA
96	96	721	721	1182	no religion	4	<1960	HACACK	1034	1038	1111	1128	1140
99	99	862	862	1181	no religion	4	1960+	HAC	1089	1105	NA	NA	NA

8.3 Exploratory Analysis

In this section, useful descriptive statistics are presented. They include summary indicators on episodes and transitions, individual and collective life histories (state sequences) and age profiles of transitions. The section also includes a Lexis diagram and state sequence plots. A separate subsection covers the estimation of occurrence-exposure rates.

8.3.1 Summary Indicators

The state space and relevant parameters are derived from the data by the function Parameters:

```
library (Biograph)
data (NLOG98)
OG <- NLOG98
param <- Parameters (OG)
```

The object param has 19 components. The number of states is param $numstates. The names of the states are stored in the vector param $namstates. The number of feasible transitions is found with param$ntrans, and the line numbers of the transitions are given by the object param$tmat:

```
         To
From  H  A  C  M  K
   H NA  1  2  3  4
   A NA NA  5  6  7
   C NA  8  9 10 11
   M NA 12 13 NA 14
   K NA NA NA NA NA
```

Transition number 9 originates and ends in the same state. If intrastate transitions are omitted, the number of transitions reduces to 13. The transition matrix can be recovered using the following code:

```
tmat <- attr(OG,"param")$tmat
```

The object param$transitions shows the transitions in different ways:

```
    Trans OR DES ORN DESN ODN
1     1   1   2   H    A   HA
2     2   1   3   H    C   HC
3     3   1   4   H    M   HM
4     4   1   5   H    K   HK
5     5   2   3   A    C   AC
6     6   2   4   A    M   AM
7     7   2   5   A    K   AK
8     8   3   2   C    A   CA
9     9   3   3   C    C   CC
10   10   3   4   C    M   CM
11   11   3   5   C    K   CK
12   12   4   2   M    A   MA
13   13   4   3   M    C   MC
14   14   4   5   M    K   MK
```

where `Trans` denotes the transition number, `OR` and `ORN` the origin, `DES` and `DESN` the destination and `ODN` the origin and destination.

The 500 respondents experience a total of 975 transitions. The number of transitions by origin and destination is given by `param$nntrans`:

```
           Destination
Origin  H    A    C    M    K
    H   0  172  106  172    6
    A   0    0  131   44    5
    C   0   46    2  132   19
    M   0   19    2    0  291
    K   0    0    0    0    0
```

The above table shows that most first births (291) occur in marriage and that 19 first-born children have mothers who cohabit, 5 have mothers living alone and 6 have mothers living at the parental home.

Individual state sequences are produced by the function `Sequences.ind`:

```
seq.ind <- Sequences.ind (OG$path,
              attr(OG,"param")$namstates)
```

The different types of episodes are obtained by the function:

```
overviewE <- OverviewEpisodes(OG,seq.ind)
```

The information on the episodes is stored in object `overviewE`. Four types of episodes are distinguished:

(a) LROpen: episodes that start before or at the onset of observation and end when the observation is discontinued at survey date. A total of 44 episodes belong to

8.3 Exploratory Analysis

Table 8.2 Overview of episodes observed in OG data

```
A. Number of episodes, by type
                    Type
Episode  LROpen  LOpen  ROpen  Closed  Total
   H        44    456      0       0    500
   A         0      0     57     180    237
   C         0      0     42     199    241
   M         0      0     36     312    348
   K         0      0    321       0    321
 Total      44    456    456     691   1647

B. Total duration of episodes, by type
                    Type
Episode  LROpen  LOpen   ROpen  Closed   Total
   H     11431  114882      0       0  126313
   A         0       0   3075    7916   10991
   C         0       0   1905    7348    9253
   M         0       0   3915   10402   14317
   K         0       0  55637       0   55637
 Total   11431  114882  64532   25666  216511
```

this class. They refer to respondents who occupy a single state throughout the observation window and are still living at the parental home at survey date.

(b) LOpen: episodes that start before or at the onset of observation and end during the observation. The 456 episodes refer to respondents who experience at least one transition during the observation period.

(c) ROpen: episodes that start during the observation period and continue at the end of observation. The total is 456. Of them, 42 women are cohabiting and childless at survey date and 321 have at least one child.

(d) Closed: episodes that start and end during the observation period. The number of episodes of this type is 691. Note that, since K represents an absorbing state, an individual who enters that state remains in that state and occupies it at survey date.

The numbers of episodes and the total durations of episodes are shown in Table 8.2. The overall observation time is 216.5 thousand months, and the average duration of an episode is 131.5 months. Note that open episodes are considerably longer than closed episodes.

The number of transitions by origin and destination and the number of censored cases by state are computed by the function `OverviewTransitions`. The function requires the ages at transition, which are computed by function `AgeTrans`:

```
agetrans <- AgeTrans (Bdata=OG)
```

Table 8.3 Number of transitions and mean ages, by origin and destination. OG

```
A. Number of transitions
                    Destination
Origin   H    A    C    M    K  Total  Censored  TOTAL
  H      0  172  106  172    6   456        44    500
  A      0    0  131   44    5   180        57    237
  C      0   46    2  132   19   199        42    241
  M      0   19    2    0  291   312        36    348
  K      0    0    0    0    0     0       321    321
Total    0  237  241  348  321  1147       500   1647

B. Mean age at transition
                    Destination
Origin   H      A      C      M      K    censored
  H    NaN  19.05  20.70  20.62  19.83      20.64
  A    NaN    NaN  24.33  23.14  25.70      27.31
  C    NaN  25.26  22.00  25.49  24.39      29.12
  M    NaN  28.50  28.00    NaN  25.04      34.47
  K    NaN    NaN    NaN    NaN    NaN      39.35
```

The object `agetrans` has five components:

(a) `agetrans`: ages at transition
(b) `ageentry`: age at entry into observation (in this case 0)
(c) `agecens`: age at censoring
(d) `st_entry`: state at entry into observation (in this case H)
(e) `st_censoring`: state at survey date

The function `OverviewTransitions` produces numbers of transitions and mean ages at transition:

```
overviewT <- OverviewTransitions
                (Bdata=OG,
                 seq.ind=seq.ind,
                 agetrans=agetrans)
```

The transitions are direct transitions. They should not be confused with discrete-time transitions that are obtained by comparing states occupied at two points in time. The number of transitions by origin and destination, the number of censored cases and the mean ages at transition and censoring are stored in `overviewT $Ttrans`, shown in Table 8.3:

From the direct transitions in Table 8.3 and the exposure times in Table 8.2, aggregate transition rates may be computed by dividing the numbers of transitions and the exposure times (in years):

8.3 Exploratory Analysis

Table 8.4 Aggregate yearly transition rates. OG

```
                        Destination
Origin        H         A         C         M         K
   H      -0.04332   0.01634   0.01007   0.01634   0.00057
   A       0.00000  -0.19652   0.14303   0.04804   0.00546
   C       0.00000   0.05966  -0.25548   0.17119   0.02464
   M       0.00000   0.01593   0.00168  -0.26151   0.24391
   K       0.00000   0.00000   0.00000   0.00000   0.00000
```

```
d <- solve(diag(overviewE$sojourn[1:5,5]/12))
M <- d%*%overviewT$Ttrans[1:5,1:5]
```

These transition rates are the off-diagonal elements of the **M**-matrix, which is the matrix of transition rates used in multistate modelling (see Chap. 2). The diagonal elements are minus the total rate of leaving a state (exit rate). They are obtained by the following expressions:

```
diag(M) <- 0
diag(M) <- -apply(M,1,sum)
dimnames(M) <- dimnames (overviewT$Ttrans[1:5,1:5])
```

The **M**-matrix is shown in Table 8.4:

8.3.2 State Sequences

The function

```
sequences <- Sequences (OG,mean_median="mean")
```

identifies the different sequences or trajectories recorded during the observation period. The object sequences has two components. The first indicates the measure used to display the central age at transition: the mean age or the median age. In this case, it is the mean age. The second component contains the sequences. The OG data reveal 48 different sequences. The 10 most prevalent sequences are shown in Table 8.5. The first column shows the trajectory number. The number of respondents experiencing the trajectory is shown in column 2. The share in the total sample population of that particular trajectory and the cumulative percentages are shown next. The mean ages at entry into and exit from observation are shown in columns 5 and 6. Column 7 shows the number of states in the trajectory. The trajectory is displayed in column 8. The next columns show the mean (or median) ages at transition and the destination states. The pathway HMK is most prevalent. Thirty percent of the subsample population leaves the parental home for marriage

Table 8.5 Event and state sequences in OG

```
     ncase    %  cum% M_age_entry M_age_exit ns  case       tr1      tr2      tr3      tr4
1      151 30.2 30.2           0       42.84  3   HMK  21.62>M  24.63>K
2       50 10.0 40.2           0       34.88  4  HCMK  21.77>C  24.62>M  26.86>K
3       44  8.8 49.0           0       21.65  1     H
4       39  7.8 56.8           0       25.42  2    HA  20.37>A
5       39  7.8 64.6           0       43.89  4  HAMK  19.05>A  23.02>M   25.9>K
6       33  6.6 71.2           0       38.05  5 HACMK  19.34>A  22.63>C  26.48>M  28.55>K
7       17  3.4 74.6           0       31.75  3   HAC  21.64>A  27.33>C
8       17  3.4 78.0           0       26.47  2    HC  22.78>C
9       12  2.4 80.4           0       31.47  3   HCK  21.16>C  24.75>K
10      12  2.4 82.8           0       35.32  2    HM  22.83>M
```

and have their first child in their first marriage. More than 80 % of the subsample population experiences one of the ten trajectories shown in Table 8.5.

The pathways by birth cohort and the median ages at transition are obtained by the following commands:

```
z1 <- Sequences (OG[OG$cohort=="<1960",])
z2 <- Sequences (OG[OG$cohort=="1960+",])
```

The most prevalent pathways are shown in Table 8.6. In the older cohort, born before 1960, 50 % of the women experience the HMK sequence. In the younger cohort, born in 1960 or later, it is 16 %.

Among women born before 1960, those who do not practise a religion are less likely to experience the HMK sequence than women who practise a religion. The figure is obtained by the following code:

```
z1 <- Sequences (OG[OG$cohort=="<1960"
                    &OG$kerk=="no religion",])
```

The proportion of women in the sample experiencing the HMK sequence is 41 % for women not practising a religion, 52 % for Protestants and 64 % for Roman Catholics.

The age profile at first marriage by birth cohort is obtained by the code:

```
z.c1 <- TransitionAB(OG[OG$cohort=="<1960",],"*M")
z.c2 <- TransitionAB(OG[OG$cohort=="1960+",],"*M")
```

The object produced by TransitionAB has eight components. The first (z.c1$ncase) identifies the origin and destination states of the transition. The second (z.c1$n) is the number of transitions (marriages). It is 193 in the oldest cohort and 146 in the youngest cohort. The third (z.c1$id) lists the identification numbers of respondents who experience the transition. The fourth (z.c1$pos) gives the position of first marriage in the state sequence. The fifth (z.c1$date)

8.3 Exploratory Analysis

Table 8.6 Pathways in OG, by birth cohort

```
a. Born before 1960
   ncase    %   cum% M_age_entry M_age_exit ns  case    tr1        tr2        tr3        tr4
1  106  50.24  50.24           0      47.17   3  HMK  20.88>M    23.5>K
2   30  14.22  64.45           0      47.17   4  HAMK 18.5>A  22.75>M  25.67>K
3   16   7.58  72.04           0      42.29   5  HACMK 18.42>A 22.25>C  25.79>M  29.54>K
4   12   5.69  77.73           0      39.25   4  HCMK 22.25>C 23.67>M  26.08>K
5    4   1.90  79.62           0      45.21   3  HAC  27.25>A 32.62>C

b. Born in 1960 or later
   ncase    %   cum% M_age_entry M_age_exit ns  case    tr1        tr2        tr3        tr4
1   45  15.57  15.57           0      33.83   3  HMK  22.17>M  26.42>K
2   44  15.22  30.80           0      20.75   1  H
3   38  13.15  43.94           0      33.83   4  HCMK 20.79>C 24.25>M  27.46>K
4   37  12.80  56.75           0      23.67   2  HA   19.17>A
5   17   5.88  62.63           0      32.58   5  HACMK 19.17>A 21.83>C  27.58>M  28.83>K
```

contains for each respondent in the group the date of marriage (in CMC), the sixth (z.c1$age) the age at marriage, the seventh (z.c1$year) the year of marriage and the last one the birth cohort to which a respondent belongs.

The life path of respondent 8 is shown in Box 8.1. The respondent is born in CMC 707, which is November 1958. She left the parental home in June 1974 at age 15 to cohabit. She married 1 year later and had a child in October 1975 at age 16. The observation ended at age 39.

Box 8.1: Life Path of Respondent with ID 8. OG

```
[[1]]
[[1]]$ID
[1] 8

[[1]]$born
[1] "Subject ID =  8   Date of birth 707 (01Nov58)"

[[1]]$path
  Episode State EntryDate1 EntryDate2 EntryAge Durat OR DE
1       1     H        707   01Nov58     0.00   187  0  1
2       2     C        894   01Jun74    15.58    12  1  3
3       3     M        906   01Jun75    16.58     4  3  4
4       4     K        910   01Oct75    16.92   270  4  5
5       5  Cens       1180   01Apr98    39.41    NA  5  0
```

The life path is produced by SamplePath(OG,8).

To produce the life paths for a selection of individuals, the IDs must be given, e.g.

    subjectsID <- c(8,96,980,1056,1496,2883)

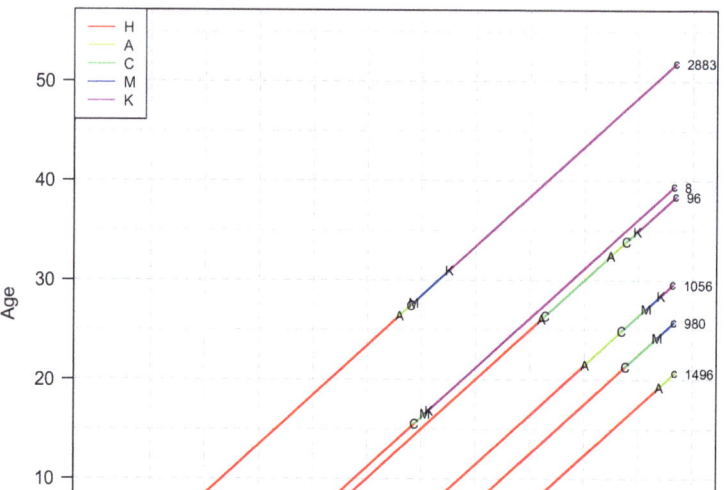

Fig. 8.2 Lifelines for selected subjects. OG

To display the lifelines, the data should be in the long format (episode data structure). The long format is produced by

```
Dlong <- Biograph.long(OG)
```

and stored in `Dlong$Depisode`.

Figure 8.2 shows the lifelines of a selection of subjects, including subject with ID 8. The code is:

```
title1 ="Living arrangements. OG98"
z<- Lexislines.episodes (OG,Dlong$Depisode,
                subjectsID,title=title1)
```

The function `Lexislines.episodes` uses functions of the *Epi* package developed by Carstensen (2007, 2009). Colours represent stages of life. Transitions are marked and the identification number of a subject is added to the lifeline. Subjects 980 and 1,496 do not have a child at survey date. Subjects 8 and 1,056 have a child, which they both received soon after marriage. Respondent 96 got a child while cohabiting.

8.3 Exploratory Analysis

Fig. 8.3 Lexis diagram: leaving parental home for marriage, by age and calendar year. OG

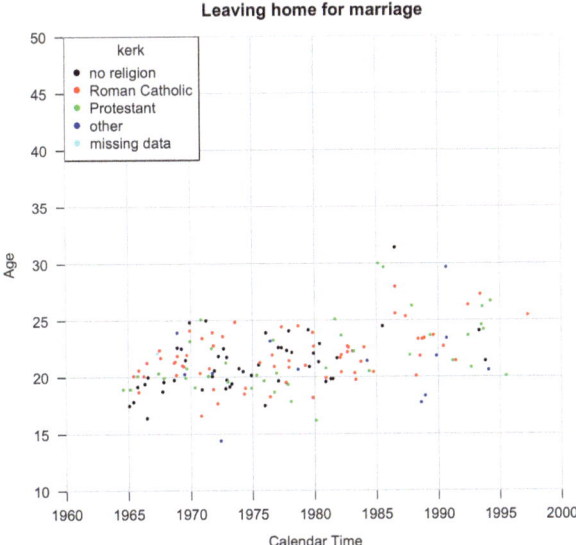

The following command plots the Lexis diagram showing the ages at leaving the parental home for marriage and the years of leaving home, by religious denomination:

```
z<- Lexispoints (Bdata=OG,transition="HM",
        title="Leaving home for marriage",
        cov="kerk",legend="topleft")
```

The result is shown in Fig. 8.3.

The cohort biography, i.e. the average life course of cohort members, is represented by state occupancies of the sample population at consecutive ages. The state occupancies are contained in the object occup$state_occup produced by the function

```
occup <- Occup (OG)
```

The data processing may take relatively long (few minutes) if the sample size is large. The object occup has four components. The state occupancies (occup $state_occup) are shown in Table 8.7 for selected ages and in Fig. 8.4 for all ages.

The following code produces Fig. 8.4:

Table 8.7 State occupancies by age. Selected ages. OG

age	H	A	C	M	K	Censored	Total
0	500	0	0	0	0	0	500
12	500	0	0	0	0	0	500
15	498	1	0	1	0	0	500
16	494	3	3	0	0	0	500
17	483	9	2	2	4	0	500
18	452	26	9	8	5	0	500
19	374	75	16	15	10	10	500
20	295	97	29	34	22	23	500
21	216	108	46	57	41	32	500
22	165	94	57	91	52	41	500
23	112	75	77	104	82	50	500
24	74	63	78	110	111	64	500
25	46	49	78	112	135	80	500
30	8	31	29	45	243	144	500
35	1	9	10	20	230	230	500
40	0	5	4	15	159	317	500
50	0	1	1	1	44	453	500
54	0	0	0	0	0	500	500

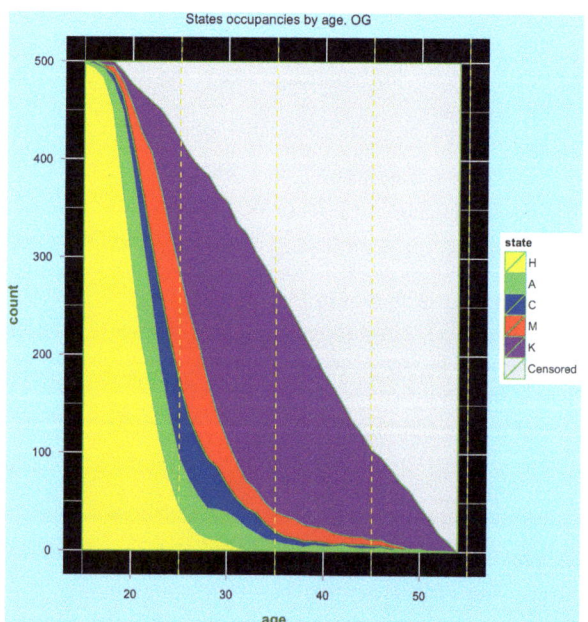

Fig. 8.4 State occupancies by age. OG

8.3 Exploratory Analysis

```
z<- plot (x=occup$state_occup,
      namstates.desired=c("H","A","C","M","K",
                "Censored"),
      colours=c("yellow","green","blue","red",
                "purple","lightgrey"),
      title="States occupancies by age. OG",
      area=TRUE,
      xmin=15,
      xmax=55)
```

The component `occup$st_age_1[,]` gives for each respondent the states occupied at consecutive birthdays. The object can be used as an input to the *TraMineR* package. In the *TraMineR* terminology, the format of `occup$st_age_1[,]` is the extended format. The extended format can be converted to a compressed format by the `seqconc` function of the *TraMineR* package:

```
library (TraMineR)
DTraMineR <- seqconc (occup$st_age_1,sep="-")
```

In the object `occup$st_age_1[,]` the states are identified by numbers. The state of a person who no longer is under observation is denoted by +.

A state sequence object is the main object of the *TraMineR* package. Most *TriMineR* functions require a state sequence object as an input argument. It is produced by the `seqdef` function of the *TraMineR* package:

```
namst <- c(param$namstates,"-")
og.seq <- seqdef(occup$st_age_1,
         1:ncol(occup$st_age_1),
         informat='STS',
         alphabet=c(param$namstates,"+"))
```

where `param` is produced in Sect. 8.3.1. The expression shows that the *Biograph* object `occup$st_age_1` can easily be converted into a state sequence object to be used as input in *TraMineR*. The labels of the states included in the state sequence object are given by the *TriMineR* function `alphabet(og.seq)`.

TraMineR has functions to produce several types of plots such as the state index plot, which displays the state sequence for selected respondents; the state frequency plot, which displays the most frequent sequences; and the state distribution plot, which displays the state distribution (state occupancies) by age. Suppose we want to graph the state sequences for selected respondents. The code is:

Fig. 8.5 State sequences of selected respondents, produced by *TraMineR*. OG

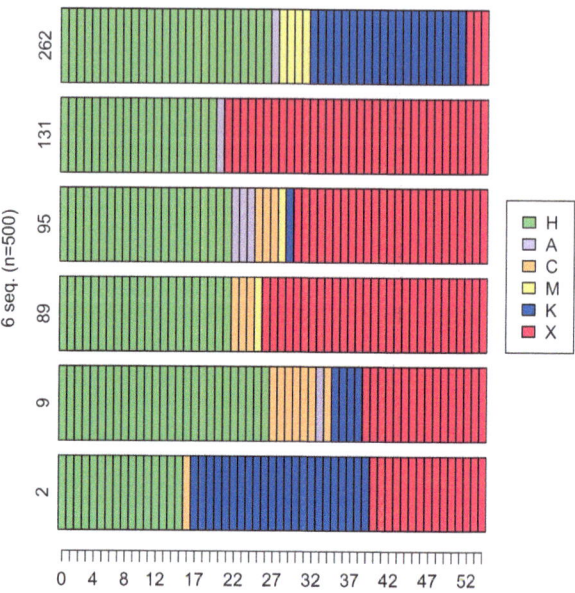

```
namstatest <- c("H","A","C","M","K","X")
subjectsID <- c(8,96,980,1056,1496,2883)
ids <- which (OG$ID%in%subjectsID)
seqplot(og.seq,type="i",
        tlim=ids,
        ltext=namstatest,
        xtlab=c(0:54),
        withlegend="right")
```

where tlim is a vector of seven respondents with selected IDs. The figure is shown in Fig. 8.5. The number on the left of each sequence is the line number of the record associated with a particular identification number.

The state frequency plot considers the frequencies of state sequences taking into account the ages at transition. The *TraMineR* command

```
seqplot(og.seq, type="f")
```

plots the 10 most frequent sequences. They comprise 11 % of all sequences. The frequency table is computed by the function seqtab. The share of these sequences is:

```
sum(attr(seqtab(og.seq),"freq")$Percent)
```

The frequency table produced by *TraMineR* differs from that produced by the Sequences function of *Biograph*, which disregards the ages at transition in determining the frequency of a state sequence. Figure 8.6 shows the state distribution by age. It is produced by the following code:

8.3 Exploratory Analysis

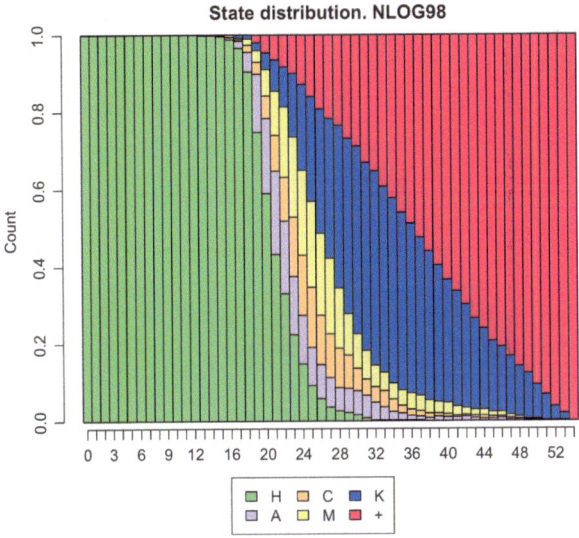

Fig. 8.6 Observed state occupancies by age, produced by *TraMineR*. OG sample population

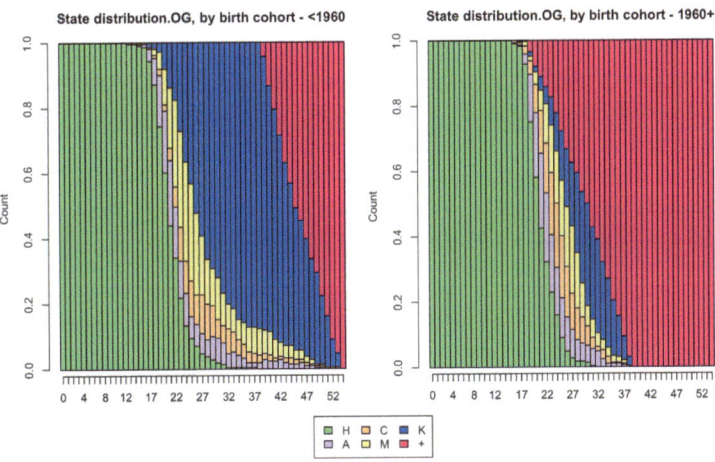

Fig. 8.7 Observed state occupancies by age and cohort, produced by *TraMineR*. OG sample population

```
seqplot(og.seq, type="d",
        title="State distribution. NLOG98",
        ylab="Count",
        xtlab=0:54)
```

The state distributions by age for the two birth cohorts are shown in Fig. 8.7. The code is:

Table 8.8 Rates (probabilities) of transition between marital status/living arrangement, produced by *TraMineR*. OG

```
         [-> H]   [-> A]   [-> C]   [-> M]   [-> K]   [-> +]
[H ->] 0.95369  0.01519  0.00917  0.01565  0.00157  0.00472
[A ->] 0.00000  0.76030  0.12148  0.04881  0.00868  0.06074
[C ->] 0.00000  0.05277  0.72329  0.12741  0.04376  0.05277
[M ->] 0.00000  0.01340  0.00335  0.73786  0.21441  0.03099
[K ->] 0.00000  0.00000  0.00000  0.00000  0.93199  0.06801
[+ ->] 0.00000  0.00000  0.00000  0.00000  0.00000  1.00000
```

```
seqplot(og.seq, type="d",
        group=OG$cohort,
        title="State distribution.OG, by birth
        cohort",ylab="Count",xtlab=0:54)
```

Here, we see that very few members of the youngest cohort have children, partly due to censoring. Members of the youngest cohort are at most 37 years of age at survey date and about half is less than 30.

The seqrtrate function of *TraMineR* computes transition rates. Note that these 'rates' are probabilities and not occurrence-exposure rates. They are 'probabilities of transition from one state to another observed in the sequence data' (see documentation of the seqtrate function). The transition probabilities (called rates in *TraMineR*) are obtained by comparing the state occupied at time t and the state occupied at time t+1 (Gabadinho et al. 2011, p. 17). They also include probabilities of leaving states due to censoring. However, those probabilities have no particularly useful meaning in the analysis of transition data. Table 8.8 shows the empirical transition probabilities produced by the code:

```
tr <- round(seqtrate(og.seq),5)
```

Transition probabilities may also be computed by taking the exponent of matrix **M** of occurrence-exposure rates (see above):

```
Require (msm)
P <- MatrixExp(M,t=1)
P <- round(P,5)
dimnames(P) = dimnames(M)
```

where MatrixExp is a function of the *msm* package and **M** is the transition rate matrix shown in Table 8.9.

8.3 Exploratory Analysis

Table 8.9 Probabilities of transition between marital status/living arrangement, derived from occurrence-exposure rates. OG

```
                        Destination
Origin        H        A        C        M        K
     H   0.9576  0.01490  0.00971  0.01517  0.00262
     A   0.0000  0.82538  0.11433  0.04793  0.01236
     C   0.0000  0.04875  0.77808  0.13354  0.03963
     M   0.0000  0.01273  0.00220  0.77035  0.21472
     K   0.0000  0.00000  0.00000  0.00000  1.00000
```

8.3.3 Age Profiles

The function `TransitionAB` gives characteristics of subjects who experience a selected transition. The following commands select data on the event from the *Biograph* object OG:

```
z1<- TransitionAB(OG,"MK")
z2<- TransitionAB(OG,"*K")
z3<- TransitionAB(OG,"H*")
```

The first command focuses on transitions from marriage to first birth. It produces information on the 291 married women who have their first child in their first marriage. The second produces information on the 321 women who have a first birth before survey date, irrespective of the marital status and living arrangement. The third produces information on the 456 persons who leave the parental home before the survey date, regardless of destination. The * indicates any state. The object produced by the function has seven components:

(a) `z1$case`: The transition selected.
(b) `z1$n`: The number of subjects experiencing the transition selected.
(c) `z1$id`: Identification numbers of subjects who experience the selected transition.
(d) `z1$pos`: For each subject experiencing the transition, the position of the transition in the character variable `path`.
(e) `z1$date`: For each subject, the date at the transition. The date is given in the time unit used in the original data. An NA indicates that a subject did not experience the transition.
(f) `z1$age`: For each subject, the age at the transition.
(g) `z1$year`: For each subject, the calendar year in which the transition occurs.
(h) `z1$cohort`: The birth cohort of the subject experiencing the transition.

Note that a respondent may have reported several occurrences of the given transition. For instance, a person may experience the transition from cohabitation to marriage (CM) more than once during the period of observation. *Biograph* selects the first occurrence.

The mean age at which married women with children have their first child is obtained by using the following two commands:

```
z<- TransitionAB(OG,"MK")
meanage <- mean(z$age,na.rm=TRUE)
```

The resulting mean age is 26.44 years. Married women born before 1960 had their first child at age 25.79 on average. That figure is produced by:

```
mean(z$age[OG$cohort=="<1960"],na.r=TRUE)
```

The younger cohort of married women had the first child at a higher age (26.88 years):

```
mean(z$age[OG$cohort=="1960+"],na.r=TRUE)
```

The mean age at first birth for the 291 married women who have their first child in their first marriage, differentiated by birth cohort and religion, is obtained as follows:

```
meanages <- aggregate(z$age,
          list(cohort=OG[OG$ID%in%z$id,]$cohort,
               Religion=OG[OG$ID%in%z$id,]$kerk),
          mean,na.rm=TRUE)
```

The `aggregate` function, which is part of the *stats* package, splits the data in subsets and computes summary statistics for each. The results are not shown for space reasons.

The mean age at first birth for all women, irrespective of marital status, is 26.32 years. It is produced by the code:

```
z<- TransitionAB(OG,"*K")
meanage <- mean(z$age,na.rm=TRUE)
```

The function `table(trunc(z$age))` tabulates the ages at first birth, and the command `hist(z$age,breaks=50)` produces the histogram, with `breaks` the number of cells for the histogram. An alternative is to use a Trellis plot, i.e. a panel of graphic displays. The age distribution of the 172 respondents in the subsample who leave the parental home for first marriage, by birth cohort and level of education, is shown in Fig. 8.8. Of the 172 respondents, 11 did not report level of education (`table(zzz$educ,zzz$cohort,useNA="always")`). The code to produce the plot, which is a density plot, is:

8.3 Exploratory Analysis

```
library (lattice)
transition <- "HM"
z <- TransitionAB(OG,transition)
     # ages at leaving home for marriage
zzz <- data.frame(cbind
 (ID=OG[OG$ID%in%z$id,]$ID,cohort=OG[OG$ID%in%z$id,]$cohort,ed
 uc=OG[OG$ID%in%z$id,]$educ,trans=z$age))
zzz$cohort <- factor(zzz$cohort,
     labels=c("Born <1960","Born 1960+"))
zzz$educ <- ifelse (zzz$educ>4,5,zzz$educ)  # recode
zzz$educ <- factor (zzz$educ,
     labels=c("Primary","Secondary lower",
     "Secondary higher","High"))
table(zzz$educ,zzz$cohort)
densityplot (~trans|educ,data=zzz,plot.points="rug",
     # main="Age at first marriage",
       sub= paste("Total number of first marriages with known
 covariates is ",length (na.omit(zzz$educ)),sep=""),
         xlab="Age",
         scale=list(x=list(alternating=FALSE)),
                   groups=cohort,ref=TRUE,
                   auto.key=TRUE)
```

Figure 8.8 shows that members of the younger cohort marry later, except for those with primary education. The figure clearly reveals that, for a given birth cohort and level of education, the age profile of first marriage is a mixture of two age profiles. Note that the density shows the proportion of women in a particular covariate class that marries at a given age. To display the number of marriages by age (and covariate class), a histogram should be used rather than a density plot.

8.3.4 Occurrence-Exposure Rates

The basic table for the estimation of age-specific transition rates is produced by the RateTable function, which requires objects produced by the Occup and Trans functions:

```
          occup <- Occup (OG)
          trans <- Trans (OG)
          ratetable <- RateTable (OG, occup,trans)
```

The basic table is ratetable$Stable. A selection of the table is presented in Table 8.10.

On their 20th birthday, 295 respondents in the subsample live at the parental home. At that age, 97 live alone, 29 cohabit and 34 are married. Finally, 22 respondents have a first child. The total number of years the sample populations spend in marriage between exact ages 20 and 21 is 51.58 years. That number is the result of

240   8 Application to the Netherlands Family and Fertility Survey

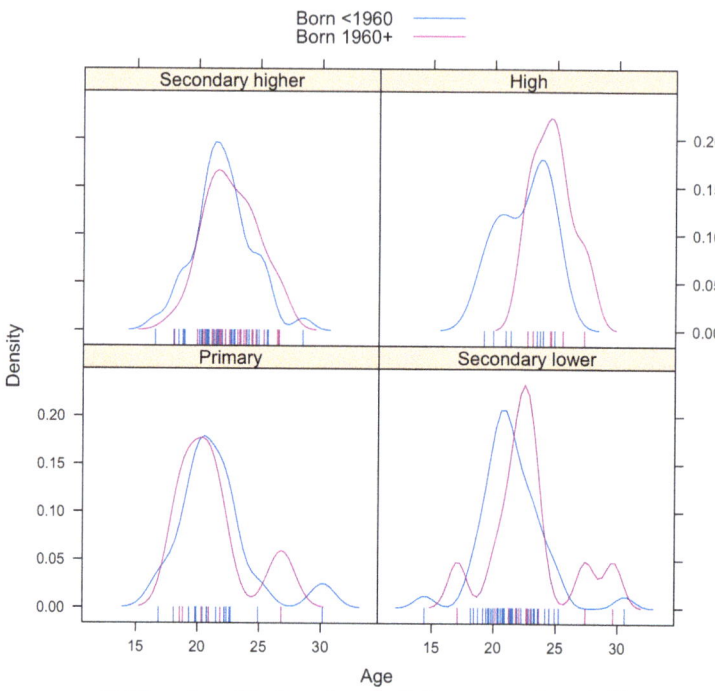

Fig. 8.8 Trellis plot of age at first marriage, by birth cohort and level of education. OG

(1) persons married at age 20 and remaining married and without children throughout the year, (2) persons who enter marriage at age 20 in completed years and remain childless at least until their next birthday, (3) persons married at age 20 who dissolve the marriage before reaching age 21, (4) persons married at age 20 who have a first child before age 21 and (5) married persons who are aged 20 at survey date. The transitions are shown in Table 8.10. The origin state is shown as the layer variable, and the destination is shown as the column variable. For instance, between ages 20 and 21, there were 26 respondents who left the parental home to live alone and 34 who left home for marriage.

The object `ratetable$Stable` is probably the most useful one produced by *Biograph*. The table is the basis for the occurrence-exposure rates. Consider the situation of respondents at age 25. Of the respondents in the subsample, 46 were living at their parental home, 49 were living alone, 78 were cohabiting, 112 were married (without children) and 135 had at least one child. The number of years lived at the parental home between the 25th and the 26th birthday by all respondents combined is 34.17 years. The number of years spent living alone is 47.17, in cohabitation is 69.42, in marriage (without children) is 113.08 and with at least

8.3 Exploratory Analysis

Table 8.10 Data for estimation of occurrence-exposure rates, by age. OG

```
, , State = H
    Case
Age  Occup     PY  Leaving H A  C  M  K Censored
 0   500   500.00        0 0  0  0  0 0       0
15   498   496.58        4 0  1  3  0 0       0
20   295   252.83       79 0 26 13 34 1       5
25    46    34.17       18 0  5  3  6 0       4

, , State = A
    Case
Age  Occup     PY  Leaving H A  C  M  K Censored
 0     0     0.00        0 0  0  0  0 0       0
15     1     2.00        0 0  0  0  0 0       0
20    97   103.58       20 0  0 10  4 2       4
25    49    47.17       12 0  0  8  1 0       3
30    31    29.50        5 0  0  2  1 0       2

, , State = C
    Case
Age  Occup     PY  Leaving H A C  M K Censored
20    29    36.92        6 0 3 0  1 2       0
25    78    69.42       25 0 2 0 16 3       4
30    29    24.67       12 0 3 0  7 1       1
35    10     9.50        3 0 0 0  3 0       0
40     4     3.58        2 0 0 0  0 0       2

, , State = M
    Case
Age  Occup     PY  Leaving H A C M  K Censored
20    34    51.58       16 0 1 0  0 15       0
25   112   113.08       29 0 0 0  0 25       4
30    45    39.75       17 0 1 0  0 14       2
35    20    20.33        3 0 0 0  0  2       1
40    15    13.58        3 0 1 0  0  0       2

, , State = K
    Case
Age  Occup     PY  Leaving H A C M K Censored
20    22    28.58        0 0 0 0 0 0        0
25   135   146.83        2 0 0 0 0 0        2
30   243   244.83       14 0 0 0 0 0       14
35   230   224.58       13 0 0 0 0 0       13
40   159   151.92       10 0 0 0 0 0       10
```

one child is 146.83 years. Of the persons at the parental home on their 25th birthday, 18 left the parental home within a year, 5 to live independently, 3 to cohabit, 6 because of marriage and 4 were lost to observation because they were aged 25 at time of interview. The age-specific transition rates (occurrence-exposure rates) can be determined directly from these data. For instance, the marriage rate of a 25-year-old living at the parental home is 6/34.17 = 0.1756, and the marriage rate for someone of the same age but cohabiting is not much different: 16/69.42 = 0.2305. The transition rates for selected ages are shown later in the chapter.

The ages at transition are stored in object agetrans$ages, produced by the function AgeTrans. The following command tabulates the age profile of the transitions:

```
agetrans <- AgeTrans(OG)
ztab <- apply(agetrans$ages,2,function(x)
              table(trunc(x)))
```

with ztab$tr1 representing the age profile of the first transition, ztab$tr2 representing the age profile of the second transition, etc.

The sojourn times in the different states by age are contained in object occup $tsjt. The total number of years of observation in each state is apply (occup $tsjt,2,sum). The total number of years of observation is 27,500 years. A large part (38 %) relates to time spent at the parental home.

Sojourn times and other measures that are recorded in the survey can be displayed for each individual. For example, the following command displays for individual with ID = 8 the sojourn time in each state and at each age. The time is with three decimal digits:

```
print (round(occup$sjt_age_1[OG$ID==8,,],3))
```

The transition rates by age, state of origin and state of destination are computed by dividing the number of occurrences by the exposure time, i.e. the sojourn time in the origin state. Table 8.11 shows the transition rates for selected ages. The off-diagonal elements of the transition matrix **M(x)** show the rates. The figures shown on the diagonal (e.g. from H to H) are minus the sum of the rates of leaving the state.

8.3 Exploratory Analysis

Table 8.11 Occurrence-exposure rates (M-matrix: age-cohort rates). OG

```
, , origin = H        destination
age       H            A            C            M            K
 15 -0.008055097 0.002013774 0.006041323 0.0000000 0.000000000
 20 -0.292686786 0.102835898 0.051417949 0.1344777 0.003955227
 21 -0.246318608 0.037483266 0.058902276 0.1499331 0.000000000
 22 -0.372439479 0.059590317 0.141527002 0.1638734 0.007448790
 23 -0.390243902 0.097560976 0.108401084 0.1842818 0.000000000
 24 -0.410256410 0.068376068 0.153846154 0.1880342 0.000000000
 25 -0.409716125 0.146327188 0.087796313 0.1755926 0.000000000
 26 -0.472366556 0.188946623 0.094473311 0.1889466 0.000000000
 27 -0.189513582 0.000000000 0.063171194 0.1263424 0.000000000
 28 -0.169061708 0.169061708 0.000000000 0.0000000 0.000000000
 29 -0.300000000 0.000000000 0.000000000 0.2000000 0.100000000
 30 -0.545454545 0.000000000 0.363636364 0.1818182 0.000000000

, , origin = A        destination
age  H     A            C            M            K
 15  0  0.00000000  0.00000000  0.00000000  0.00000000
 20  0 -0.15446997  0.09654373  0.03861749  0.01930875
 21  0 -0.23150381  0.16398187  0.06752194  0.00000000
 22  0 -0.33949895  0.16389604  0.17560290  0.00000000
 23  0 -0.25092251  0.16236162  0.07380074  0.01476015
 24  0 -0.29357798  0.25688073  0.03669725  0.00000000
 25  0 -0.19079924  0.16959932  0.02119992  0.00000000
 26  0 -0.34146341  0.26829268  0.07317073  0.00000000
 27  0 -0.26865672  0.26865672  0.00000000  0.00000000
 28  0 -0.13258204  0.09943653  0.03314551  0.00000000
 29  0 -0.09730782  0.03243594  0.06487188  0.00000000
 30  0 -0.10169492  0.06779661  0.03389831  0.00000000

, , origin = C        destination
age  H     A            C            M            K
 15  0  0.00000000   0.0000000  0.00000000  0.00000000
 20  0  0.08125677  -0.1625135  0.02708559  0.05417118
 21  0  0.11940299  -0.3184080  0.15920398  0.03980100
 22  0  0.02853881  -0.1426941  0.09988584  0.01426941
 23  0  0.06500260  -0.2340094  0.16900676  0.00000000
 24  0  0.02566735  -0.2181725  0.17967146  0.01283368
 25  0  0.02881014  -0.3025065  0.23048113  0.04321521
 26  0  0.01673640  -0.2677824  0.21757322  0.03347280
 27  0  0.05504587  -0.2752294  0.18348624  0.03669725
 28  0  0.13043478  -0.1956522  0.06521739  0.00000000
 29  0  0.09022556  -0.4210526  0.33082707  0.00000000
 30  0  0.12160519  -0.4458857  0.28374544  0.04053506

, , origin = M        destination
age  H     A            C            M            K
 15  0  1.204819277  0.000000000 -1.2048193  0.0000000
 20  0  0.019387359  0.000000000 -0.3101978  0.2908104
 21  0  0.000000000  0.000000000 -0.1228669  0.1228669
 22  0  0.020761964  0.000000000 -0.3114295  0.2906675
 23  0  0.000000000  0.000000000 -0.2712308  0.2712308
 24  0  0.008816787  0.000000000 -0.2116029  0.2027861
 25  0  0.000000000  0.000000000 -0.2210824  0.2210824
 26  0  0.029460866  0.009820289 -0.2651478  0.2258666
 27  0  0.000000000  0.000000000 -0.3481490  0.3481490
 28  0  0.015484670  0.000000000 -0.4180861  0.4026014
 29  0  0.020374898  0.000000000 -0.4686227  0.4482478
 30  0  0.025157233  0.000000000 -0.3773585  0.3522013
```

8.4 Transition Rate Models

The packages *survival*, *mvna* and *mstate* are illustrated using data from the subsample of the Netherlands Family and Fertility Survey (NLOG98), included in the *Biograph* package. The subsample is a random selection of 500 women. Three subsections are distinguished. The first subsection covers data preparation. The estimation of cumulative hazard rates is covered in the second subsection. The third subsection illustrates the estimation of regression models to determine covariate effects.

8.4.1 Data Preparation

The first step in the implementation of transition rate models is the preparation of data in the long format. *Biograph* has several utilities that facilitate the conversion. Biograph.long is a generic function. It produces a long format accepted by the *survival* and *eha* packages. Biograph.mvna produces the long format required by the *mvna* package, and Biograph.mstate produces the format for the *mstate* package.

Intrastate transitions are removed since they are not of interest:

```
OGd <- Remove.intrastate(OG)
```

The packages *mvna* and *mstate* require that intrastate transition is omitted. The object OGd has 13 possible transitions. The transition matrix is part of the parameters:

```
param <- Parameters (OGd).
```

The transition matrix is (param$tmat):

```
             To
  From  H   A   C   M   K
     H  NA   1   2   3   4
     A  NA  NA   5   6   7
     C  NA   8  NA   9  10
     M  NA  11  12  NA  13
     K  NA  NA  NA  NA  NA
```

The number of transitions is included in the object param$nntrans:

8.4 Transition Rate Models

```
             Destination
   Origin H    A    C    M    K
        H 0  172  106  172    6
        A 0    0  131   44    5
        C 0   46    0  132   19
        M 0   19    2    0  291
        K 0    0    0    0    0
```

Of the 500 respondents, 321 have at least one child, most during marriage. 44 respondents are still living at the parental home at time of interview.

The 'missing data' category of the covariate religious denomination (kerk) is replaced by NA to exclude the respondents from the assessment of effects of religion:

```
OGd$kerk[OGd$kerk=="missing data"] <- NA
OGd$kerk <- factor(OGd$kerk,exclude="missing data")
```

In the subsample, one person did not report religious denomination (ID 289). The following expression converts the data in wide format to data in long format.

```
Dlong <- Biograph.long(OGd)
```

The Dlong object has two components: Dlong$Devent and Dlong$Depisode. The latter object is used in the survival package. It is renamed for convenience:

```
Depisode <- Dlong$Depisode
```

The object Depisode carries two attributes: the parameters (attr(Depisode,"param")) and the date format (attr(Depisode, "format.date")). The format of the birth date is included in the param attribute. An additional variable is defined:

```
Depisode$one <- rep(1,nrow(Depisode))
```

The object Depisode contains information on 13 different transitions. The number of respondents included in the analysis is 494.

The function Biograph.mvna converts a *Biograph* object into an object that is accepted by the *mvna* package:

```
Dmvna <- Biograph.mvna (OG)
```

The function removes intrastate transitions, calls the Parameters function, creates data in a long format using the Biograph.long function and adjusts that data file to meet the *mvna* requirements. The *mvna* package requires a data set that includes the following variables: id, from, to, entry and exit. The variable names are not free. They must be id, from, to, entry and exit. The origin and destination are character variables.

The object Dmvna has three components: Dmvna$D, Dmvna$Dcov and Dmvna$cens. The first omits the covariates, the second includes the covariates and the third is the label used to indicate censoring.

The package *mvna* requires that absorbing states receive special attention (in this example, state K). In *mvna* entry into an absorbing state is treated as censoring. State K needs to be marked as an absorbing state, and *episodes censored in state K need to be removed from the data set*. If the package encounters a respondent who is censored in an absorbing state, the following error message is generated: "There is an undefined transition in the data set" and the computation stops. The following code is used to remove redundant records:

```
zz1 = attr(Dmvna$D,"param")
zz2 = attr(Dmvna$D,"format.date")
Dmvna$D <- subset (Dmvna$D,Dmvna$D$from!="K")
attr(Dmvna$D,"param") = zz1
attr (Dmvna$D,'format.date') <- zz2
```

The subset function removes attributes of the object. Hence the attributes need to be added later.

The function Biograph.mstate converts a *Biograph* object into an object that is accepted by the *mstate* package:

```
Dmstate <- Biograph.mstate (OG)
```

The function removes intrastate transitions, calls the Parameters function, creates data in a long format using the Biograph.long function and adjusts that data file to meet the *mstate* requirements. The object Dmstate carries three attributes: the parameters (attr(Dmstate, "param")), the data format used in the data (attr(Dmstate, "format.date")) and the transition matrix (attr(Dmstate, "trans")), which is the same as attr (Dmstate,"param")$tmat. The dates of transitions are expressed in CMC. Ages at transitions are included too.

8.4.2 Cumulative Transition Rates

The *mvna* package implements a non-parametric estimation of the cumulative transition rates (Nelson-Aalen estimates). The following code computes the cumulative transition hazards for each possible transition in the multistate model:

8.4 Transition Rate Models

```
na <- mvna(data=Dmvna$D,
        state.names=c("H","A","C","M","K"),
        tra=attr(Dmvna$D,"param")$trans_possible,
        cens.name=Dmvna$cens)
```

The object na has a large number of components. For each of the 13 transitions, it gives the cumulative hazard and two variance estimators: the Aalen estimator and the Greenwood estimator. The cumulative hazards are computed at the ages at which transitions occur. The cumulative transition rates from H to A produced by *mvna* are in object na$'H A'$na.

Consider the first respondent (ID = 2). She left the parental home at exact age 28 to live independently. That age is shown in Dmvna$D and can be derived from the original data OGd by the function cmc_as_age(OGd$Tr1[1],OGd$born[1],"cmc"). It is the 693rd element of na$time (obtained by which(na$time==28.00)). She was the only person in the sample who left home at exact age 28.00. At age 28, 13 persons are at risk of leaving home (na$n.risk[693,1]). It is the number of persons living at home just before the event (see the definition of n.risk in the documentation of the *mvna* function and the theory in Beyersmann et al. 2012, p. 57 and Aalen et al. 2008, p. 71). The rate of transition from state H to state A at age 28.00 is $1/13 = 0.07692$. The cumulative transition rate at age 28 includes the transition rate at exact age 28. The cumulative transition rate at that age is 0.9865. The cumulative transition rate from H to A at the age at which the previous HA transition occurred (age 26.499) is 0.9096. The difference is 0.0769. The cumulative HA transition rates by age are displayed by the expression

```
k<- cbind(time=na$'H A'$time,na=na$'H A'$na)
```

The risk set and numbers of transitions by age are displayed by the expression:

```
z<- cbind(Age=na$time,
        RiskSet=na$n.risk[,1],
        Trans=aperm(na$n.event,c(3,1,2))[,1,],
        Cens=na$n.cens)
```

Note that in na$n.risk and na$n.cens, age is the first dimension, whereas in na$n.event age is the third dimension. That explains the aperm function in the expression. Note that the object k has 900 rows, whereas z has 938 rows. In both objects, row 693 shows data for age 28.00. For that age the two objects may be combined to produce an object that contains all the relevant information:

```
x<- cbind (z[690:695,],k[690:695,])
```

Table 8.12 shows, for selected ages around age 28.00, the risk set, the number of transitions and the cumulative hazard rate. At age 28.00, one female leaves the

Table 8.12 Risk set and transition count for estimating (cumulative) rate of leaving parental home to live independently at age 28. Data produced by *mvna*. OG

```
               Leave home    Censored
               to state      in state
Age     RiskSet 1 2 3 4 5    1 2 3 4 5            cumHazard
27.91530    14  0 0 0 0 0    0 0 0 0 0  27.91530  0.9096176
27.91781    14  0 0 0 0 0    1 0 0 0 0  27.91781  0.9096176
27.91803    13  0 0 0 0 0    0 0 0 0 0  27.91803  0.9096176
28.00000    13  0 1 0 0 0    0 1 0 0 0  28.00000  0.9865407
28.08219    12  0 0 0 0 0    0 0 0 0 0  28.08219  0.9865407
28.08470    12  0 0 0 0 0    0 0 0 0 0  28.08470  0.9865407
```

parental home, and one is interviewed and the observation censored. At time of survey, that woman lives independently.

Figure 8.9 shows the cumulative transition rates and their 95 % confidence intervals for the 13 transitions considered in this illustration. The figure is produced by the xyplot.mvna function, which uses the *lattice* package:

```
xyplot(na,tr.choice=c("H A","H C","H M",
          "H K","A C","A M","A K","C A",
          "C M","C K","M A","M C","M K"),
       aspect=1,
       strip=strip.custom(bg="white",
          factor.levels=c("HC","HA","HM",
          "HK","CA","CM","CK","AC","AM",
          "AK","AC","MA","MK"),
       par.strip.text=list(cex=0.9)),
       scales=list(alternating=1),
       xlab="Age in years",
       xlim=c(10,60),
       ylab="Nelson-Aalen estimates")
```

The Nelson-Aalen estimates of the cumulative transition rates, produced by *mvna*, may be compared with the cumulative transition rates produces by the *survival* and *mstate* packages. The Cox model in *survival* produces results that are considerably different. To obtain the cumulative hazard for each of the 13 transitions, the Cox model is estimated with the line numbers of transitions as stratification variables:

```
coxa <- coxph(Surv(Depisode$Tstopa,status)
              ~strata(trans),
              data=Depisode,method="breslow")
```

The cumulative transition rates are produced by the expression:

```
zh<- basehaz(coxa)
```

8.4 Transition Rate Models

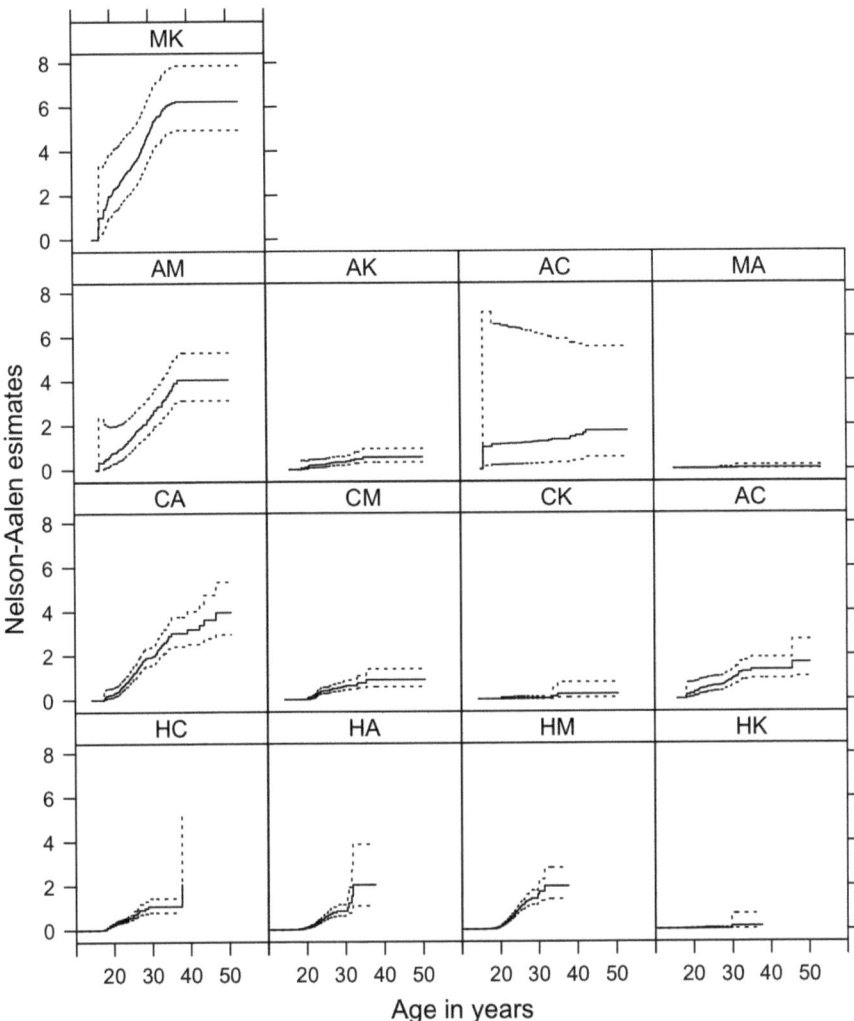

Fig. 8.9 Trellis plot of cumulative transition rates (Nelson-Aalen estimator), 13 transitions. OG

The object zh has three components: the cumulative hazard rate at each transition (zh$hazard), the time at each transition (zh$time) and the strata used (zh$strata). The cumulative transition rates from H to A produced by the Cox model are contained in the object:

```
zh1 <- zh[zh$strata=="trans=1",]
```

To illustrate the difference, consider the lowest age at HA transition. In the OG data, the minimum age at leaving home is 12.00 years, which is produced by:

```
min(Depisode$Tstopa[Depisode$trans==1])
```

The respondent leaves home to live independently. The age of 12.00 is probably misreported, but that is not a concern in this particular discussion. The information about the respondent who left home at that age, including her ID (4922), is:

```
aa<- min(Depisode$Tstopa[Depisode$trans==1])
Depisode[Depisode$Tstopa==aa,]
```

At age 12.00, the HA transition rate is 0.0020 in *mvna*. Since all respondents live at the parental home just before that age, the risk set is 500. The transition rate is $1/500 = 0.002$. To see all elements of the calculation, use:

```
cbind (z[1:10,],k[1:10,]).
```

In the stratified Cox model, the HA transition rate at age 12.00, produced by the function basehaz(coxb), is $1/216 = 0.0046$. The risk set consists of the 172 respondents who leave home to live independently and the 44 respondents who live at the parental home at time of survey. The transition of the latter category is coded as 1. The cumulative hazard for transition HA produced by mvna should be compared to the cumulative hazard produced by the Cox model with the transitions as factors rather than strata. Notice that the rates produced by the Cox model differ slightly from the empirical rates produced by *mvna*.

The *mstate* package uses the stratified Cox proportional hazard model to compute the empirical cumulative hazard by age for each of the 13 transitions. Age is used as duration variable, and 13 strata are distinguished, one stratum for each transition:

```
c1 <- coxph(Surv(Tstarta,Tstopa,status) ~
                        strata(trans),
                        data=Dmstate,
                        method="breslow")
fit1 <- msfit (c1,trans=attr(Dmstate,"trans"),
                        vartype="aalen")
```

The function msfit of *mstate* computes cumulative transition hazards for each of the possible transitions. It also estimates the variance by using the method proposed by Aalen. The object fit1 has three components: the cumulative hazard (fit1 $Haz), the variance of the cumulative hazard (fit1$varHaz) and the transition matrix with the line numbers of the transitions (fit1$trans). The cumulative hazard at exact age 12 is 0.002. The value is contained in the object fit1$Haz [1,]. The cumulative hazard produced by the basehaz function of the *survival* package gives the same result, if the object c1 is used:

8.4 Transition Rate Models

```
ch3 <- basehaz(c1)
ch3[ch3$strata=="trans=1",]
```

To select the cumulative hazards for the MK transition, use `fit1$Haz[fit1$Haz$trans==13,]`. The first column shows the age; the second, the cumulative hazard; and the third, the transition. The maximum of the cumulative hazard is `max(fit1$Haz[fit1$Haz$trans==13,2])`=6.257. Compare this with the maximum produced by the *mvna* package: `max(na$'MK'$na)`=6.242. The cumulative hazard produced by the `basehaz` function of the *survival* package gives the same result, if the object c1 is used:

```
ch3 <- basehaz(c1)
ch3[ch3$strata=="trans=13",]
```

The maximum of the cumulative hazard is `max(ch3[ch3$strata=="trans=13",1])`, which is 6.257.

To plot the 13 cumulative hazards estimated in the *mstate* package, use `plot(fit1)`.

Summary information on the strata is given by:

```
kk <- survfit(c1)
```

The following code displays more detailed output of the Cox model. It includes for each of the possible transitions the ages at transition, the risk set at each transition (number of respondents at risk just prior to a transition), the value of the survival function and the cumulative hazard.

```
zhh <- cbind(Time=kk$time,
             RiskSet=kk$n.risk,
             Trans=kk$n.event,
             Surv=kk$surv,
             CumHaz=ch3$hazard,
             Strata=ch3$strata)
```

The object zhh has all the necessary information to compute empirical transition rates. The object is comparable to the object Stable produced by the *Biograph* function `RateTable`.

8.4.3 Regression Models

In this section, two applications are presented. The first is the effect of reason for leaving home on the rate of leaving home. The second is the effect of birth cohort and religious denomination on the rate at which cohabitating and married couples have a first child. The substantive question is whether the concepts of cohabitation and marriage vary between cohorts and religious denominations.

Suppose we are interested in the effect of reason for leaving home on the rate of leaving home and on the shape of the age pattern of leaving home. The reasons for leaving home are independent living, cohabitation and marriage. Do young adults who leave home to live independently leave home earlier than those who leave for marriage or to cohabit? The model is essentially a competing risks model (Beyersmann et al. 2012). Six respondents have their first child while living at the parental home; they are excluded from the analysis.

```
H. <- subset (Depisode,Depisode$OR=="H" &
              Depisode$trans!=4)
```

The remaining 494 respondents are divided in three strata: those experiencing the HA transition, those experiencing the HC transition and those with the HM transition.

A Cox proportional hazards regression model of the *survival* package is applied to study the effect of the reason for leaving home on the rate of leaving home:

```
coxa<- coxph(Surv(H.$Tstopa,status)
             ~as.factor(trans),
             data=H.,
             method="breslow")
```

The transitions 1 (HA), 2 (HC) and 3 (HM) are specified as categorical variable. The first category is the reference category. Box 8.2 shows the results. The rate of leaving home for respondents who leave home to cohabit is 82 % of the rate of leaving home to live independently. The rate of leaving home for marriage is 14 % lower than the rate of leaving home to live independently.

Box 8.2: Effect Reason for Leaving Home on Rate of Leaving Parental Home. Cox Competing Risks Model. OG

```
Call:
coxph(formula = Surv(H.$Tstopa, status) ~ as.factor(trans),
    data = H., method = "breslow")

                   coef exp(coef) se(coef)     z    p
as.factor(trans)2 -0.194    0.824    0.124 -1.56 0.12
as.factor(trans)3 -0.148    0.863    0.109 -1.36 0.17

Likelihood ratio test=2.96  on 2 df, p=0.228  n= 494, number
of events= 450
```

8.4 Transition Rate Models

This model assumes that the age profile of leaving home (baseline hazard) is the same for the three reasons, implying that the effect of reason on the rate of leaving does not vary with age. The expression z<- basehaz(coxa) produces a table with the cumulative baseline hazard at ages at which transitions occur. The function plot(z$time,z$hazard,type="l") plots the baseline hazard. The assumption that the baseline hazard is the same for all three reasons, i.e. that the effects are proportional, may be tested graphically. The Schoenfeld residual plot is produced by the following code:

```
coxa.zph <- cox.zph(coxa,
            transform="identity",global=TRUE)
plot (coxa.zph[1])
```

The rate of leaving home for cohabitation or marriage is not proportional to the baseline hazard, which is the rate of leaving home to live independently (reference category). The effects of cohabitation (coxa.zph[1]) and marriage (coxa.zph[2]) increase with age, up to about age 25.

The following model yields separate cumulative hazard rates for each of the reasons for leaving home:

```
coxb<- coxph(Surv(H.$Tstopa,status)
          ~ strata(trans),
            data=H.,method="breslow")
```

The cumulative transition rates are produced by the expression:

```
zh<- basehaz(coxb)
```

Note that the rates are specified per year. If rates are expressed per month, the cumulative hazard is considerably lower.

The following code plots the baseline hazards with their 95 % confidence intervals:

```
zz <- survfit (coxb)
plot(zz,fun="cumhaz",
    xlim=c(15,30),
    main="Leaving parental home. OG.",
    xlab="Age",ylab="Cumulative hazard",
    col=c("red","blue","green"),
    conf=TRUE)
legend(15,5,legend=c("HA","HC","HM"),
        fill=c("red","blue","green"))
```

The plot is not shown. Persons who leave home to live independently leave at younger ages than those who leave home for another reason. The rate of leaving home to live independently is relatively constant, i.e. does not vary with age. Persons who leave home for cohabitation or marriage leave at higher ages, but, if the reason is marriage, they catch up with respondents who leave home to live alone.

To address the second question, I use *mstate*. Two transitions are of interest: the CK transition (transition number 10) and the MK transition (transition number 13). To facilitate model specifications, two expanded (transition-specific) covariates are created: birth cohort and religious denomination (kerk):

```
Dcov <- expand.covs(data=Dmstate,covs=c("cohort","kerk"))
```

Dcov is the expanded covariate data set. The expanded covariates are a combination of (1) the covariate name, (2) the level and (3) the transition number. If the use of the function expand.covs produces an error message, a likely cause is that the transition matrix has at least one non-missing diagonal element (check with attr(Dmstate,"trans")).

The effect of birth cohort and religion on the rate at which cohabiting and married couples have a first child is obtained by the model:

```
ck <- coxph(Surv(Tstarta,Tstopa,status) ~
+cohort1960..10+cohort1960..13
+kerkRoman.Catholic.10+kerkRoman.Catholic.13
+kerkProtestant.10+kerkProtestant.13
+kerkother.10+kerkother.13
+strata(trans),
data=Dcov,
method="breslow")
```

Notice that respondent with ID 558 ends cohabitation in CMC 1975 to live independently and has a first child in that same month. The coxh function gives a warning: 'Stop time must be>start time, NA created', which means that the case is omitted.

The model specification implies that the covariates cohort and kerk affect the CK and MK transitions but not the other transitions. The cumulative hazards associated with other transitions (1 to 9, 11 and 12) are not affected by the covariates. They differ between strata, however. It implies that for these transitions the cumulative hazards are the same for all respondents.

The rate at which cohabiting and married women enter motherhood depends on birth cohort and religious denomination. Box 8.3 shows the results of the Cox regression, stored in object ck. The reference category of the covariate 'cohort' is the cohort born before 1960, and the reference category for 'kerk' consists of persons without a religion. The rate at which married women have a first child is about the same in the two birth cohorts. In the younger cohort born in 1960 or later, it is 20 % lower than in the cohort born before 1960. The finding is consistent with a lower marital fertility and postponement in recent birth cohorts. Among cohabiting women, the rate is quite different: those born in 1960 or later have a rate that is 53 % higher than the rate for cohabiting women born before 1960. It shows that in the Netherlands, cohabitation has become more similar to marriage. Protestant women who cohabit become mothers at a rate that is 4 % higher than cohabiting women without a religion. Protestant women who are married become mothers at a rate that is 27 % higher than the rate for married women without a religion. Among Protestant women, the marriage institution remains an important factor in fertility.

Box 8.3: Effect of Birth Cohort and Religion on First Birth Rate for Cohabiting and Married Women. Cox Model, Using *mstate* Package. OG

```
Call:
coxph(formula = Surv(Tstarta, Tstopa, status) ~ +cohort1960..10 +
    cohort1960..13 + kerkRoman.Catholic.10 + kerkRoman.Catholic.13 +
    kerkProtestant.10 + kerkProtestant.13 + kerkother.10 + kerkother.13
    + strata(trans), data = Dcov, method = "breslow")

                         coef  exp(coef)  se(coef)      z        p
cohort1960..10         0.42438    1.529    0.595   0.71364   0.480
cohort1960..13        -0.22951    0.795    0.124  -1.85813   0.063
kerkRoman.Catholic.10  0.55840    1.748    0.535   1.04437   0.300
kerkRoman.Catholic.13  0.07330    1.076    0.139   0.52608   0.600
kerkProtestant.10      0.03682    1.038    0.782   0.04710   0.960
kerkProtestant.13      0.23948    1.271    0.160   1.49494   0.130
kerkother.10          -0.00769    0.992    1.071  -0.00718   0.990
kerkother.13          -0.06997    0.932    0.288  -0.24294   0.810

Likelihood ratio test=7.97  on 8 df, p=0.436  n= 4462,
number of events= 1142 (10 observations deleted due to missingness)
```

Transition rate models predict transition rates from information on transitions and covariates. In this section, the semi-parametric Cox model is applied, using functions of the *survival* package. Since our interest is in transition rates, the Cox model needs to be combined with the baseline hazard to produce age-specific transition rates. The Cox model and other transition rate models estimate effects of covariates on transition rates. In multistate modelling, several transitions are distinguished and covariates may affect transitions differently. The *mstate* package incorporates a method to flexibly specify transition rate models and to test different hypotheses about the impact of covariates on transitions. By way of example, the effects of birth cohort and religious denomination on birth rates of cohabiting and married women are estimated. The analysis sheds light on the evolving concept of marriage and the impact of religious denomination on the pace of change.

8.5 The Multistate Life Table

A multistate life table describes the biography of a cohort of people moving between states. Transitions are governed by transition rates estimated from data. Since the empirical rates are estimated from data on different people passing through different segments of life, the cohort is a *synthetic* cohort (for details, see Chap. 2). Three classes of indicators describe the cohort biography: counts, probabilities and durations (state occupation times; sojourn times). Two types of probabilities are distinguished: state probabilities and transition probabilities. The state probability at a given age is the probability of being in a given state at that age. The transition probability is the probability that an individual who is in a state (i) at a given reference age (x) is in another state (j) at a given later age (y). The state probability at a given age may be conditional on being present (alive) at a previous age and on the state occupied at that age. Probabilities and sojourn times may be conditional or unconditional.

The first step in computing the multistate life table consists of estimating age-specific (cumulative) transition rates. The subsample of 500 respondents in the Netherlands Family and Fertility Survey 1998 is used for the estimation. The function Cumrates is used to obtain Nelson-Aalen estimates and occurrence-exposure rates.

The following function produces Nelson-Aalen estimates of the cumulative hazard (irate = 1):

```
cumrates <- Cumrates(irate=1,Bdata=OGd)
```

where OGd is the data with intrastate transitions removed.

The function Cumrates uses the mvna function of the *mvna* package. Cumrates returns an object with seven components: the data (cumrates$D), the value of irate (cumrates$irate), the Nelson-Aalen estimates (cumrates$NeAa), the predicted transition rates and their 95 % confidence intervals (cumrates$predicted), the age-specific transition rates computed from the Nelson-Aalen estimates (cumrates$astr), the cumulative occurrence-exposure rates (cumrates$oeCum) (NULL in this case) and the occurrence-exposure rates (cumrates$oe) (NULL in this case). Since in this illustration, occurrence-exposure rates are not computed, their values are zero. For our analysis, we use the expected value (cumrates$NeAa[,,,1]) of the

8.5 The Multistate Life Table

cumulative hazards. The cumulative HA transition rates by age are cumrates $predicted$"H A".

Transition rates may also be computed as occurrence-exposure rates using:

```
cumrates.oe <- Cumrates(irate=2,Bdata=OGd)
```

The transition rates are stored in object cumrates.oe$oe. The function uses the Rates.ac function of *Biograph*. An alternative is to use the Rates.ac function directly:

```
rates <- Rates.ac(Stable=ratetable$Stable)
```

where ratetable is the object produced by the RateTable function.

The multistate survival function is one of the multistate life table indicators. It is shown in Fig. 8.10. The multistate survival function is a stack diagram. At a given age, the distance between two curves gives the probability that a member of the synthetic cohort is in a given state. The function MSLT.S computes the multistate survival function. The argument of the function is a set of transition rates, in this case Nelson-Aalen estimators:

```
s <- MSLT.S (cumrates$astr[,,,1])
```

Notice that the arguments are transition rates and not cumulative transition rates.

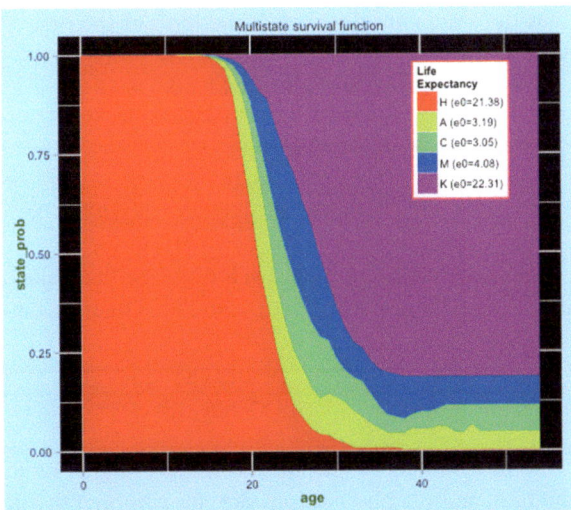

Fig. 8.10 Multistate survival function: state occupation probabilities by age. OG

The figure also shows the expected sojourn time in each state. The expected sojourn time in a state is the area between two curves in the multistate survival function. The function MSLT.e computes the expected sojourn times in the different states. The arguments are the multistate survival function and the radix. The radix gives the number of cohort members by state occupied at the initial age. Since at birth, all persons live at the parental home, the radix is:

```
radix <- c(10000,0,0,0,0)
```

The expected sojourn times are computed as follows:

```
e <- MSLT.e (s,radix)
```

The total time a newborn may expect to spend in each state is contained in the component e$e0. These figures may also be computed from the sojourn times by state and age interval: apply(e$L[,,1],2,sum). In this illustration, the total expected sojourn time is 54 years. That figure is a consequence of *truncating* observations at age 54 and omitting mortality. In the absence of mortality, every member of the synthetic cohort is followed for 54 years. The expected age at which a cohort member leaves the parental home is 21.4 years. The expected duration of independent living is 3.2 years, the expected number of years of cohabitation is 3.0 and the expected duration of marriage before marriage dissolution or birth of a child is 4.1 years. The durations in these states depend on the ages at which states are entered and the reasons for leaving. In this state space, cohabitation is ended because of marriage, separation (to live alone) and childbirth. In this example no transitions are considered after the birth of the first child. Hence the mean age at birth of the first child is $54 - 22.3 = 31.7$ years.

The following code draws Fig. 8.10:

```
z<- plot (x=s$S,e$e0,
         title="Multistate survival function",
         area=TRUE,order=c("H","A","C","M","K"))
```

In the sample the mean age at birth of the first child, irrespective or marital status and living arrangement, is 26.3 years. That figure is obtained by the following code:

```
z<- TransitionAB (OGd,"*K")
mean(z$age,na.rm=TRUE)
```

In the synthetic cohort, the mean age is higher because (1) some women remain childless and (2) observations are not censored at survey date but continue until cohort members reach age 54. The mean age at censoring (survey date) is 36 years: mean(AgeTrans(OGd)$agecens) or:

8.5 The Multistate Life Table

```
agetrans <- AgeTrans(OGd)
mean (agetrans$agecens)
```

Transition probabilities are informative life table indicators. Transition probabilities are computed for a reference period, usually 1 or 10 years. The period may also be variable, e.g. remaining lifetime. The probability that a woman who cohabits at age 20 is married at age 21 is obtained by solving the matrix exponent. The function MatrixExp is part of the *msm* package. The transition probabilities are:

```
P <- MatrixExp(
     cumrates$astr[namage="20",,,1],
     t=1,n=5,k=3,method="series")
```

where cumrates$astr are age-specific transition rates, produced by the following code:

```
library(mvna)
zz<- Cumrates (irate=1,OGd)
rates.na <- zz$astr[,,,1]
```

The transition probabilities may also be computed from the age-specific occurrence-exposure rates:

```
rates <- Rates.ac(Stable=ratetable$Stable)
library(msm)
P <- MatrixExp(rates$M[namage="20",,],
               t=1,n=5,k=3,method="series")
```

Transition probabilities are shown in Table 8.13.

The probability that a woman, who cohabits on her 20th birthday, is married exactly 1 year later and has not yet a child at that age is a little less than 2 %. The probability that a 20-year-old married woman has a first child within a year is 25 %.

In comparing of Nelson-Aalen estimates of transition rates with occurrence-exposure rates, one should note differences in the treatment of age. Consider an example. One respondent left the parental home exactly at age 12. The Nelson-Aalen estimator of the cumulative transition rate exactly at age 12 is nonzero, because the transition is related to the population at risk just before age 12. If the difference between the cumulative transition rate at exact age x and the cumulative transition rate at exact age x−1 is computed to determine the transition rate at age x−1, then the transition rate at age 11 is nonzero. It should be zero because the transition takes place at age 12. The occurrence-exposure rate at age 11 is zero. The difference is due to the definition of an age interval. In the first method, the lowest age is excluded and the highest age is included. In the second method, which is common in demography, the lowest age is included and the highest age is excluded.

Table 8.13 One-year probabilities of transition between marital status/living arrangement for females aged 20. Comparison of Nelson-Aalen estimator and occurrence-exposure rates. OG

a. Based on occurrence-exposure rates

```
             origin
destination    H       A       C       M     K
          H 0.7463  0.0000  0.0000  0.0000   0
          A 0.0851  0.8605  0.0697  0.0154   0
          C 0.0451  0.0825  0.8534  0.0008   0
          M 0.1016  0.0318  0.0227  0.7336   0
          K 0.0218  0.0252  0.0543  0.2502   1
```

b. Based on Nelson-Aalen estimator

```
             origin
destination    H       A       C       M     K
          H 0.7504  0.0000  0.0000  0.0000   0
          A 0.0819  0.8839  0.0763  0.0144   0
          C 0.0423  0.0749  0.8279  0.0006   0
          M 0.1031  0.0247  0.0233  0.7332   0
          K 0.0223  0.0164  0.0724  0.2518   1
```

Table 8.14 Ten-year probabilities of transition between marital status/living arrangement for females aged 20, based on Nelson-Aalen estimator combined with assumption of time-invariant rates. OG

```
                              origin
destination       H            A            C            M         K
          H 0.04119894  0.0000000   0.00000000  0.000000000   0
          A 0.09337932  0.1673202   0.08049936  0.010627939   0
          C 0.11139482  0.1869962   0.14072561  0.008747751   0
          M 0.15906774  0.1699861   0.15203619  0.060643236   0
          K 0.59495918  0.4756975   0.62673884  0.919981075   1
```

The 10-year transition probabilities based on the Nelson-Aalen estimators, for persons aged 20, can be obtained with the following code:

```
P <- MatrixExp(cumrates$NeAa[namage="30",,,1]-
               cumrates$NeAa[namage="20",,,1],
               t=1,n=5,k=3,method="series")
```

The function MatrixExp, which is from the *msm* package, computes the exponent of a matrix. Table 8.14 shows the probabilities of being in a state at age 30 by state occupied at age 20. The cumulative transition rates are Nelson-Aalen estimators. The probability that a childless and cohabiting woman aged 20 has at least one child at age 30 is 63 %. The percentage is considerably higher if the woman is married at age 20 (92 %). To obtain the probability that she will ever have a child (at least one), age 30 should be replaced by age 54, which is the maximum age.

The probabilities differ slightly when cumulative occurrence-exposure rates are used (rate = 2). One could easily introduce covariates to determine the probabilities

8.5 The Multistate Life Table

for women with given attributes. For example, the probability that a woman of age 20, born before 1960, Protestant, married and childless has at least one child at age 30 is 95.5 % if the Nelson-Aalen estimator is applied and 95.8 % if the probability is derived from the occurrence-exposure rates. They are obtained using the following code:

```
OGdd <- OGd[OGd$cohort=="<1960"&
OGd$kerk=="Protestant",]
OGdd <- OGdd[!is.na(OGdd$ID),]
zz<- Cumrates (irate=1,OGdd)
Pna10 <- MatrixExp(zz$NeAa[namage="30",,,1]-
              zz$NeAa[namage="20",,,1],
              t=1,n=5,k=3,method="series")
oe <- Cumrates (irate=2,OGdd)
Poe10 <- MatrixExp(oe$oeCum[namage="30",,]-
              oe$oeCum[namage="20",,],
              t=1,n=5,k=3,method="series")
```

An alternative method for estimating x-year transition probabilities is to use the `probtrans` function of the *mstate* package. Consider the Cox model that determines the effect of birth cohort and religion on the rate at which cohabiting and married couples have a first child. It is given in the previous section. The cumulative transition rates for each of the possible transitions are computed by the msfit function of the *mstate* package. We fit a different cumulative hazard for each possible transition and assume that the population is homogeneous, i.e. no covariates are considered. The Cox model is:

```
Dmstate <- Biograph.mstate (OGd)
c1 <- coxph(Surv(Tstarta,Tstopa,status) ~
                  strata(trans),
                  data=Dmstate,
                  method="breslow")
```

The cumulative hazard rates are produced by the msfit function:

```
fit1 <- msfit (c1,
           trans=attr(Dmstate,"param")$tmat,
           vartype="aalen")
```

The following code predicts the state probabilities:

```
Prob0 <- probtrans(fit1,direction="forward",predt=20)
```

The prediction starts at age 20 (`predt=20`) and yields state probabilities for successive ages at which transitions occur (direction forward). For example, the probability that a childless woman of age 20 who cohabits has at least one child at age 30 is 64 %. The probability that a married childless woman of age 20 has at least one child at age 30 is 92 %. A woman who lives at the parental home at age 20 has a probability of 62 %, and a woman who lives alone has a probability of 54 %. These probabilities are comparable to those given in Table 8.14. The probabilities are produced by the following code:

```
for (i in 1:5)
{ z<- cbind(Age=Prob0[[i]]$time,
             ProbK = Prob0[[i]]$pstate5)[121,]
  print (c(i,z)) }
```

The probabilities associated with age 30 are in the 120th line of Prob0[[1]] which shows the time at which a transition occurs and the probability that a 20-year-old woman in state i has at least one child at that age, i.e. is in state 5 (pstate5).

Consider the effect of birth cohort and religion on the probability that a woman of age 20 has at least one child at age 30. Since we are not interested in effects on other transitions, the covariates are defined for transition 10 (CK) and 13 (MK) only. Consider a woman born before 1960, with a religion other than Roman Catholic or Protestant. The relevant characteristics are defined in the newdata data frame:

```
newdat <- data.frame(trans=1:13,
    cohort1960..10=c(0,0,0,0,0,0,0,0,0,0,0,0,0),
    kerkRoman.Catholic.10=c(0,0,0,0,0,0,0,0,0,0,0,0,0),
    kerkProtestant.10=c(0,0,0,0,0,0,0,0,0,0,0,0,0),
    kerkother.10=     c(0,0,0,0,0,0,0,0,0,1,0,0,0),
    cohort1960..13=c(0,0,0,0,0,0,0,0,0,0,0,0,0),
    kerkRoman.Catholic.13=c(0,0,0,0,0,0,0,0,0,0,0,0,0),
    kerkProtestant.13=c(0,0,0,0,0,0,0,0,0,0,0,0,0),
    kerkother.13=     c(0,0,0,0,0,0,0,0,0,1,0,0,0),
    strata=1:13)
attr(Dcov,"param") <- Parameters (OGd)
msck <-msfit(ck,newdata=newdat,
             trans=attr(Dcov,"param")$tmat)
```

where ck was estimated using *mstate* (Sect. 8.4.3). The following code predicts the state probabilities:

```
probck <- probtrans(msck,direction="forward",predt=20)
```

The probability that a cohabiting woman of age 20, who is born before 1960 with a religion other than Roman Catholic or Protestant, has at least one child at age 30 is 62 %, with standard deviation of 6.95 % (line 120 of probck[[3]]). The probability is 93 % with a standard deviation of 2.65 % if she is married at age 20 (line 120 of probck[[4]]). The probability of having at least one child during a lifetime is 81.5 %, with a standard deviation of 4.52 %, if the woman cohabits at

8.5 The Multistate Life Table

Fig. 8.11 Multistate survival function: state occupation probabilities for women born before 1960 and with a religion other than Roman Catholic or Protestant. Produced by *mstate* package. OG

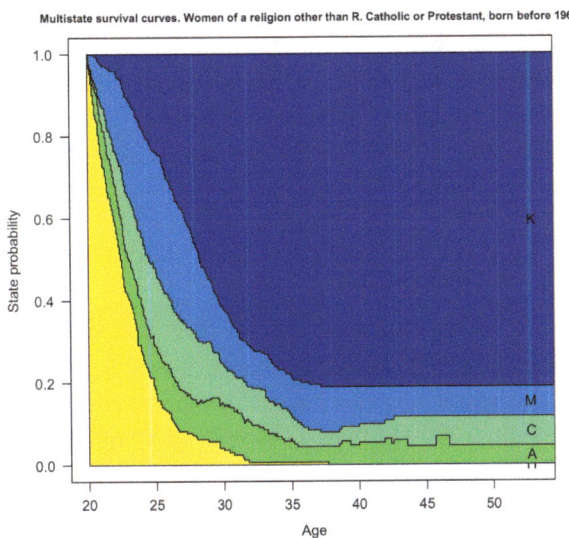

age 20 and 97 %, with standard deviation of 1.05 %, if she is married at age 20. If she lives at the parental home at age 20, the probability is also 81 %, but the standard deviation is larger (3.63 %).

The multistate survival function for a woman born before 1960 having a religion other than Roman Catholic or Protestant is shown in Fig. 8.11. The figure is produced by the plot.probtrans function, which plots an object of class 'probtrans'. The code is:

```
plot (probck,type="filled",ord=c(1:5),las=1,
    xlab="Age",
    ylab="State probability",
    main="Multistate survival curves. Women of a
    religion other than R. Catholic or Protestant, born
    before 1960",
    cex.main=0.8)
```

The multistate life table describes the life history that results from age-specific rates of transition. Transition rates are estimated from data, in this illustration a subsample of the Netherlands Family and Fertility Survey of 1998. In this section, two approaches to estimating transition rates are considered: the non-parametric method, which estimates transition rates any time a transition occurs (Nelson-Aalen estimator), and the method that defines age intervals and estimates transition rates for each interval separately (occurrence-exposure rate). The transition rates are very similar. Transition rates are input to the estimation of life history indicators. Three classes of indicators are considered: state occupation probabilities, transition probabilities and expected state occupation times. State occupation probabilities by age define the multistate survival function. They extend the conventional survival function, which gives probabilities of being alive at consecutive ages. The multistate survival function shows how state occupancies evolve with age. Transition probabilities may be viewed as state occupation probabilities that are conditional on the state occupancy at a reference age. Expected state occupation times summarise multistate survival functions in terms of expected years spent in each state.

8.6 Conclusion

In this chapter, *Biograph* was used to investigate the path women in the Netherlands follow between leaving parental home and motherhood. The chapter is based on a subsample of 500 women. The original sample was more than 5,000 women. The life course is described in terms of marital status and living arrangement. After leaving the parental home, a person may live alone (independently), cohabit (non-married cohabitation) or be married. In any of these states, a child may be born. Of the 500 respondents, one third does not have a child before the end of the observation period. That is considerably higher than one would expect from the official statistics on the proportion remaining childless. The reason is that respondents are relatively young.

About 90 % of the respondents with a child had their first child in marriage. Women who left the parental home to marry had their first child at age 24, and those who lived independently and cohabited before marriage had the child at 28 or later. The trajectory of living arrangements has a considerable influence on the age at birth of the first child. Pathways to motherhood differ greatly among women. *Biograph* identifies 48 different pathways in the subsample of 500 women, but the pathways are not evenly distributed among women. Two thirds of women in the subsample experienced one of 5 pathways.

The analysis reveals that women born in 1960 or later have a much larger variety of pathways than women born before 1960. Half of the women born before 1960 left the parental home for marriage (HMK), and they had a first child at a median age of 23.5 years. In the younger cohort, only 15 % experienced the HMK trajectory, and those who did had the first child at a median age of 26.4 years, mostly as a result of postponement of marriage. Women with an HACMK trajectory had the first child around age 29; the difference between the two cohorts is small, about half a year.

If respondents who were interviewed at relatively young age would experience the rates of transition that were observed among the older women in the sample, then about 18 % of the sample population would remain childless, and those who have a child would give birth on age 29.7, on average.

The meaning of marriage as an institution for raising children has eroded. The fertility rate of cohabiting women is tending to the fertility rate of married couples. The rate at which married women have a first child is about the same in the two birth cohorts. In the younger cohort born in 1960 or later, it is 20 % lower than in the

8.6 Conclusion

cohort born before 1960. The finding is consistent with a lower marital fertility and postponement in recent birth cohorts. Among cohabiting women, the rate is quite different: those born in 1960 or later have a rate that is 53 % higher than the rate for cohabiting women born before 1960. It shows that in the Netherlands, cohabitation has become more similar to marriage. Religious denomination influences the trend, however. For instance, among protestant women the meaning of marriage is much stronger than among women without a religion. Protestant women who cohabit become mothers at a rate that is 4 % higher than cohabiting women without a religion. Protestant women who are married become mothers at a rate that is 27 % higher than the rate for married women without a religion.

The findings illustrate the types of insight that can be obtained using *Biograph* and related packages in CRAN.

Chapter 9
Summary

As life unfolds people move between states and enter new stages of life. The path taken depends on personal characteristics, early life experiences, context and chance. The life course can be represented as a sequence of states and modelled as a multistate process, governed by transition rates. In this book, the continuous-time Markov process is used to model life histories. Transition rates may depend on covariates.

Biograph is designed to facilitate the study of the life course as a multistate process. The package serves three important purposes. The first is to assist the user who tries to comprehend life history data. The second is to document, as fully as possible, the computation of transition rates. The third is to facilitate the use of advanced statistical techniques for life history analysis.

Graphics and summary measures are useful means to characterise data. Life histories of individuals and sets of individuals can be displayed and patterns identified. Summary indicators of transitions, episodes and state sequences can be produced for the entire sample population or for a subset of people with similar characteristics. It should facilitate a comparison of subpopulations.

Observations on life histories are usually incomplete. Information on the entire life span is usually not available; information is limited to parts of the life course and relevant transitions may occur before observation starts or after observation ends. Transitions outside of the observation window are not recorded. For each individual under observation, *Biograph* identifies which segment of life is observed and when, i.e. in which calendar years, it is observed. For instance, information on persons in their thirties may be available for a few years only or for many years, enabling the study of cohort effects. The Lexis diagram is used to display segments in an age-time framework.

A particularly useful feature of *Biograph* is the information it provides on exposure time during periods of observation. In order to comprehend how transition rates are estimated from data and to determine the contribution of each individual observation to the transition rate, transitions during a period of observation should be related to exposure time during that same period. An individual is exposed to the risk of a transition if he occupies a state that may end in that transition. *Biograph* tracks individual transitions and episodes of state occupancy and exposure. That ability to track transitions and exposure time for individuals and user-defined groups of individuals is an important feature of the package. One could, for instance, identify which subjects are under observation at a given age or time and contribute to the likelihood function, which expresses the likelihood of the data given a probability model of the transition rate. One could identify the types of episodes (open or closed) at that time. The distinction between open and closed intervals is important in the maximum likelihood estimation of multistate models. *Biograph* also identifies common state sequences and how state sequences are affected by changes in the observation window.

Biograph facilitates the reconstruction of life histories from the empirical evidence in the sample population. The package uses the multistate life table (MSLT) method to produce synthetic biographies by combining information on different individuals. Since the observation usually records the experience of people of different ages during a relatively short period of time, 5 or 10 years say, information on different individuals should be combined to produce an entire life history. *Biograph* estimates transition rates for use as inputs to the multistate life table. Two estimation methods are considered in the multistate life table: the non-parametric method, which yields the Nelson-Aalen estimator, and the partly parametric method, which produces occurrence-exposure rate. The MSLT generates a number of useful measures: discrete-time transition probabilities, state probabilities, expected state occupancies (number of cohort members by age and state occupied at that age) and expected state occupation times (sojourn times, exposure times). The indicators are given by age and selected covariates. They may be conditioned on the state occupied at a reference age. The synthetic biographies produced by the MSLT are the basis for a range of life history indicators.

The package also facilitates the use of advanced statistical techniques for life history analysis. *Biograph* does not include advanced statistical methods but provides links to packages in R that implement advanced statistical methods. These packages require data in a particular long format that usually vary between packages. Users often spend much time to prepare data in the required format. *Biograph* reduces the burden on the user by providing functions that convert data to a desired format. *Biograph* includes conversion utilities for several packages: *survival*, *msm*, *mvna*, *etm*, *mstate*, *Epi* and *TraMineR*. Because of the adaptors it is sufficient to convert the data only once.

Biograph accepts data in a particular wide format. A *Biograph* object has that data structure. The preparation of the data in the right format and the creation of a *Biograph* object can be cumbersome. Five steps are required. First, the state space and the possible transitions are defined. Second, relevant covariates are selected. Third, the observation window is set for each subject. Fourth, the state sequence is determined and the dates at transition are recorded. In the fifth and final step, all data are stored in a data frame and three data attributes are attached to the data frame. A utility included in *Biograph* may be used for steps four and five.

9 Summary

In the book two data sets are used to illustrate the *Biograph* package. The first is a subsample of the German Life History Survey (GLHS). The subsample was used by Blossfeld and Rohwer (2002) to illustrate event history modelling. That data set is used in Chaps. 2, 3, 4, 5, 6 and 7. In Chap. 8, another data set is used: a subsample of the Netherlands Family and Fertility Survey 1998 (NLOG98). An additional six data sets are used to demonstrate the creation of a *Biograph* object. Two are very simple and hypothetical data sets to demonstrate the steps as clearly as possible. One data set consists of simulated life histories. The other data sets are real retrospective surveys and follow-up studies: the Survey of Health, Ageing and Retirement in Europe (SHARELIFE), conducted in 2010; the National Family Healthy Survey of India (2005–2006); and a subset of the European Group for Blood and Marrow Transplantation (EBMT). The subset was used by Putter and colleagues (see de Wreede et al. 2011) to illustrate the *mstate* package.

Annexes

Annex A: How to Create a *Biograph* Object

A.1 Introduction

The purpose of this annex is to show how to create a *Biograph* object. The R code is included in the online documentation of the *Biograph* package (Version 2). In this book, several data sets are used to illustrate the method. The preparation of a *Biograph* object starting from the published GLHS data is described in Chap. 3 and the preparation of a *Biograph* object starting from the public use file of the Netherlands Family and Fertility Survey 1989 (NLOG98) in Chap. 8. In this annex, the conversion of another six data sets is documented. Two are hypothetical data sets, the first carries information on three subjects and the second on 22 subjects. In the third example of how to prepare a *Biograph* object, data from the Survey of Health, Ageing and Retirement in Europe (SHARE) are used. The SHARE survey is modelled after the US Health and Retirement Survey (HRS). Data from the National Family Health Survey of India are used in the fourth example. The NFHS is one of the many Demographic and Health Surveys (DHS) organised in Third World countries and countries in transition. In the fifth example, medical data are used. They are included in the *mstate* package for multistate modelling in R, developed by Putter and colleagues at Leiden University Medical Centre. The data cover 2,279 leukaemia patients who had a bone marrow transplant. The final example consists of simulated life histories. A separate R programme is written for each data set. The source code is distributed with the *Biograph* package. The code is included in the documentation file (inst/doc) of the package source (extension .tar.gz).

The *Biograph* object carries information on (1) subjects, (2) transitions and (3) observation period. The subject data consist of dates of birth and covariates, which may include time-varying covariates. In the GLHS data, marital status is a time-varying attribute. The age at marriage is included in the data. Information on transitions includes state sequences and dates of transition or ages at transition. The state sequence is the sequence of states occupied by a subject during the period of observation. The dates or ages are ordered chronologically, with the date or age at the first transition displayed first, followed by the date or age at the second transition, etc.

A *Biograph* object is created in five steps. The first is the specification of the state space and the transitions between states. Transitions that are not possible or not relevant for the study are excluded. The transitions that are included are feasible and relevant. The second step is the selection of covariates. The observation window for each subject in the observation is specified in the third step. It requires the dates at start and end of observation. In the fourth step, the state sequence is determined, and the dates or ages at transition are determined. In the fifth and final step, data are stored in a data frame and three data attributes are attached. The first is the object produced by the `Parameters` function of the *Biograph* package. The object includes the state space. The second indicates how dates at transition are represented (e.g. calendar time, CMC or age). The third indicates how dates of birth are represented.

A.2 Hypothetical Data A

Consider three individuals, one male and two females. Two have medium levels of education and one completed higher education. The three individuals are born in 1986. The first person is born on 5 April 1986, the second on 8 August 1986 and the third on 28 November 1986. Assume that during an interview on 9 May 2012, life history data were collected on living arrangements. Consider four living arrangements: living at the parental home (H), living alone (A), cohabiting (C) and married (M). The set of possible living arrangements constitutes the state space, which is denoted as {H, A, C, M}. The first person starts living independently on 20 August 2004 at the age of 18. It is her first transition, i.e. she leaves the parental home to live independently. She starts cohabitation on 1 December 2011 and is still cohabiting at the time of interview. The second person starts living independently in September 2011. The exact date is not known. He is still living independently at survey date. The third person starts living independently on 10 August 2006 and marries on 16 March 2012. If the month of transition is known, but not the date, it is assumed that the transition takes place on the 15th of that month. The information on the transitions is shown in Table A.1. A row carries information on an individual. A column has the date of entry in a given state.

The covariates are sex and level of education. The observation period differs between individuals. Observation starts at birth and ends at interview. The data are shown in Table A.2

The first column is the line number. The second column is the subject's identification number (ID). The third and fourth columns delineate the observation window. The dates are objects of class 'Date', which enables arithmetic and logical

Table A.1 Transition dates for three hypothetical individuals

```
            A          C          M
1  2004-08-20  2011-12-1       <NA>
2  2011-09-15       <NA>       <NA>
3  2006-08-10       <NA>  2012-03-16
```

Table A.2 Data on three hypothetical individuals

```
   ID       start         end  sex    educ
1   1  1986-04-05  2019-05-09    F    High
2   2  1986-08-08  2019-05-09    M  Medium
3   3  1986-11-28  2019-05-09    F  Medium
```

operations on the dates. The fifth and sixth columns show the covariates. The covariates are factors.

The code to produce a *Biograph* object is shown in create.Simple1a.r and create.Simple1b.r. The first step in the creation of a *Biograph* object is the specification of the state space. The state space is {H, A, C, M}. The second step is the selection of covariates. They are sex and education. The third step is the specification of the observation period for each individual in the study. They are shown in Table A.2. In the fourth step, state sequences and the transition dates are determined. To determine the state sequence, the transition dates need to be ordered chronologically, i.e. the event that occurred first is listed first. The subsequent event is listed second, etc. The second event is not the same for everyone. In the data above, it is cohabitation for the first person and marriage for the third person. The function Sequences.ind.0 orders the dates chronologically and derives state sequences. The raw transition dates (shown above) are stored in a data frame with the dates as character variables. The function as.Date of base R is used to convert the character dates in Julian dates. The function is evoked using the code:

```
f <- Sequences.ind.0(d=dd,namstates=namstates,absorb=NULL)
```

where dd is the data frame with the transition dates and namstates is the state space. The function produces an object with three components, but two are of particular importance. They are the state sequence (f$path) and the sorted transition dates (f$d). Table A.3 shows the object produced by the function Sequences.ind.0.

The Julian dates are converted back to calendar dates (class 'Date') using the as.Date function. The results is a data frame, which in the code is called dates. The code is:

Table A.3 Object produced by the *Biograph* function Sequences.ind.0

```
$namstates
[1] "H" "A" "C" "M"

$d
     [,1]  [,2] [,3]
[1,] 12650 15309   NA
[2,] 15232    NA   NA
[3,] 13370 15415   NA

$path
[1] "HAC" "HA"  "HAM"
```

Table A.4 *Biograph* object: hypothetical data A

```
  ID       born      start        end sex educ path         Tr1        Tr2
1  1 1986-04-05 1986-04-05 2019-05-09   F High  HAC  2004-08-20 2011-12-01
2  2 1986-08-08 1986-08-08 2019-05-09   M Medium HA  2011-09-15       <NA>
3  3 1986-11-28 1986-11-28 2019-05-09   F Medium HAM 2006-08-10 2012-03-16
```

```
dates <- data.frame (f$d)
for (i in 1:3)
     {dates[,i] <- as.Date(dates[,i],origin="1970-01-01")}
path <- as.character(f$path)
```

The final step is to assemble the data in a data frame and to add the date format and the parameters as attributes. The following code produces the *Biograph* object (Table A.4):

```
bio   <- data.frame (
           ID=id,
           born=born,
           start=start,
           end=interview,
           sex=sex,educ=educ,
           path=as.character(path),
           dates[,1:(max(nchar(path))-1)]1)],
              stringsAsFactors=FALSE)
attr(bio,"format.date") <- "%Y-%m-%d"
attr(bio,"format.born") <- "%Y-%m-%d"
param <- Parameters (bio)
attr (bio,"param") <- Parameters (bio)
```

The data frame has different data types. The function str(bio) displays the data types (Table A.5):

Note that the path variable must be a character variable. It should not be a factor variable. The covariates are factor variables.

Table A.5 *Biograph* object: data types

```
'data.frame':     3 obs. of  9 variables:
 $ ID    : num  1 2 3
 $ born  : Date, format: "1986-04-05" "1986-08-08" "1986-11-28"
 $ start : Date, format: "1986-04-05" "1986-08-08" "1986-11-28"
 $ end   : Date, format: "2019-05-09" "2019-05-09" "2019-05-09"
 $ sex   : Factor w/ 2 levels "F","M": 1 2 1
 $ educ  : Factor w/ 2 levels "High","Medium": 1 2 2
 $ path  : chr  "HAC" "HA" "HAM"
 $ Tr1   : Date, format: "2004-08-20" "2011-09-15" "2006-08-10"
 $ Tr2   : Date, format: "2011-12-01" NA "2012-03-16"
 - attr(*, "format.date")= chr "%Y-%m-%d"
 - attr(*, "format.born")= chr "%Y-%m-%d"
 - attr(*, "param")=List of 18
  ..$ nsample        : int 3
  ..$ numstates      : int 4
  ..$ namstates      : chr [1:4(1d)] "H" "A" "C" "M"
  ..$ absorbstates   : chr [1:2(1d)] "C" "M"
  ..$ iagelow        : num 0
  ..$ iagehigh       : num 34
  ..$ namage         : int  0 1 2 3 4 5 6 7 8 9 ...
  ..$ nage           : num 35
  ..$ maxtrans       : num 2
  ..$ ntrans         : int 3
  ..$ trans_possible: logi [1:4, 1:4] FALSE FALSE FALSE FALSE TRUE FALSE
  .. ..- attr(*, "dimnames")=List of 2
  .. .. ..$ Origin     : chr [1:4(1d)] "H" "A" "C" "M"
  .. .. ..$ Destination: chr [1:4(1d)] "H" "A" "C" "M"
  ..$ tmat           : num [1:4, 1:4] NA NA NA NA 1 NA NA NA 2 ...
  .. ..- attr(*, "dimnames")=List of 2
  .. .. ..$ From: chr [1:4(1d)] "H" "A" "C" "M"
  .. .. ..$ To  : chr [1:4(1d)] "H" "A" "C" "M"
  ..$ transitions    :'data.frame':  3 obs. of  6 variables:
  .. ..$ Trans: Factor w/ 3 levels "1","2","3": 1 2 3
  .. ..$ OR   : Factor w/ 2 levels "1","2": 1 2 2
  .. ..$ DES  : Factor w/ 3 levels "2","3","4": 1 2 3
  .. ..$ ORN  : Factor w/ 2 levels "A","H": 2 1 1
  .. ..$ DESN : Factor w/ 3 levels "A","C","M": 1 2 3
  .. ..$ ODN  : chr "HA" "AC" "AM"
  ..$ nntrans        : num [1:4, 1:4] 0 0 0 0 3 0 0 0 0 1 ...
  .. ..- attr(*, "dimnames")=List of 2
  .. .. ..$ Origin     : chr [1:4(1d)] "H" "A" "C" "M"
  .. .. ..$ Destination: chr [1:4(1d)] "H" "A" "C" "M"
  ..$ locpat         : int 7
  ..$ ncovariates    : num 2
  ..$ covariates     : chr "sex" "educ"
  ..$ format.date    : chr "%Y-%m-%d"
  ..$ format.born    : chr "%Y-%m-%d"
```

The *Biograph* function Parameters can be invoked to check whether the *Biograph* object is correctly specified: Parameters(bio). The function produces an object that lists the states in the state space and identifies absorbing states. The latter are states that are entered but not left during the observation period. The Parameters function also shows the lowest age and the highest age in the observation period. It also shows the transition matrix, which consists of logical values: a 'TRUE' indicates the transitions that occur during the observation period, and a 'FALSE' identifies the transitions that do not occur during the observation period. It shows the line numbers of the transitions and the frequency of transitions

Table A.6 *Biograph* object with dates in CMC

	ID	born	start	end	sex	educ	idim	ns	path	Tr1	Tr2
1	1	1036	1036	1433	F	High	1	3	HAC	1256	1344
2	2	1040	1040	1433	M	Medium	1	2	HA	1341	NA
3	3	1043	1043	1433	F	Medium	1	3	HAM	1280	1347

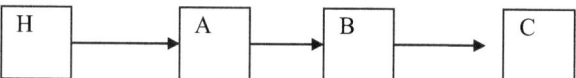

Fig. A.1 State space and transitions. Hypothetical case B

($nntrans). Finally, it lists the covariates and displays the format of dates of birth and dates at transition. In this case, the dates are of class 'Date', and a character string "%Y-%m-%d" gives the date format.

Dates are often expressed in CMC. The preparation of a *Biograph* object requires the same procedure. Let's convert the calendar dates to CMC, using the function Date_as_cmc of the *Biograph* package:

```
bio.cmc <- date.b (
    Bdata=bio,
    format.in="%Y-%m-%d",
    selectday=15,
    format.out="cmc",
    covs=NULL)
```

The *Biograph* object is shown in Table A.6.

A.3 Hypothetical Data B

Suppose we have information on 22 individuals. The state space consists of four fictitious states {H, A, B, C}. C is an absorbing state. Suppose that three transitions are possible: HA, AB and BC. Return transitions are not allowed (Fig. A.1).

Assume that the information is collected retrospectively as part of a cross-sectional survey. The date of interview is the end of the observation period. Since the data are collected retrospectively, no one drops out during observation. The respondents are born in 1991 and start in state H. The exact date of birth is unknown, but it is assumed that births are uniformly distributed throughout the year. The date of birth is obtained by adding a random number between 0 and 365 to 1 January 1991. For each individual, six dates are given: the date of birth, the date at entry into observation, the date of interview and the dates of transitions between the states. Of the 22 individuals, 10 do not experience a transition during the observation period, 4 experience one transition, 2 experience 2 transitions and 6 three.

Annexes

Respondent 1 is born on 31 July 1991 and enters observation on 2 January 2007. He experiences the first event on 11th February of that year, when he leaves H and enters A. On 23rd March, he experiences the second event to state B. On 5th May, he makes a transition to state C. He stays in that state until the end of observation on 25 May 2007. The data are shown in Table A.7.

The function Sequences.ind.0 orders the dates chronologically and derives the state sequence. The components f$d and f$path are included in the *Biograph object*. The following code produces the *Biograph* object:

```
RS <- data.frame (ID=id,
    born=birth,
    start=as.Date(entry,"%d/%m/%Y"),
    end=as.Date(interview,"%d/%m/%Y"),
    cov=cov,
    path=as.character(path),
    dates[,1:(maxns-1)],
    stringsAsFactors=FALSE)
attr(RS,"format.date") <- "%Y-%m-%d"
attr(RS,"format.born") <- "%Y-%m-%d"
attr(RS,"param") <- Parameters (RS)
```

The *Biograph* object is shown in Table A.8. The data types in the data frame are shown in Table A.9. The code to produce the *Biograph* object is shown in create.Simple2.r.

Table A.7 Hypothetical survey data: multiple transitions

	ID	Born	Start	Stop	A	B	C
1	1	31/07/1991	02/01/2007	25/05/2007	11/02/2007	23/03/2007	05/05/2007
2	2	31/12/1991	17/01/2007	17/05/2007	04/05/2007	NA	NA
3	3	21/04/1991	18/01/2007	10/05/2007	NA	NA	NA
4	4	11/08/1991	22/01/2007	13/05/2007	28/02/2007	10/04/2007	10/05/2007
5	5	17/07/1991	10/02/2007	23/05/2007	17/05/2007	NA	NA
6	6	28/06/1991	30/01/2007	15/05/2007	12/02/2007	05/03/2007	17/04/2007
7	7	01/09/1991	04/04/2007	06/05/2007	NA	NA	NA
8	8	06/11/1991	29/04/2007	27/05/2007	NA	NA	NA
9	9	24/01/1991	18/05/2007	29/05/2007	NA	NA	NA
10	10	25/03/1991	20/05/2007	31/05/2007	NA	NA	NA
11	11	29/04/1991	15/05/2007	18/05/2007	NA	NA	NA
12	12	14/11/1991	05/02/2007	19/05/2007	25/02/2007	01/04/2007	02/05/2007
13	13	07/01/1991	05/02/2007	10/05/2007	18/04/2007	30/04/2007	NA
14	14	14/02/1991	06/02/2007	28/05/2007	18/05/2007	20/05/2007	NA
15	15	27/04/1991	26/02/2007	22/05/2007	NA	NA	NA
16	16	08/08/1991	10/03/2007	25/05/2007	NA	NA	NA
17	17	04/02/1991	11/03/2007	12/05/2007	08/05/2007	NA	NA
18	18	05/11/1991	28/03/2007	29/05/2007	NA	NA	NA
19	19	09/04/1991	15/03/2007	10/05/2007	23/03/2007	08/04/2007	20/04/2007
20	20	24/12/1991	13/04/2007	20/05/2007	NA	NA	NA
21	21	16/04/1991	04/04/2007	11/05/2007	09/05/2007	NA	NA
22	22	31/03/1991	25/04/2007	31/05/2007	16/05/2007	20/05/2007	26/05/2007

Table A.8 *Biograph* object: hypothetical data B

```
   ID       born      start        end cov path      Tr1        Tr2        Tr3
1   1 1991-05-14 2007-01-02 2007-05-25   X HABC 2007-02-11 2007-03-23 2007-05-05
2   2 1991-05-22 2007-01-17 2007-05-17   X   HA 2007-05-04       <NA>       <NA>
3   3 1991-12-27 2007-01-18 2007-05-10   X    H       <NA>       <NA>       <NA>
4   4 1991-01-01 2007-01-22 2007-05-13   X HABC 2007-02-28 2007-04-10 2007-05-10
5   5 1991-02-02 2007-02-10 2007-05-23   X   HA 2007-05-17       <NA>       <NA>
6   6 1991-06-08 2007-01-30 2007-05-15   X HABC 2007-02-12 2007-03-05 2007-04-17
7   7 1991-06-23 2007-04-04 2007-05-06   X    H       <NA>       <NA>       <NA>
8   8 1991-09-14 2007-04-29 2007-05-27   X    H       <NA>       <NA>       <NA>
9   9 1991-10-06 2007-05-18 2007-05-29   X    H       <NA>       <NA>       <NA>
10 10 1991-03-10 2007-05-20 2007-05-31   X    H       <NA>       <NA>       <NA>
11 11 1991-06-24 2007-05-15 2007-05-18   X    H       <NA>       <NA>       <NA>
12 12 1991-02-07 2007-02-05 2007-05-19   X HABC 2007-02-25 2007-04-01 2007-05-02
13 13 1991-06-01 2007-02-05 2007-05-10   X  HAB 2007-04-18 2007-04-30       <NA>
14 14 1991-06-14 2007-02-06 2007-05-28   X  HAB 2007-05-18 2007-05-20       <NA>
15 15 1991-10-07 2007-02-26 2007-05-22   X    H       <NA>       <NA>       <NA>
16 16 1991-04-07 2007-03-10 2007-05-25   X    H       <NA>       <NA>       <NA>
17 17 1991-10-21 2007-03-11 2007-05-12   X   HA 2007-05-08       <NA>       <NA>
18 18 1991-05-07 2007-03-28 2007-05-29   X    H       <NA>       <NA>       <NA>
19 19 1991-07-20 2007-03-15 2007-05-10   X HABC 2007-03-23 2007-04-08 2007-04-20
20 20 1991-09-05 2007-04-13 2007-05-20   X    H       <NA>       <NA>       <NA>
21 21 1991-09-15 2007-04-04 2007-05-11   X   HA 2007-05-09       <NA>       <NA>
22 22 1991-07-07 2007-04-25 2007-05-31   X HABC 2007-05-16 2007-05-20 2007-05-26
```

A.4 Survey of Health, Ageing and Retirement in Europe (SHARE)

The Survey of Health, Ageing and Retirement in Europe (SHARE) (http://www.share-project.org/) is a multidisciplinary and cross-national panel database of individual data on health, socio-economic status and social and family networks of more than 55,000 individuals aged 50 or over from 20 European countries. SHARE is harmonised with the US Health and Retirement Study (HRS) and the English Longitudinal Study of Ageing (ELSA). The SHARE baseline study (wave 1) was carried out in 2004. The third wave of data collection for SHARE (2008–2009) focused on people's life histories from birth to survey date. The survey is referred to as SHARELIFE. Almost 30,000 men and women across 13 European countries took part in this round of the survey. The respondents are representative for the European population aged 50 and over in Scandinavia (Denmark and Sweden), Central Europe (Austria, France, Germany, Switzerland, Belgium and the Netherlands) and the Mediterranean (Spain, Italy and Greece), as well as two transition countries (the Czech Republic and Poland). The SHARELIFE questionnaire covers different domains of life, ranging from partners and children over housing and work history to health and health care. The SHARELIFE questionnaire has several modules. The data from each module are stored in a different data file. The following modules and data files are distinguished:

- ac   Accommodation section
- cs   Childhood section
- dq   Disability
- fs   Financial history
- gl   General life questions
- gs   Grip strength

Table A.9 *Biograph* object: data types

```
'data.frame':    22 obs. of  9 variables:
 $ ID   : int  1 2 3 4 5 6 7 8 9 10 ...
 $ born : Date, format: "1991-07-06" "1991-10-03" "1991-12-05" ...
 $ start: Date, format: "2007-01-02" "2007-01-17" "2007-01-18" ...
 $ end  : Date, format: "2007-05-25" "2007-05-17" "2007-05-10" ...
 $ cov  : chr  "X" "X" "X" "X" ...
 $ path : chr  "HABC" "HA" "H" "HABC" ...
 $ Tr1  : Date, format: "2007-02-11" "2007-05-04" NA ...
 $ Tr2  : Date, format: "2007-03-23" NA NA ...
 $ Tr3  : Date, format: "2007-05-05" NA NA ...
 - attr(*, "format.date")= chr "%Y-%m-%d"
 - attr(*, "format.born")= chr "%Y-%m-%d"
 - attr(*, "param")=List of 19
  ..$ nsample        : int 22
  ..$ numstates      : int 4
  ..$ namstates      : chr [1:4(1d)] "H" "A" "B" "C"
  ..$ absorbstates   : chr "C"
  ..$ iagelow        : num 15
  ..$ iagehigh       : num 17
  ..$ namage         : int  15 16 17
  ..$ nage           : num 3
  ..$ maxtrans       : num 3
  ..$ ntrans         : int 3
  ..$ trans_possible: logi [1:4, 1:4] FALSE FALSE FALSE FALSE TRUE FALSE ...
  .. ..- attr(*, "dimnames")=List of 2
  .. .. ..$ Origin     : chr [1:4(1d)] "H" "A" "B" "C"
  .. .. ..$ Destination: chr [1:4(1d)] "H" "A" "B" "C"
  ..$ tmat           : num [1:4, 1:4] NA NA NA NA 1 NA NA NA 2 ...
  .. ..- attr(*, "dimnames")=List of 2
  .. .. ..$ From: chr [1:4(1d)] "H" "A" "B" "C"
  .. .. ..$ To  : chr [1:4(1d)] "H" "A" "B" "C"
  ..$ transitions    :'data.frame':   3 obs. of  6 variables:
  .. ..$ Trans: Factor w/ 3 levels "1","2","3": 1 2 3
  .. ..$ OR   : Factor w/ 3 levels "1","2","3": 1 2 3
  .. ..$ DES  : Factor w/ 3 levels "2","3","4": 1 2 3
  .. ..$ ORN  : Factor w/ 3 levels "A","B","H": 3 1 2
  .. ..$ DESN : Factor w/ 3 levels "A","B","C": 1 2 3
  .. ..$ ODN  : chr  "HA" "AB" "BC"
  ..$ nntrans        : num [1:4, 1:4] 0 0 0 0 12 0 0 0 8 ...
  .. ..- attr(*, "dimnames")=List of 2
  .. .. ..$ Origin     : chr [1:4(1d)] "H" "A" "B" "C"
  .. .. ..$ Destination: chr [1:4(1d)] "H" "A" "B" "C"
  ..$ locpat         : int 6
  ..$ ncovariates    : num 1
  ..$ covariates     : chr "cov"
  ..$ format.date    : chr "%Y-%m-%d"
  ..$ format.born    : chr "%Y-%m-%d"
```

hc	Childhood health care
hs	Childhood health section
iv	Interviewer
rc	Retrospective children
re	Work history
rp	Partner section
st	Demographics
wq	Work quality
xt	End of life interview

The data are available for download after registration. Data are available as SPSS and STATA files.

For the illustration of *Biograph*, I selected data on partnerships and living arrangement and downloaded the STATA files. The code to prepare the *Biograph* object is shown in `create.SHARElife.r`. The code to read the downloaded data, with the STATA files in the current directory, is:

```
d.st <- data.frame(read.dta ("sharew3_rel1_st.dta",
       convert.dates=TRUE,convert.underscore=TRUE))
d.rp <- data.frame(read.dta ("sharew3_rel1_rp.dta",
       convert.dates=TRUE,convert.underscore=TRUE))
d.ac <- data.frame(read.dta ("sharew3_rel1_ac.dta",
       convert.dates=TRUE,convert.underscore=TRUE))
d.re <- data.frame(read.dta (" / sharew3_rel1_re.dta",
       convert.dates=TRUE,convert.underscore=TRUE))
d.rc <- data.frame(read.dta ("sharew3_rel1_rc.dta",
       convert.dates=TRUE,convert.underscore=TRUE))
```

Consider the following state space:

- Living at parental home (H)
- Living alone (independently) (A)
- Cohabiting (C)
- Married (M)

In the SHARELIFE data file, the following transitions and their dates are relevant:

(a) Year in which separate household was established, i.e. first household after leaving parental home (d.ac$sl.ac003)
(b) Date of marriage (first to 6th marriage) (d.rp$sl.rp008.k), with k = 1 to 6
(c) Year started living with a partner who was later married (first to 6th cohabitation) (d.rp$sl.rp004b.k, with k = 1 to 6)
(d) Year stopped living with partner (first to 6th cohabitation) (d.rp$sl.rp012.k)
(e) Year of divorce (first to 4th divorce) (d.rp$sl.rp014.k)
(f) Year started living with a partner (not related to marriage) (d.rp$sl.rp003.k, with k = 11 to 18)

Five covariates are considered:

- Country: country of residence at survey date
- Sex
- Education: year in which full-time education is ended
- Year in which respondent starts first job
- Birth cohort: four birth cohorts, <1930, 1930–1939, 1940–1949, 1950+

The variables that are extracted from the raw data are identification number, date of birth, date of interview, dates of transitions and selected covariates. The variable name is the name in the STATA file. The variables are as follows.

Annexes

Dates

Variable name	Meaning
d.st$mergeid	Identification number
d.st$sl.st007	Year of birth
d.st$sl.st006	Month of birth
d.ac$sl.ac003.	Year of leaving parental home
d.rp$sl.rp008.1	Year of first marriage
d.rp$sl.rp008.k	Year of k-th marriage (k = 1 to 6)
d.rp$sl.rp013.k	Divorce (k = 1 to 4) (yes/no)
d.rp$sl.rp014.k	Year of k-th divorce (k = 1 to 4)
d.rp$sl.rp004b.k	Year in which k-th cohabitation before a marriage started (k = 1 to 6)
d.rp$sl.rp012.k	Year in which k-th cohabitation ended (k = 1 to 4)
d.rp$sl.rp003.n	Year in which cohabitation NOT related to marriage started (n = 11 to 18)
d.rp$sl.rp012.n	Year in which cohabitation NOT related to marriage ended

Covariates:

Variable name	Meaning
d.st$country	Country
d.st$sl.st011.	Sex
d.re$sl.re002.	Year in which full-time education is finished
d.rc$sl.rc023.	Number of children at survey date
d.re$sl.re011.1	Year of entry in labour market

First, a data frame of transition dates is constructed. The dates of transitions are taken from the SHARELIFE data files. A new transition label is added to indicate the destination state. Leaving the parental home and the dissolution of marriage or cohabitation are assumed to be followed by independent living (living alone), unless cohabitation or marriage starts in the same month. Table A.10 shows the years at transition for a selected number of respondents. The person identification number is shown in the column, and the destination state is shown in the row.

The first respondent, who is the seventh respondent in the data file and has identification number AT-010768-01, married in 1960 and started a separate household in 1962. The marriage was dissolved (divorce) in 1973. The person lived alone after the divorce until the start of a cohabitation in 1977 (unrelated to marriage). That cohabitation ended in 1979 and was followed by a new cohabitation (related to marriage) in the same year. The respondent married for the second time in 1981.

Table A.10 Changes in living arrangements. SHARELIFE. A selection of respondents

	AT-010768-01	AT-010904-02	AT-015615-01	AT-020895-01	AT-024225-01
A	NA	NA	NA	NA	NA
M	1960	1964	1965	1973	1983
M	1981	NA	NA	NA	NA
M	NA	NA	NA	NA	NA
M	NA	NA	NA	NA	NA
M	NA	NA	NA	NA	NA
M	NA	NA	NA	NA	NA
C	1962	1963	NA	1974	NA
C	1979	NA	NA	NA	NA
C	NA	NA	NA	NA	NA
C	NA	NA	NA	NA	NA
C	NA	NA	NA	NA	NA
C	NA	NA	NA	NA	NA
A	NA	NA	NA	NA	NA
A	NA	NA	NA	NA	NA
A	NA	NA	NA	NA	NA
A	NA	NA	NA	NA	NA
A	1973	NA	1976	NA	NA
A	NA	NA	NA	NA	NA
A	NA	NA	NA	NA	NA
A	NA	NA	NA	NA	NA
C	1977	NA	1980	1971	1969
C	NA	NA	1986	NA	NA
C	NA	NA	NA	NA	NA
C	NA	NA	NA	NA	NA
C	NA	NA	NA	NA	NA
C	NA	NA	NA	NA	NA
C	NA	NA	NA	NA	NA
A	1979	NA	1980	1971	1979
A	NA	NA	1987	NA	NA
A	NA	NA	NA	NA	NA
A	NA	NA	NA	NA	NA
A	NA	NA	NA	NA	NA
A	NA	NA	NA	NA	NA
A	NA	NA	NA	NA	NA
A	NA	NA	NA	NA	NA

The transitions have to be ordered chronologically and the state sequence (path) needs to be determined. The function Sequence.ind.0 is used. For the selected respondents, the result is shown in Table A.11.

These respondents experience the following state sequences: HMACACCAM, HACM, HMACACA, HCAMAC and HACAM.

These data, the covariates, the years of birth and the year of survey are stored in a *Biograph* data frame. Three attributes are added to the data frame: the format of the transition dates (year), the format of the dates of birth (year) and the object produced by the Parameters function. For one respondent, the date of birth is missing; he is removed from the data. Table A.12 shows a selection of rows of the SHARELIFE data in the *Biograph* format.

Table A.11 Sorted transition dates. Selection of respondents

	AT-010768-01	AT-010904-02	AT-015615-01	AT-020895-01	AT-024225-01
[1,]	1960	1963	1965	1971	1969
[2,]	1962	1964	1976	1971	1979
[3,]	1973	NA	1980	1973	1983
[4,]	1977	NA	1980	1974	NA
[5,]	1979	NA	1986	NA	NA
[6,]	1979	NA	1987	NA	NA
[7,]	1981	NA	NA	NA	NA
[8,]	NA	NA	NA	NA	NA
[9,]	NA	NA	NA	NA	NA
[10,]	NA	NA	NA	NA	NA

Table A.12 Biograph object (transposed) with SHARELIFE data. Selected respondents

ID	8	14	26	28
born	1942.333	1946.333	1952.417	1947.000
start	1942.333	1946.333	1952.417	1947.000
end	2008.5	2008.5	2008.5	2008.5
country	Austria	Austria	Austria	Austria
IDc	AT-010904-02	AT-015615-01	AT-020895-01	AT-024225-01
cohort	1940-49	1940-49	1950+	1940-49
sex	female	female	female	male
eduf	1959	1964	1971	1961
job1	1959	1964	1971	1961
children	1	2	3	2
path	HCM	HMACACA	HCAMC	HCAM
Tr1	1963	1965	1971	1969
Tr2	1964	1976	1971	1979
Tr3	<NA>	1980	1973	1983
Tr4	<NA>	1980	1974	<NA>
Tr5	<NA>	1986	<NA>	<NA>
Tr6	<NA>	1987	<NA>	<NA>
Tr7	<NA>	<NA>	<NA>	<NA>
Tr8	<NA>	<NA>	<NA>	<NA>

A.5 National Family Health Survey of India 2005–2006 (NFHS): Andhra Pradesh

The National Family Health Survey (NFHS) (http://www.nfhsindia.org/) is a large-scale, multi-round survey conducted in a representative sample of households throughout India. In total, 109,041 households were interviewed. The survey provides state and national information for India on fertility, infant and child mortality, the practice of family planning, maternal and child health, reproductive health, nutrition, anaemia, utilisation and quality of health and family planning services. NFHS surveys are conducted under the stewardship of the Ministry of Health and Family Welfare (MOHFW), Government of India. The agency, responsible for coordination and technical guidance is the International Institute for Population Sciences (IIPS) in Mumbai.

Three rounds of surveys have been conducted since the first survey in 1992–1993. The second survey was organised in 1998–1999 and the third in 2005–2006.

The third survey (NFHS-3) covered all 29 states in India, which comprise more than 99 % of India's population. The survey included 124,385 women and 74,369 men with completed interview (married and unmarried). Women interviewed were between ages 15 and 49, while men were between 15 and 54. All dates are in Century Month Code (CMC).

The data are available from the Demographic and Health Survey (DHS) data distribution system (http://www.measuredhs.com). Data files are available in user-friendly formats for SPSS, SAS and STATA users. For the illustration of *Biograph*, I used the 2005–2006 data file named APIR42RT.SAV and more particularly the data for women from the state of Andhra Pradesh (AP). The survey covered 5,153 women. The number of variables is 4,386. For the main survey report, see IIPS and Macro International (2007).

Suppose we are interested in the fertility career of women: when they marry, whether and when they have children, and whether and when they opt for sterilisation. The state space is:

- Never married (N)
- Married without children (M)
- One child (a)
- Two children (b)
- Three children up to 20 children (c, d, e, ..., m)
- Sterilised (S)

The following variables are extracted from the raw data.
Dates

Variable name	Meaning
v011	Date of birth
v008	Date of interview
v509	Date of first marriage
b3.*	Date of birth of child (from youngest to oldest)
bord.*	Birth order of child
v312	Contraceptive method (sterilisation = 6 (female) or 7 (male))
v317	Date of sterilisation

Covariates

Variable name	Meaning
v106	Level of education
v190	Wealth index
v102	Place of residence (urban/rural)
v201	Number of children ever born (nCEB)

In addition, three birth cohorts (COH) are distinguished: born before 1970, between 1970 and 1979 and in 1980 or later.

Annexes

The observation window starts at birth and ends at time of interview. The date of interview is given in CMC. I assume that the interview takes place at the beginning of the month. Therefore, one is added to variable v008.

The raw data present the months of birth of the children starting with the youngest child. In *Biograph*, the dates should be ordered chronologically, i.e. from the birth of the oldest child to the birth of the youngest and last child. The first step is to arrange the CMCs at birth of children from the oldest child to the youngest child. The result is the object `cmc_k06`. The CMC at first marriage and the CMC at sterilisation of the woman or her spouse are added next. A missing value (NA) indicates the absence of sterilisation. The dates are stored in the data frame `cmc`. The next step is to sort the dates at transitions, using the standard `Sequence.ind.0` function. The function produces state sequences and the sequence of dates at transition.

The data are stored in a data frame (AP). Table A.13 shows a selection of rows. The code is shown in `create.NFHS.r`.

A.6 European Registry for Blood and Marrow Transplantation (EBMT)

(a) Introduction

The EBMT data are included in the *mstate* package, developed by Putter and colleagues (see de Wreede et al. 2011).

The haematopoietic stem cells in bone marrow in large bones produce new blood cells. Bone marrow transplantation is a treatment for people with certain forms of cancer such as leukaemia and lymphoma. High doses of chemotherapy or radiation therapy can effectively kill cancer cells but they also destroy bone marrow, where blood cells are made. The purpose of a bone marrow transplant is to replenish the body with healthy bone marrow after a high-dose chemotherapy or radiation therapy. Transplanted cells are able to rebuild the patient's bone marrow. After a successful transplant, the bone marrow will start to produce new blood cells. Engraftment is the process of transplanted stem cells reproducing new cells. Bone marrow transplantation is also a treatment of acute leukaemia patients whose bone marrow contains malignant cells.

The goal of cancer therapy is to bring the disease into remission. Remission is when the patient's blood counts return to normal and (in case of leukaemia) bone marrow samples show no sign of disease. Patients may fail to attain a complete remission (CR) because of drug resistance or death. A percentage of patients who initially attain a CR will relapse. Relapse is the reoccurrence of the cancer. If the doses of therapy are not sufficiently high, they are not generally curative. They induce remission but the patient usually relapses. The purpose of bone marrow transplants is to provide the patient with healthy marrow so as to allow massive, and hopefully, curative doses of therapy.

Table A.13 *Biograph* object: NFHS-AP

	ID	born	start	end	COH	EDU	WEAL	U_R	CEB	path	Tr1	Tr2	Tr3	Tr4	Tr5	Tr6
1	1	709	709	1274	<1970	0	2	2	4	HMabcdS	936	937	964	1006	1045	1045
2	2	997	997	1274	>=1980	1	2	2	2	HMabS	1200	1210	1238	1238	NA	NA
3	3	1033	1033	1276	>=1980	0	2	2	1	HMa	1172	1197	NA	NA	NA	NA
4	4	1009	1009	1274	>=1980	0	3	2	2	HMabS	1193	1202	1221	1221	NA	NA
5	5	973	973	1274	>=1980	2	3	2	2	HMabS	1169	1200	1211	1211	NA	NA
6	6	733	733	1274	<1970	0	4	2	3	HMabcdS	919	949	997	1040	1046	NA
7	7	985	985	1274	>=1980	2	4	2	2	HMabS	1241	1250	1262	1263	NA	NA
8	8	1011	1011	1274	>=1980	0	3	2	1	HMa	1205	1238	NA	NA	NA	NA

There are two types of bone marrow transplants:

- *Autologous bone marrow transplant* – The donor of the bone marrow (haematopoietic stem cells) is the person himself/herself.
- *Allogeneic bone marrow transplant* – The donor is another person whose tissue has the same genetic type as the person needing the transplant (recipient). Because tissue types are inherited, it is more likely that the patient's brother and sister are suitable donors. If a family member does not match the recipient, the Marrow Donor Program Registry database is searched for an unrelated individual whose tissue type is a close match. If the donor and recipient are compatible, the infused cells will then travel to the bone marrow and initiate blood cell production.

The European Group for Blood and Marrow Transplantation (EBMT) (http://www.ebmt.org/) maintains a patient database known as the EBMT Registry. The Registry goes back to the beginning of the 1970s and contains patient clinical data. The population covered consists of patients who have undergone a haematopoietic stem cell transplantation (HSCT) procedure; patients with bone marrow failures receiving immunosuppressive therapies; and patients receiving non-haematopoietic cell therapies. Patients are followed up indefinitely. The database has data on close to 400 thousand patients. The data cover aspects of the diagnosis, first-line treatments, HSCT (haematopoietic stem cell transplantation) or cell therapy-associated procedures, complications and outcome. The transplant data are submitted to the central registry by EBMT member centres performing any of the above treatments. The purpose of the Registry is to provide a pool of data to perform retrospective studies, assess epidemiological trends or prepare prospective trials.

(b) The Data

The data, in a file name ebmt4 included in the *mstate* package, are from 2,279 acute lymphoid leukaemia (ALL) patients who had an allogeneic bone marrow transplant from an HLA-identical sibling donor between 1985 and 1998. An HLA-identical donor is a donor who shares the same human leukocyte antigens (HLA). The data were extracted from the EBMT database in 2004. All patients were transplanted in first complete remission. Events recorded during the follow-up of these patients were:

(i) Acute graft-versus-host disease (AGvHD). AGvHD is a GvHD of grade 2 or higher, appearing before 100 days posttransplant.
(ii) Platelet recovery. A platelet is a particle in the blood that is an important part of blood clotting. The bone marrow produces a large number of platelets per mm^3 of blood daily. During chemotherapy, the platelet count drops significantly. Platelet recovery is the recovery of platelet count.
(iii) Relapse and death.

Four prognostic factors are known at baseline for all patients. They are: donor-recipient gender match (where gender mismatch is defined as female donor, male recipient), prophylaxis, year of transplant and age at transplant in years. All these covariates are treated as time-fixed categorical covariates. Younger patients have a better prognosis and transplantation before 1990 had a worse prognosis. Donor-recipient gender mismatch seems to be of minor importance, while T-cell depletion (TCD) shows a clear negative effect on failure-free survival.

The data were used in Fiocco et al. (2008) and van Houwelingen and Putter (2008). The included variables are

id	Patient identification number
Rec	Time in days from transplantation to recovery or last follow-up
rec.s	Recovery status; 1 = recovery, 0 = censored
ae	Time in days from transplantation to adverse event (AE) or last follow-up
ae.s	Adverse event status; 1 = adverse event, 0 = censored
recae	Time in days from transplantation to both recovery and AE or last follow-up
plag.s	Recovery and AE status; 1 = both recovery and AE, 0 = no recovery or no AE or censored
rel	Time in days from transplantation to relapse or last follow-up
rel.s	Relapse status; 1 = relapse, 0 = censored
srv	Time in days from transplantation to death or last follow-up
srv.s	Relapse status; 1 = dead, 0 = censored
year	Year of transplantation; factor with levels '1985–1989', '1990–1994' and '1995–1998'
agecl	Patient age at transplant; factor with levels '<=20', '20–40' and '>40'
proph	Prophylaxis; factor with levels 'no' and 'yes'
match	Donor-recipient gender match; factor with levels 'no gender mismatch' and 'gender mismatch'

(c) The Model

In their research, the authors opt for a multistate approach because it enables the distinction between disease-related and the treatment-related morbidity and mortality. Information on the occurrence of two intermediate events (recovery and an adverse event) is used to update the prognoses of the patients. An example of an adverse event is an acute graft-versus-host disease (AGVHD). It is a complication that can occur after a bone marrow transplant in which the newly transplanted material attacks the transplant recipient's body. Instead of recovery, engraftment or platelet recovery can be included. The multistate model considers six states (with the multicharacter state labels used in *mstate* and the single-character state labels used in *Biograph* in parentheses):

- Alive and in remission, no recovery or adverse event (Tx, T)
- Alive in remission, recovered from the treatment (Rec, P)
- Alive in remission, occurrence of the adverse event (AE, A)
- Alive, both recovered and adverse event occurred (Rec+AE, Z)
- Alive, in relapse (treatment failure) (Rel, R)
- Dead (treatment failure) (Death, D)

All patients start in state Tx. States Rel and Death are called absorbing: once the patient has entered one of them, she/he stays there. This leaves us with a model with 12 transitions. Time is measured in days since transplant. Status variables (.s) indicate the (non)occurrence of a transition. For instance, patient 2 experiences the adverse event after 12 days (transition from state Tx to state AE), then recovery after 29 days (transition from state AE to state 'Rec+AE') and a relapse after 422 days (transition from state 'Rec+AE' to state Rel). Finally, he/she dies after 579 days. The last event is not relevant to the model because the patient has already reached an absorbing state.

Putter et al. make a few adjustments of the data for a multistate analysis. Since the model does not allow patients to enter two states at the same time, a patient who experiences relapse and death on the same day is assumed to have entered the absorbing state of relapse rather than death because the patients experience relapse before death. Patients who experience the adverse event and recovery on the same day are assumed to experience the AE half a day before Rec. Two new variables have been created to express the time of entry in state 'Rec+AE' and the accompanying status indicator: recae and recae.s, respectively.

For modelling, the events relapse and death are combined into a single event 'failure'. Three intermediate events are included in the model: recovery (Rec), an adverse event (AE) and a combination of the two (AE and Rec). To avoid misinterpretation, the authors have abstracted from the actual disease, covariate values and intermediate events. The data include four covariates: year at transplantation, age at transplantation, donor-recipient gender match and prophylaxis.

(d) Preparation of *Biograph* Object

The preparation of a *Biograph* object involves the five steps listed in previous sections of the annex. The code is shown in `create.ebmt.r`. The state space includes the six states shown above: {T, P, A, Z, R, D}. All patients start in state T. In *Biograph*, transitions are specified a little different from the specification of transitions in the data (`ebmt4`). In case an event occurs, both an *mstate* object and a *Biograph* object show the date of the event. In case an event does not occur, the *mstate* object lists the date at censoring, which is the end of exposure to the risk of

Table A.14 Data frame with event dates in days since transplantation. EBMT

	P	A	Z	R	D
1	22	NA	NA	NA	NA
2	NA	12.0	29	422	NA
3	NA	27.0	NA	NA	NA
4	NA	42.0	50	84	NA
5	22	NA	NA	114	NA

experiencing that event. A *Biograph* object shows NA for not applicable. The preparation of a *Biograph* object involves the removal of censoring dates in cases of nonoccurrence of transitions. Note that in *Biograph*, a transition is defined by the state of destination. The transition dates are stored in the data frame `days`. Table A.14 shows the first rows of the data frame. The maximum number of transitions patients experience is 3.

The first patient recovers 22 days after transplantation. The second patient experiences an adverse event 12 days after transplantation, recovers at 29 days and experiences a relapse 422 days after transplantation. Patient 4 enters relapse 84 days after transplantation. The observation ends at that time.

The covariates are

Variable name	Meaning
match	Donor-recipient gender match
proph	Prophylaxis
year	Year of transplantation
agecl	Patient age at transplant

The observation window is from date of transplantation to date of entry into the absorbing state. Time is measured in days since transplantation. The function `Sequences.ind.0` arranges event dates chronologically and determines the state sequence:

```
f<- Sequences.ind.0 (days,namstates,absorb=c("R","D"))
```

Note the two absorbing states. The output component `f$path` gives for each patient the state sequences. The event dates in days since transplantation are given in `f$d`.

The data frame with all the data is produced by the code:

Table A.15 *Biograph* object: EBMT data

```
   ID born start  end     year agecl proph              match path  Tr1 Tr2 Tr3
1   1   0    0    995 1995-1998 20-40 no no gender mismatch   TP  22.0  NA  NA
2   2   0    0    422 1995-1998 20-40 no no gender mismatch TAZR  12.0  29 422
3   3   0    0   1264 1995-1998 20-40 no no gender mismatch   TA  27.0  NA  NA
4   4   0    0     84 1995-1998 20-40 no    gender mismatch TAZR  42.0  50  84
5   5   0    0    114 1995-1998   >40 no    gender mismatch  TPR  22.0 114  NA
6   6   0    0   1427 1995-1998 20-40 no no gender mismatch  TAZ  27.0  33  NA
7   7   0    0    775 1995-1998   >40 no no gender mismatch TAZD  28.5  29 775
8   8   0    0   1618 1995-1998 20-40 no no gender mismatch   TP  31.0  NA  NA
9   9   0    0   1111 1995-1998 20-40 no    gender mismatch  TAZ  29.0  87  NA
10 10   0    0    255 1995-1998 20-40 no no gender mismatch   TR 255.0  NA  NA
```

```
EBMT <- data.frame (ID=id,
                    born=rep(0,nsample),
                    start=rep(0,nsample),
                    end=end,
                    year=year,
                    agecl=agecl,
                    proph=proph,
                    match=match,
                    path=as.character(path),
                    f$d[,1:(max(ns)-1)])
```

Three attributes are added: the format of the event dates (days), the format of the date of birth and the set of parameters. Table A.15 shows the first rows of the data frame.

A.7 Simulated Life Histories

Life histories of 200 individuals are simulated from age 20 to age 40. Individuals can occupy one of three states, labelled A, B and C. A state is selected randomly for each of the 200 individuals. Transition rates are constant between ages 20 and 40. The transition matrix **M**, with origin in column and destination in row, is:

$$\mathbf{M} = \begin{bmatrix} 0.15 & -0.07 & -0.02 \\ -0.10 & 0.10 & -0.05 \\ -0.05 & -0.03 & 0.07 \end{bmatrix}$$

To generate the life history of a single individual, the function sim.msm of the *msm* package is used. The function simulates an individual trajectory from a continuous-time Markov model (Jackson 2014b). The function requires the transition matrix in a different format than shown above and used in this book. The row variable should indicate origin and the column variable destination. The off-diagonal elements should be transition rates rather than minus transition rates. The required format is produced by −t(**M**), where t() denotes transpose. The function also requires that a numeric value rather than a character denotes a state.

Table A.16 *Biograph* object: simulated life histories

ID	born	start	end	cov1	path	Tr1	Tr2	Tr3	Tr4	Tr5
1	0	20	40	X	AB	28.14	NA	NA	NA	NA
3	0	20	40	X	AB	23.69	NA	NA	NA	NA
4	0	20	40	X	BA	24.56	NA	NA	NA	NA
5	0	20	40	X	ACBC	20.73	27.79	37.81	NA	NA
6	0	20	40	X	BACABC	30.15	33.33	34.29	35.87	38.00
7	0	20	40	X	CAC	29.44	34.39	NA	NA	NA
8	0	20	40	X	CBCB	34.32	35.56	39.44	NA	NA
9	0	20	40	X	B	NA	NA	NA	NA	NA
10	0	20	40	X	ABABA	22.80	25.29	26.73	39.37	NA

A is replaced by 1, B by 2 and C by 3. The simulation is an application of dynamic microsimulation in continuous time. For background information, see, e.g. Willekens (2009).

The following code generates a trajectory for an individual starting in state A (state 1) at age 20:

```
bio <- sim.msm (-t(M),mintime=20,maxtime=40,start=1)
```

The object produced by `sim.msm` has three components. The first is the state sequence. The second provides information on the start of the observation window, transition times and end of the observation window. The third is the matrix of transition rates. The result is:

```
$states
[1] 1 3 1 2 2
$times
[1] 20.00000 21.57682 38.39406 39.17881 40.00000
$qmatrix
        destination
origin    A     B      C
     A -0.15  0.10   0.05
     B  0.07 -0.10   0.03
     C  0.02  0.05  -0.07
```

The subject starts in A, moves to C, back to A and continues to B. At the end of the observation period, the individual is in B. The first transition is at age 21.58, the second at 38.39 and the third at 39.18. The character string showing the state sequence is ACAB.

The code `Create.simul.r` generates trajectories for 200 individuals. Table A.16 shows the data for the first 10 individuals.

Annex B: List of Biograph Functions and Data

This annex lists (a) all Biograph functions and their main task and (b) the data sets included in the package.

Biograph function	Task
age_as_year	Converts age to decimal year (utility)
age_as_Date	Converts age to object of class 'Date' (utility)
Agetrans	Computes ages at transition from transition dates
Biograph.long	Converts Biograph object to long format
Biograph.msm	Converts Biograph object to msm format
Biograph.mstate	Converts Biograph object to mstate format
Biograph.mvna	Converts Biograph object to mvna format
ChangeObservationWindow.e	Changes observation window to period between two transitions
ChangeObservationWindow.t	Changes observation window to period between two points in time
check.par	Checks major characteristics of Biograph object (utility)
cmc_as_age	Converts dates in Century Month Code (CMC) to age (utility)
cmc_as_Date	Converts dates in Century Month Code (CMC) to object of class 'Date' (utility)
cmc_as_year	Converts dates in Century Month Code (CMC) to dates in decimal year (calendar year and fraction of year) (utility)
Cumrates	Computes cumulative hazard rates (Nelson-Aalen estimator and occurrence-exposure rates)
Date_as_age	Converts dates (class 'Date') to age (utility)
Date_as_year	Converts dates (class 'Date') to decimal years (calendar years and fraction of year) (utility)
Date_as_cmc	Converts dates (class 'Date') to CMC (utility)
date_b	Converts dates in Biograph object to dates in a desired format (utility)
date_convert	A generic function that converts dates in one format to another format (utility)
GLHS.IllnessDeath	Illness-death model of job transitions
GLHS.trans	Obtains transition matrix of illness-death model
Lexis.lines	Draws Lexis diagram with lifelines for selected subjects (using ggplot2 package)
Lexislines.episodes	Draws Lexis diagram with lifelines for selected subjects (using EPI package)
LexisOccExp	Displays event counts, exposure times and transition rates in Lexis diagram (using EPI package)
Lexis.points	Plots observations in Lexis diagram (scatter plot) (using ggplot2 package)
Lexispoints	Plots observations in Lexis diagram (scatter plot) (using EPI package)

(continued)

Biograph function	Task
Locpath	Determines location of state sequence in Biograph object (utility)
MSLT.S	Computes multistage life table: multistage survival function (MSLT.S)
MSLT.e	Computes multistage life table: exposure function (MSLT.e)
Occup	Determines state occupancies and sojourn times by age for each subject under observation and groups of subjects
OverviewEpisodes	Displays summary information on episodes
OverviewTransitions	Displays summary information on transitions
Parameters	Derives several indicators from the data, e.g. sample size, state space, absorbing states and transition matrix
plot.cumrates	Plots cumulative hazard rates
plot.MSLT.S	Plots the multistage survival function
plot.occup.S	Plots state occupancies by age for the sample population (subjects under observation)
pos.char	Determines the position of a character in a string variable (utility)
pos.charstr	Determines the position of a character string in a string variable (utility)
Rates.ac	Computes occurrence-exposure rates (age-cohort rates)
RateTable	Produces a table with necessary information to compute occurrence-exposure rates
Remove.intrastate	Removes intrastate transitions from Biograph object (utility)
SamplePath	Obtains the life path for a selection of subjects under observation
Sequences	Determines the state sequences in the data
Sequences.ind	Determines for each subject under observation the state trajectory from onset to end of observation
Sequences.ind.0	Determines for each subject under observation event dates sorted in ascending order and generates state sequence (this function is used to produce a Biograph object)
state_age	Determines for given individuals state occupied at given ages
state_time	Determines for given individuals state occupation times by single years of age (in years)
StateSpace	Gets the state space from the data. This function allows the user to change the sequence of states in the state space
string.blank.omit	Removes blanks in character string, including leading and trailing white spaces (utility)
Stringf	Converts a character string to a character vector (utility)
Trans	Computes the number of transitions by origin and destination (total and by age)
TransitionAB	Computes for a selected transition (by origin and destination) the number of occurrences by age. This function is basis for age profile of transition
Transitions	Generates several useful measures of transitions by origin and destination (utility)

(continued)

Biograph function	Task
year_as_age	Determines ages from event years and birth years (utility)
year_as_cmc	Converts decimal years to Century Month Code (CMC) (utility)
year_as_Date	Converts decimal years to dates in Gregorian calendar (utility)
YearTrans	Computes decimal years of transition from transition dates
Data	
GLHS	The German Life History Survey (GLHS) data
NLOG98	The Netherlands Family and Fertility Survey 1989 (NLOG98)
rrdat	German Life History Survey subsample (raw data)

Annex C: Biograph Functions and the Functions They Depend On

This annex lists Biograph function together with the functions they call (excluding Base R functions).

A distinction is made between main functions and utilities that are included in Biograph.

Function	Depends on
Agetrans	date.b
	locpath
Biograph.long	Parameters
	locpath
	reshape
Biograph.msm	check.par
	reshape
Biograph.mstate	check.par
	Parameters
	Biograph.long
Biograph.mvna	Remove.intrastate
	Biograph.long
ChangeObservationWindow.e	
ChangeObservationWindow.t	check.par
	locpath
Cumrates	Biograph.mvna
	mvna (mvna)
	predict (mvna)
	locpath
	Remove.intrastate
	statesequence.ind

(continued)

	Occup	
	Trans	
	RateTable	
	Rates.ac	
GLHS.IllnessDeath	locpath	
	GLHS.trans	
GLHS.Biograph	locpath	
	Parameters	
GLHS.trans		
Lexis.lines	ggplot2	
	check.par	
	date.b	
	Biograph.long	
	date.convert	
Lexislines.episodes	Lexis (Epi)	
	rainbow	
LexisOccExp	locpath	
	Parameters.check	
	Lexis (Epi)	
	splitLexis (Epi)	
	timeBand (Epi)	
	Lexis.diagram (Epi)	
	Surv (survival)	
Lexispoints	TransitionAB	
	Lexis (Epi)	
	Lexis.diagram (Epi)	
Lexis.points	ggplot2	
	check.par	
	date.b	
	TransitionAB	
MSLT.e		
MSLT.S	MatrixExp (msm)	
NLOG98		
Occup	check.par	
	Parameters	
	state_age	
	state_time	
OverviewEpisodes	locpath	
OverviewTransitions	Parameters	
SamplePath	statesequence.ind	
	locpath	
	date.b	
	AgeTrans	
Parameters	StateSpace	

(continued)

	transitions
check.par	Parameters
	StateSpace
plot.cumrates	
plot.MSLT.S	ggplot (ggplot2)
	melt (reshape)
plot.occup	ggplot (ggplot2)
	Occup
	reshape
Rates.ac	
RateTable	
Remove.intrastate	transitions
Sequences	AgeTrans
Sequences.ind	check.par
Sequences.ind.0	
state_age	Agetrans
	stringf
StateSpace	
state_time	Parameters
	AgeTrans
	state_age
Trans	AgeTrans
	statesequence.ind
TransitionAB	locpath
transitions	check.par
	stringf

Utilities

1. Dates

Function	Depends on
age_as_Date	Date_as_year
	year_as_Date
age_as_year	cmc_as_Date
	Date_as_year
cmc_as_age	cmc_as_year
	Date_as_year
cmc_as_Date	
cmc_as_year	cmc_as_Date
	Date_as_year
Date_as_age	as.interval (lubridate)
	as.period (lubridate)
	as.duration (lubridate)
	Date_as_year
Date_as_year	
Date_as_cmc	

(continued)

Annexes

date_b	locpath
	date.convert
date_convert	age_as_year
	age_as_Date
	cmc_as_age
	cmc_a-.Date
	cmc_as_year
	Date_as_age
	Date_as_cmc
	Date_as_year
	year_as_age
	year_as_cmc
	year_as_Date
year_as_age	Date_as_year
year_as_cmc	Date_as_cmc
year_as_Date	

2. Text

Function	Depends on
check.par	Parameters
	StateSpace
pos.char	stringf
pos.charstr	stringf
string.blank.omit	
stringf	

3. Other

Function	Depends on
locpath	

References

Aalen, O. O., Borgan, Ø., & Gjessing, H. K. (2008). *Survival and event history analysis. A process point of view.* New York: Springer.
Abbott, A. (2001). *Time matters. On theory and method.* Chicago: The University of Chicago Press.
Allignol, A. (2013). Package *mvna. Nelson-Aalen estimator of the cumulative hazard in multistate models.* Published on CRAN.
Allignol, A. (2014). Package *etm. Empirical transition matrix.* Published on CRAN.
Allignol, A., Beyersmann, J., & Schumacher, M. (2008). mvna: An R package for the Nelson-Aalen estimator in multistate models. *R Newsletter, 8*(2), 48–50.
Allignol, A., Schumacher, M., & Beyersmann, J. (2011). Empirical transition matrix of multistate models: The etm package. *Journal of Statistical Software, 38*(4), 15.
Alter, G., & Gutmann, M. (1999). Casting spells. Database concepts for event-history analysis. *Historical Methods, 32*(4), 165–176.
Andersen, P. K., & Gill, R. D. (1982). Cox's regression model for counting processes. A large sample study. *Annals of Statistics, 10*, 1100–1120.
Andersen, P. K., & Keiding, N. (2002). Multi-state models for event history analysis. *Statistical Methods in Medical Research, 11*, 91–115.
Andersen, P. K., Borgan, O., Gill, R. D., & Keiding, N. (1993). *Statistical models based on counting processes.* New York: Springer.
Aoki, M. (1996). *New approaches to macroeconomic modeling. Evolutionary stochastic dynamics, multiple equilibria, and externalities as field effects.* Cambridge: Cambridge University Press.
Beyersmann, J., & Putter, H. (2014). A brief note on computing average state occupation times. *Demographic Research, 30*(62), 1681–1696.
Beyersmann, J., Schumacher, M., & Allignol, A. (2012). *Competing risks and multistate models with R.* New York: Springer.
Blossfeld, H. P., & Rohwer, G. (2002). *Techniques of event history modeling. New approaches to causal analysis* (2nd ed.). Mahwah: Lawrence Erlbaum Associates.
Blossfeld, H. P., Golsh, K., & Rohwer, G. (2007). *Event history analysis with Stata.* Mahwah: Lawrence Erlbaum Associates.
Borgan, O., & Hoem, J. M. (1988). Demographic reproduction rates and the estimation of an expected total count per person in an open population. *Journal of the American Statistical Association, 83*(403), 886–891.

Borgan, O. (1998). *Three contributions to the Encyclopedia of Biostatistics: The Nelson-Aalen, Kaplan-Meier and Aalen-Johansen estimators*. Encyclopedia of Biostatistics. Chichester: Wiley.
Broström, G. (2003). New package: eha. http://tolstoy.newcastle.edu.au/R/announce/03/0029.html. Accessed 4 May 2014.
Broström, G. (2012). *Event history analysis with R*. Boca Raton: CRC Press.
Broström, G. (2014). Package *eha. Event history analysis*. Published on CRAN.
Carstensen, B. (2007). Age-period-cohort models for the Lexis diagram. *Statistics in Medicine, 26* (15), 3018–3045.
Carstensen, B. (2013). Package *Epi. A package for statistical analysis in epidemiology*. Published on CRAN.
Carstensen, B., & Plummer, M. (2011). Using Lexis objects for multi-state models in R. *Journal of Statistical Software, 38*(6), 1–18.
Chiang, C. L. (1968). *Introduction to stochastic processes in biostatistics*. New York: Wiley. Chapter 9 reprinted in Bogue, D. J., Arriage, E. E., & Anderton, E. L. (Eds.). (1993). *Readings in population research methodology* (Vol. 2, pp. 7.84–7.97). Chicago/New York: Social Development Center/UNFPA.
Chiang, C. L. (1984). *The life table and its applications*. Malabar: R.E. Krieger Publishing.
Chrysanthopoulou, S. A. (2014). Package *MILC. Microsimulation long cancer (MILC) model*. Published on CRAN.
Çinlar, E. (1975). *Introduction to stochastic processes*. Englewood Cliffs: Prentice-Hall.
Cleveland, W. S. (1993). *Visualizing data*. Summit: Hobart Press.
De Graaf, A., & Steenhof, L. (1999, December). Relatie en gezinsvorming van generaties 1945–1979: uitkomsten van het Onderzoek Gezinsvorming 1998 [Partnership and family formation of cohorts 1945–1979: Results of the Netherlands Fertility and Family Survey 1998]. *Maandstatiek Bevolking* (Statistics Netherlands), *12*, 21–36.
de Wreede, L. C., Fiocco, M., & Putter, H. (2010). The mstate package for estimation and prediction in non- and semi-parametric multi-state and competing risks models. *Computer Methods and Programs in Biomedicine, 99*, 261–274. doi:10.1016/j.cmpb.2010.01.001.
de Wreede, L. C., Fiocco, M., & Putter, H. (2011). mstate: An R package for the analysis of competing risks and multistate models. *Journal of Statistical Software, 38*(7), 1–30.
Dubin, J. A., & O'Malley, S. (2010). Event charts for the analysis of adverse events in longitudinal studies: An example from a smoking cessation pharmacotherapy trial. *The Open Epidemiology Journal, 3*, 34–41.
Dubin, J. A., Müller, H.-G., & Wang, J.-L. (2001). Event history graphs for censored survival data. *Statistics in Medicine, 20*, 2951–2964.
Fiocco, M., Putter, H., & van Houwelingen, H. C. (2008). Reduced-rank proportional hazards regression and simulation-based prediction for multi-state models. *Statistics in Medicine, 27*, 4340–4358.
Francis, B., & Fuller, M. (1996). Visualization of event histories. *Journal of the Royal Statistical Society A, 159*(2), 301–308.
Gabadinho, A., Ritschards, G., Müller, N. S., & Studer, M. (2011). Analyzing and visualizing state sequences in R with TraMineR. *Journal of Statistical Software, 40*(4), 1–37.
Gabadinho, A., Studer, M., Müller, N., Bürgin, R., & Ritchard, G. (2012). Package *TraMineR. Trajectory miner: A toolkit for exploring and rendering sequence data*. Published on CRAN.
Gampe, J., Zinn, S., Willekens, F., Van der Gaag, N., de Beer, J., Himmelspach, J., & Uhrmacher, A. (2009, June). *The microsimulation tool of the MicMac project*. Paper presented at the 2nd general conference of the international microsimulation association, Ottawa.
Goldman, A. I. (1992). EVENTCHARTS: Visualizing survival and other timed-events data. *The American Statistician, 46*(1), 13–18.
Helbing, D. (2010). *Quantitative sociodynamics. Stochastic methods and models of social interaction processes*. Berlin: Springer.

References

Hoem, J. M., & Funck Jensen, U. (1982). Multistate life table methodology: A probabilist critique. In K. C. Land & A. Rogers (Eds.), *Multidimensional mathematical demography* (pp. 155–264). New York: Academic.

Holford, T. R. (1980). The analysis of rates and of survivorship using log-linear models. *Biometrics, 36*, 299–305.

Hougaard, P. (2000). *Analysis of multistate survival data*. New York: Springer.

International Institute for Population Sciences (IIPS) and Macro International. (2007). *National Family Health Survey (NFHS-3), 2005–06: India: Volume I*. Mumbai: IIPS.

Izmirlian, G., Brock, D., Ferrucci, L., & Phillips, C. (2000). Active life expectancy from annual follow-up data with missing responses. *Biometrics, 56*(1), 244–248.

Jackson, C. (2011). Multi-state models for panel data: The msm package for R. *Journal of Statistical Software, 38*(8), 28.

Jackson, C. (2014a). Package *msm. Multi-state Markov and hidden Markov models in continuous time*. Published on CRAN.

Jackson, C. (2014b). *Multistate modeling with R: The msm package. Vignette distributed with the msm package*. CRAN repository.

Kalbfleisch, J. D., & Lawless, J. F. (1985). The analysis of panel data under a Markov assumption. *Journal of the American Statistical Association, 80*(392), 863–871.

Kalbfleisch, J. D., & Prentice, R. L. (2002). *The statistical analysis of failure time data* (2nd ed.). New York: Wiley.

Korn, E. I., Graubard, B. I., & Midthune, D. (1997). Time-to-event analysis of longitudinal follow-up of a survey: Choice of time-scale. *American Journal of Epidemiology, 145*(1), 72–80.

Laird, N., & Olivier, D. (1981). Covariance analysis of censored survival data using log-linear analysis techniques. *Journal of the American Statistical Association, 76*(374), 231–240.

Land, K. C., & Rogers, A. (Eds.). (1982). *Multidimensional mathematical demography*. New York: Academic.

Lee, J. J., Hess, K. R., & Dubin, J. A. (2000). Extensions and applications of event charts. *American Statistician, 84*, 1065–1073.

Li, Y., Gail, M. H., Preston, D. L., Graubard, B. I., & Lubin, J. H. (2012). Piecewise exponential survival times and analysis of case-control data. *Statistics in Medicine, 31*(13), 1361–1368.

Lumley, T. (2004). *The survival package*. The newsletter of the R project. 4/1, June 2004, pp. 26–28.

Mamun, A. A. (2003). *Life history of cardiovascular disease and its risk factors*. Amsterdam: Rozenberg Publishers.

Matsuo, H. (2003). *The transition to motherhood in Japan. A comparison with the Netherlands*. Amsterdam: Rozenberg Publishers.

Matsuo, H., & Willekens, F. (2003). *Event histories in the Netherlands fertility and family survey 1998. A technical report*. Research report 03-1. Population Research Centre, University of Groningen.

Meira-Machado, L. M., et al. (2009). Multi-state models for the analysis of time-to-event data. *Statistical Methods in Medical Research, 18*(2), 195–222.

Meira-Machados, L. M., & Roca-Pardinas, J. (2012). Package *p3state.msm. Analyzing survival data*. Published on CRAN.

Mills, M. (2011). *Introducing survival and event history analysis*. London: Sage.

Namboodiri, K., & Suchindran, C. M. (1987). *Life table techniques and their applications*. Orlando: Academic.

Pencina, M. J., Larson, M. G., & D'Agostino, R. B. (2007). Choice of time scale and its effect on significance of predictors in longitudinal studies. *Statistics in Medicine, 26*, 1343–1359.

Pleasant, C., Milash, B., Rose, A., Widoff, S., & Shneiderman, B. (1996). Life Lines; visualizing personal histories. In *Proceedings SIG-CHI 1996* (pp. 221–227). New York: ACM Press.

Plummer, M., & Carstensen, B. (2011). Lexis: An R class for epidemiological studies with long-term follow-up. *Journal of Statistical Software, 38*(5), 1–12.

Preston, S. H., Heuveline, P., & Guillot, M. (2001). *Demography. Measuring and modelling population processes*. Oxford: Blackwell.

Putter, H. (2014). *Tutorial in biostatistics: Competing risks and multi-state analysis using the mstate package* [Electronic resource]. http://cran.r-project.org/web/packages/mstate/vignettes/Tutorial.pdf

Putter, H. (2011a). Special issue about competing risks and multi-state models. *Journal of Statistical Software, 38*(1), 1–4.

Putter, H. (2011b). Package *dynpred. Companion package to "Dynamic prediction in clinical survival analysis"*. Chapman and Hall/CRC Publishers. Published on CRAN.

Putter, H., Fiocco, M., & Geskus, R. B. (2007). Tutorial in biostatistics: Competing risks and multi-state models. *Statistics in Medicine, 26*, 2389–2430.

Putter, H., de Wreede, L., & Fiocco, M. (2011). Package *mstate. Data preparation, estimation and prediction in multistate models*. Published on CRAN.

Reuser, M. (2010). *The effect of risk factors on compression or expansion of disability a multistate analysis of the U.S. health and retirement study*. Amsterdam: Rozenberg Publishers.

Ritschard, G. (2014). Package *TraMineR. Trajectory miner: A toolkit for exploring and rendering sequence data*. Published on CRAN.

Rogers, A. (1975). *Introduction to multiregional mathematical demography*. New York: Wiley.

Rogers, A. (1986). Parameterized multistate population dynamics and projections. *Journal of the American Statistical Association, 81*(393), 48–61.

Sarkar, D. (2008). *Lattice. Multivariate data visualization with R*. New York: Springer.

Sarkar, D. (2014). Package *lattice. Lattice graphics*. Published on CRAN.

Schoen, R. (1988). *Modeling multigroup populations*. New York: Plenum Press.

Steele, J., & Iliinsky, N. (2010). *Beautiful visualization. Looking at data through the eyes of experts*. Sebastopol: O'Reilly.

Therneau, T. M. (1999). *A package for survival analysis in S*. Published on http://www.mayo.edu/research/documents/tr53pdf/DOC-10027379. Accessed 4 May 2014.

Therneau, T. M. (2014). Package *survival. Survival analysis*. Published on CRAN.

Therneau, T. M., & Grambsch, P. M. (2000). *Modeling survival data: Extending the Cox model*. New York: Springer.

Tuma, N. B., & Hannan, M. T. (1984). *Social dynamics. Models and methods*. Orlando: Academic.

Van den Hout, A. (2013). ELECT: Estimation of life expectancies using continuous-time multi-state survival models. Available at http://www.ucl.ac.uk/~ucakadl/ELECT_Manual_13_02_2013.pdf. Accessed 4 May 2014.

Van den Hout, A., & Matthews, E. F. (2008). Multi-state analysis of cognitive ability data: A piecewise-constant model and a Weibull model. *Statistics in Medicine, 27*, 5440–5455.

Van den Hout, A., Ogurtsova, E., Gampe, J., & Matthews, F. E. (2014). Investigating healthy life expectancy using a multi-state model in the presence of missing data and misclassification. *Demographic Research, 30*(42), 1219–1244.

Van Houwelingen, H. C., & Putter, H. (2008). Dynamic predicting by landmarking as an alternative for multi-state modeling: An application to acute lymphoid leukemia data. *Lifetime Data Analysis, 14*, 447–463.

Van Houwelingen, H. C., & Putter, H. (2011). *Dynamic prediction in clinical survival analysis*. Boca Raton: Chapman and Hall/CRC Press.

Van Imhoff, E. (1990). The exponential multidimensional demographic projection model. *Mathematical Population Studies, 2*(3), 171–182.

Weidlich, W., & Haag, G. (1983). *Concepts and models of quantitative sociology: The dynamics of interacting populations*. Berlin: Springer.

Weidlich, W., & Haag, G. (Eds.). (1988). *Interregional migration. Dynamic theory and comparative analysis*. Berlin: Springer.

Wickham, H. (2009). *ggplot2. Elegant graphics for data analysis*. New York: Springer.

Wickham, H. (2010). A layered grammar of graphics. *Journal of Computational and Graphical Statistics, 19*(1), 3–28.

References

Wickham, U. (2014). Package *ggplot2*. Published on CRAN.

Wilkinson, L. (2005). *The grammar of graphics* (2nd ed.). New York: Springer.

Wilkinson, L. (2012). The grammar of graphics. In J. E. Gentle, W. K. Härdle, & Y. Mori (Eds.), *Handbook of computational statistics. Concepts and methods* (2nd ed.). Berlin/New York: Springer.

Willekens, F. J. (1987). The marital status life-table. In J. Bongaarts, T. Burch, & K. W. Wachter (Eds.), *Family demography: Models and applications* (pp. 125–149). Oxford: Clarendon Press.

Willekens, F. J. (2009). Continuous-time microsimulation in longitudinal analysis. In A. Zaidi, A. Harding, & P. Williamson (Eds.), *New frontiers in microsimulation modelling* (pp. 413–436). Surrey: Ashgate.

Willekens, F. (2013a). *Biograph*: Explore life histories.

Willekens, F. (2013b). Chronological objects in demographic research. *Demographic Research, 28*(23), 649–680.

Willekens, F., & Putter, H. (2014). Multistate event history analysis. Special collection of *Demographic Research*. www.demographic-research.org

Wolf, D. A. (1986). Simulation methods for analyzing continuous-time event history models. *Sociological Methodology, 16*, 283–308.

Zinn, S. (2011). *A continuous-time microsimulation and first steps towards a multi-level approach in demography*. PhD dissertation, University of Rostock, Faculty of Informatics and Electrotechnics.

Zinn, S. (2014). Package *MicSim. Performing continuous-time microsimulation*. Published on CRAN.

Zinn, S., Himmelspach, J., Uhrmacher, A. M., & Gampe, J. (2013). Building Mic-Core, a specialized M&S software to simulate multi-state demographic micro models, based on JAMES II, a general M&S framework. *Journal of Artificial Societies and Social Simulation, 16*(3), 5.

Index

A

Aalen–Johansen estimator, 34–37, 166, 172–173
Absorbing state, 1, 28, 29, 35, 43, 81, 83, 84, 175, 188, 220, 225, 246, 275, 288, 289, 293
Aesthetics (*ggplot2*), 111, 112, 114
At risk. *See* Risk set

B

Baseline hazard. *See* Hazard
Biographical method, 2, 5, 268
Biograph object, 3–6, 18, 25, 37, 38, 48, 53–79, 81–83, 85, 112, 189, 207, 213, 214, 217–222, 233, 237, 245, 246, 268, 269, 271–293
 create object, 4, 5, 19, 53, 54, 57–59, 69, 71, 217, 219, 271–291
Bootstrapping, 25, 26, 40, 45, 52

C

Censoring, 4, 18, 22, 23, 29, 54, 63, 65, 66, 68, 70, 73, 74, 76, 82, 85, 86, 90, 91, 99, 103, 116, 121, 128, 131, 135–137, 149, 164, 166, 174, 175, 195, 211, 222, 226, 236, 246, 258, 288, 289
Century Month Code (CMC), 4, 11, 12, 25, 54–59, 61, 62, 65, 68, 69, 71, 73, 74, 76–78, 97, 112, 136, 162–164, 175, 177, 196, 198, 199, 205, 218, 221, 222, 229, 246, 254, 272, 276, 284, 285, 292, 294
Chapman–Kolmogorov equation, 30–32
Chiang's 'a,' 45
Chronological object, 53
Clock forward approach, 65
Clock reset approach, 65
Closed episode, 82, 90, 97, 107, 116, 118, 136, 225
CMC. *See* Century Month Code (CMC)
Competing risk, 2, 7, 49, 54, 70, 71, 173, 216, 252
Counting process, 2, 8, 14–17, 19, 21–24, 28, 52, 63, 136, 195
 counting-process format, 65
Covariate
 time-dependent, 141, 173, 183, 202
 transition-specific, 177, 189, 254
Cox model. *See* Cox regression model
Cox regression model
 cumulative hazard, 145, 248, 250, 251
 stratified, 143, 145, 158, 183, 184, 194, 250
 time-dependent covariate, 183
CRAN task view 'Survival Analysis', 135
Cumulative hazard, 11, 16–18, 21, 34, 35, 49, 69–70, 143–145, 154, 157, 165, 168, 170, 171, 173, 180, 181, 184, 190, 192, 207, 212, 244, 247, 249–251, 253, 254, 256, 257, 261, 292, 293

D

Data
 European Registry of Blood and Marrow Transplantation (EBMT), 5, 285–290
 German Life History Survey (GLHS), 4, 10, 13, 269, 294

Data (cont.)
  National Family Health Survey (NFHS) of India, 5, 59, 269, 271, 283–285
  Netherlands Family and Fertility Survey (NLOG98), 5, 59, 217–265, 271, 294
  Survey of Health, Ageing and Retirement in Europe (SHARE), 5, 59, 269, 271, 278–283
Delayed entry. *See* Left-truncation
Discrete event simulation (DEV), 46, 49

E
Empirical transition matrix, 34, 35
Episode data, 63, 64, 66, 125, 137, 230
European Registry of Blood and Marrow Transplantation (EBMT). *See* Data
Event chart, 110, 111
Event data, 62–64, 66, 72, 73, 218, 219
Exponential model
  exponential transition rate model, 21, 23, 24, 42, 43, 91, 136, 138–141, 155, 197, 201, 202
  piecewise exponential model, 9, 21, 24, 26, 27, 33, 39, 42, 52, 210, 215
Exposure process. *See* Risk process

F
Faceting (*ggplot2*), 115
Framingham Heart Study (FHS), 74, 75

G
Geom. (*ggplot2*), 116
German Life History Survey (GLHS). *See* Data
Gompertz, 1, 21, 22, 155, 160
Grammar of graphics, 110, 111

H
Hazard
  baseline, 8, 142, 143, 147, 154, 155, 157–162, 173, 178–180, 182, 183, 185, 253, 255
  cumulative, 11, 16–18, 21, 34, 35, 49, 69–70, 143–145, 154, 157, 165, 168, 170, 171, 173, 180, 181, 184, 190, 192, 207, 212, 244, 247, 249–251, 253, 254, 256, 257, 261, 292, 293
  proportional hazard model (*see* Cox regression model)
  ratio, 2, 142, 179, 184
  transition (*see* Transition rate)

I
Illness-death model, 174–189, 194, 292
Intensity process, 15, 16, 22, 23

K
Kaplan–Meier estimator
  competing risk, 2, 7, 49, 54, 70, 71, 173, 216, 252
  Greenwood variance estimator, 247
  multistate model, 1, 2, 5, 10, 22, 33, 35, 71, 72, 84, 126, 135, 141, 166–173, 177, 189, 196, 216, 246, 268, 288

L
Landmark method, 29, 35, 37
Left-truncation, 63, 136, 141
Lexis diagram, 3, 5, 13, 87, 109–111, 120–129, 133, 223, 231, 267, 292, 295, 296
Lexis pencil, 111
LifePath, 49
Likelihood ratio test, 142, 179, 184, 186, 191, 193, 252, 255
Long format, 4, 25, 53, 54, 59, 63–66, 69–73, 118, 125, 136, 162, 174, 176–178, 194, 195, 230, 244–246, 268, 292

M
Markov
  Markov assumption, 211
  Markov chain, 34, 72, 174, 189–194
  Markov process
    homogeneous, 8
    multistate model (*see* Multistate model)
  reversible Markov chain, 189–194
Martingale, 16
Master equation, 32
Mean duration of transfer. *See* Chiang's 'a'
MicMac, 49
Microsimulation, 5, 6, 8, 46, 49, 51, 52, 103, 195, 205, 206, 212–216, 291
Multistate life table, 5, 8, 35, 103, 171–173, 197, 205–217, 256–265, 268
Multistate model
  Aalen–Johansen estimator (*see* Aalen–Johansen estimator)
  Cox regression model, 255

Index

Nelson–Aalen estimator, 166–172
transition rate (*see* Transition rate)
Multistate survival function, 33, 188, 206, 208–210, 212, 257, 258, 263, 264

N

National Family Health Survey (NFHS) of India. *See* Data
Nelson–Aalen estimator, 17, 18, 20, 21, 23, 33–35, 51, 154, 165–173, 206–209, 211, 216, 246, 248, 249, 256, 257, 259–261, 263, 268, 292
Netherlands Family and Fertility Survey (NLOG98). *See* Data
Non-parametric estimator, 34, 166, 215, 246

O

Observation window, 2–5, 25, 53, 55, 58, 60–63, 155, 162–165, 219, 222, 225, 267, 268, 272, 285, 289, 291, 292
Occurrence-exposure rate, 2, 21, 23, 24, 27, 33, 39, 45, 51, 91, 128, 155, 161, 164, 165, 171–173, 206–212, 215, 216, 223, 236, 237, 239–243, 256, 257, 259–261, 263, 268, 292, 293
Open-ended age group, 33, 44
Open episode, 82, 97, 106, 107, 116, 118, 136, 137, 224, 225, 268

P

Partial likelihood,
Person data, 64
Population at risk, 2, 3, 11, 16, 18, 21, 29, 167–169, 259
Population-based, 210
Product integral, 30, 31, 34, 35
Product-limit estimator, 30

R

Reference age, 29, 35, 37, 39, 41–44, 206, 209, 211, 256, 264, 268
Regression model
  Cox (*see* Cox regression model)
  proportional hazard (*see* Cox regression model)
  transition probability, 3, 7, 9, 10, 12, 15, 28–40, 43, 49, 52, 135, 165–166, 172, 195–198, 200, 203, 206, 209, 216, 236, 237, 256, 259–268
Reversible Markov chain, 189–194
Risk process, 2, 15, 16

Risk set, 11, 15, 35, 155, 166, 167, 208, 247, 248, 250, 251
R packages
  Biograph, 3, 11, 54, 55, 57, 78, 107, 121, 213, 219, 221, 244, 265, 268, 269, 271, 272, 276
  eha, 3, 5, 11, 64, 65, 135, 154–155, 157, 162, 244
  Epi, 3, 54, 65–67, 71, 110, 121, 122, 125, 129, 230, 268, 292
  etm, 5, 10, 18, 33, 35, 38, 54, 64, 71, 135–166, 172–173, 268
  ggplot2, 3, 109–121, 123, 125, 126, 130, 212, 292
  lattice, 109, 168, 248
  lubridate, 294
  msm, 3, 5, 6, 10, 11, 24, 25, 34, 48, 49, 54, 73, 135, 195–203, 213, 236, 259, 260, 268, 290
  mstate, 3, 5, 10, 11, 33, 54, 59, 60, 65, 66, 70, 71, 84, 135, 173–194, 217, 244, 246, 248, 250, 251, 255, 261, 263, 268, 269, 271, 285, 286
  mvna, 3, 5, 10, 11, 18, 54, 60, 64, 66, 68, 69, 84, 135, 165–172, 174, 206, 207, 217, 244–246, 251, 256, 268
  survival, 3, 5, 54, 60, 63, 65, 88, 135–154, 158, 173, 174, 179, 180, 184, 194, 217, 244, 245, 248, 250–252, 255, 268

S

Sample path, 81, 91–93, 189, 229, 293, 296
Schoenfeld residual, 147, 253
Simulation
  competing risk, 48, 49
  multistate model, 1–3, 5, 10, 11, 14, 16, 22, 24, 28, 33, 35, 53, 54, 59, 65, 71, 72, 84, 126, 135, 141, 165–173, 177, 189, 196, 216, 227, 246, 255, 268, 271, 288
Sojourn time. *See* Sate occupation time
State occupation probability. *See* State probability
State occupation time, 15, 28, 40–46, 51, 52, 81, 90, 95–103, 206, 212, 216, 256, 293
  expected state occupation time, 3, 10, 12, 40–46, 51, 52, 196, 202, 206, 210–212, 263, 264, 268
State probability, 3, 209, 256
State space, 1, 7, 29, 41, 45, 55, 57, 58, 60, 79, 81–84, 92, 189, 219–220, 222, 223, 258, 268, 272, 273, 275, 276, 280, 284, 288, 293, 296, 297

Status-based, 35, 41, 44, 210
Status data, 62, 63
Survey of Health, Ageing and Retirement in Europe (SHARE). *See* Data
Survival analysis, 1, 8, 14, 15, 54, 55, 60, 63, 135, 154
Survival function, 10, 33, 34, 45, 138, 141, 143, 144, 147, 149, 172, 180–182, 188, 206, 208–210, 212, 215, 251, 257, 258, 263–264, 293
Survival object, 54, 65, 128, 136–137, 163, 164
Synthetic biography, 3, 5, 8, 9, 46, 51, 52, 268
Synthetic life history. *See* Synthetic biography

T
Theme system (*ggplot2*), 111, 117
Tied transition times, 19, 21, 42
Time-dependent covariate
  connection to mulstitate model, 141, 173
Time origin, 41, 63, 70, 102, 226, 242
Time scale, 1, 8, 10, 11, 17, 30, 61, 63, 65, 66, 69, 110, 121, 131, 136, 196, 199
Transient state, 1, 29, 35, 45, 195, 201
Transition hazard. *See* Transition rate
Transition probability, 3, 7, 9, 10, 12, 15, 28–40, 43, 49, 52, 135, 165–166, 172, 195–198, 200, 203, 206, 209, 216, 236, 237, 256, 259–268
Transition rate, 2–4, 6–34, 39–52, 81, 91, 97, 102, 103, 107, 121, 126, 128, 135–142, 147, 155–157, 160, 161, 165, 168, 171–173, 176, 178–180, 183–185, 187, 190, 192–194, 196–203, 205–217, 226, 227, 236, 239–242, 244–257, 259–261, 263, 264, 267, 290W
Weibull
  Weibull function, 156
  Weibull model, 22, 155, 157, 158, 161
  Weibull regression, 154–156, 159
Wide format, 3, 4, 53, 54, 59, 63, 64, 71, 72, 162, 174–176, 195, 245, 268

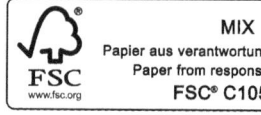

If you have any concerns about our products,
you can contact us on
ProductSafety@springernature.com

In case Publisher is established outside the EU,
the EU authorized representative is:
**Springer Nature Customer Service Center GmbH
Europaplatz 3, 69115 Heidelberg, Germany**

Printed by Libri Plureos GmbH
in Hamburg, Germany